CU00854687

ROYAL HISTORICAL SOCIETY

STUDIES IN HISTORY

New Series

THE ROYAL TOUCH
IN EARLY MODERN ENGLAND

To Anna and Lora,

With much love,

Stephen

xo xo

30 - 8- 17

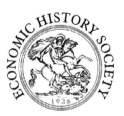

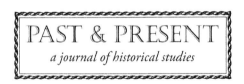

PAST & PRESENT
a journal of historical studies

THE ROYAL TOUCH
IN EARLY MODERN ENGLAND

POLITICS, MEDICINE AND SIN

Stephen Brogan

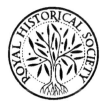

THE ROYAL HISTORICAL SOCIETY

THE BOYDELL PRESS

First published 2015
Reprinted 2016

A Royal Historical Society publication
Published by The Boydell Press
an imprint of Boydell & Brewer Ltd
PO Box 9, Woodbridge, Suffolk IP12 3DF, UK
and of Boydell & Brewer Inc.
668 Mt Hope Avenue, Rochester, NY 14620–2731, USA
website: www.boydellandbrewer.com

ISBN 978–0–86193–337–2

ISSN 0269–2244

A CIP catalogue record for this book is available
from the British Library

Contents

Illustrations

Tables

Illustrations acknowledgements

The author and publisher are grateful to the following for permission to reproduce copyright material:
Bedfordshire and Luton Archives, Bedford, for figure 14; the British Library, London, for plate 2; the British Museum for figures 10, 13, 16, and plates 6 and 7; the estate of the late Profesor Howard Erskine-Hill, for figure 17 and plates 8 and 9; the National Portrait Gallery, London, for figure 12; the Science Museum, London, for plate 4; the Society of Antiquaries, London, for figure 4; Surrey History Centre, Woking, for figure 7; The Wellcome Library, London, for the cover illustration, figures 1, 2, 3, 6, 11 and plates 1 and 4; and Westminster Cathedral, London, for plates 3 and 5

This volume was published with the help of a grant from the late Miss Isobel Thornley's Bequest to the University of London. A further generous grant was made on behalf of the Jacobite Studies Trust.

Acknowledgements

I have incurred many debts whilst working on this book. The initial research was funded by The Arts and Humanities Research Council, after which The Jacobite Studies Trust awarded me a Research Fellowship at The Institute of Historical Research for 2011–12. Further assistance came from The Oxford Centre for Methodism and Church History, where I was a Visiting Research Fellow. I am extremely grateful to these organisations for their financial support and encouragement.

As this is my first book I must record a debt of thanks to three exceptional teachers from my school years in Welwyn Garden City. Mr Jones at Blackthorn School, and Mr Ellis and Mrs Bates at Heronswod School, all encouraged me to think for myself, and to enjoy doing so, especially in relation to the early modern period. An even bigger debt is owed to Birkbeck College, where I studied as a mature student between 2000 and 2010. Three gifted academics took an interest in my work: Michael Hunter, Julian Swann and the late Barry Coward. Their enthusiasm and encouragement has been stimulating and heartening. Michael Hunter supervised much of my postgraduate research and was patient, generous, meticulous and inspiring. I have benefitted no end from his vast knowledge of early modern England. He kindly read an earlier draft of this book, providing insightful comments for which I am very thankful. Studying at Birkbeck was a life-affirming and life-changing experience as the college is full of hard-working and enthusiastic lecturers and mature students, many of whom are happy to continue seminars in the bar after formal teaching has ceased for the evening. I have made many friends there, especially the members of the Birkbeck Early Modern Society, none of whom looked bored when I turned the conversation around yet again to the royal touch.

During the last three years I have been extremely fortunate to have Alexandra Walsham as my advisory editor for the RHS Studies in History series. She has been an outstanding editor and mentor during the process of revision for publication. The royal touch is a subject that is close to her heart and consequently the process has been both enlightening and enjoyable. I have learned a huge amount whilst working with her, both in terms of the early modern period itself and how to present interpretations of it. I must thank her for her patience, generosity, vigilance and helpfulness. The scope and priorities of this book owe much to her expertise. At the Royal Historical Society Christine Linehan and Sue Carr have both been very helpful and encouraging.

It has been a privilege and a joy to teach early modern history at Birkbeck and at Royal Holloway. Teaching has helped me to contextualise my research and to make links to related subjects that otherwise would have escaped me. I have learned a great deal from my colleagues and students, who have encouraged my work while often forcing me to think harder about what I am trying to say. This is especially true of the students at Royal Holloway who studied the course 'Killing the king: England in an age of revolutions, 1603–1714', which has been a delight to teach.

Whilst working on the royal touch I have been invited to speak at a number of research seminars and conferences and I wish to express my gratitude to both the conveners and the audiences for their support and engagement. The details are as follows: 12 September 2008 at the British Printed Images to 1700 Conference, Victoria and Albert Museum, London; 5 March 2009 at the Society, Culture and Belief, 1400–1800 seminar, Institute of Historical Research, London; 25 February 2010 at the British History in the Seventeenth Century seminar, Institute of Historical Research, London; 28 May 2010 at the Society for Court Studies conference to mark the 350th anniversary of the Stuart Restoration, University of Greenwich; 30 June 2010 at the Ecclesiastical History Colloquium, Oxford Centre for Methodism and Church History, Oxford Brookes University; 24 August 2010 at the conference '"The Burthen of the Mortal Body": Life, Death, Sickness and Health in the Early Modern Period', University of Exeter; 15 July 2011 at the British Society for the History of Science Conference, University of Exeter; 7 December 2011 at the Director's Seminar, Institute of Historical Research, London; 6 February 2012 at the European History 1500–1800 seminar, Institute of Historical Research, London; 4 April 2012 at The Royal Body Conference, at Royal Holloway, University of London; 26 June 2012 at The British Numismatic Society at the British Museum; 2 February 2013 at the Birkbeck Early Modern Society's conference 'Science, Magic and Religion'; 20 February 2013 at the Early Modern British and Irish History Seminar, Trinity College, Cambridge; 20 March 2013 at the round table discussion at the History of Health and Medicine Seminars, King's College, London.

Within academia I have benefited greatly from conversations, both real and electronic, with John Arnold, Phil Baker, Andrew Barclay, Kate Billington, Peter Burke, Anne Byrne, Justin Champion, Nikki Clarke, Eveline Cruickshanks, Nick Dew, Robin Eagles, Peter Elmer, William Gibson, Vanessa Harding, Karen Hearn, John Henderson, Andrew Hopper, Ludmilla Jordanova, Marilyn Lewis, Diarmaid MacCulloch, Angela McShane, Kate Meaden, Roger Mettam, Michael Prestwich, Matthew Shaw, Richard Sharp, David Smith, Adam Smyth, John Spurr, Laura Stewart, Julian Swann and Anna Whitelock.

I have been helped by librarians and archivists around England, and particularly want to thank staff at the Bedfordshire and Luton Archives, Birkbeck Library, the British Library, The National Archives, the Senate House Library, and the Wellcome Library; in America I have been helped by librarians at the National Library of Medicine, Washington. At the British

Museum Barrie Cook in the Department of Coins and Medals has been especially helpful and generous concerning touch-pieces. Richard Sharp arranged for the late Professor Howard Erskine-Hill's touch-pieces to be photographed by George Skipper, and I am beholden to both. Marilyn Polan translated much of William Tooker's *Charisma sive donum sanationis* from Latin into English for me, and I am very grateful for her help.

I am very lucky that the royal touch elicits much interest outside academia, and I have had many helpful and enjoyable conversations about it with friends. Special thanks go to Dean Bright, Tony Bull, Philip Carter, Karen Chester, Sue Dale, Laura Jacobs, Danny McCosh, Anna Minogue, Meg Russell, Carole Semaine, Sue Tilley, Thomas Turner and David Walls.

My family has been especially kind, understanding and good humoured. Heart-felt thanks go to my mum Pat and her husband Madhu, my sister Suzy and her daughter Lulu, my uncle Bob and Wen, and all the Brogans in Hertfordshire and Melbourne, Australia. Geraint Edwards encouraged me to enrol for a degree when I really thought it was beyond me and has been a tower of strength, wisdom and fun. His parents Dave and Edna, his brother Rhodri, and his grandmother Margaret have all been kind and helpful.

No one has saved me from myself, however, and I take full responsibility for the parts of this book that are in such poor health that even a miracle-working healer would shy away from them.

Stephen Brogan,
June 2015

Abbreviations

MS Add.	BL, Additional Manuscript
BL	British Library, London
BM	British Museum, London
Bodl. Lib.	Bodleian Library, Oxford
CUL	Cambridge University Library
HMC	Historical Manuscripts Commission
PRO	Public Record Office, London
TNA	The National Archives, London
BNJ	*British Numismatic Journal*
CSPD	*Calendar of state papers, domestic series*
CSPV	*Calendar of state papers and manuscripts, relating to English affairs, existing in the archives and collections of Venice: and in other libraries of northern Italy*, ed. Rawden Brown, London 1864–1947
EHR	*English Historical Review*
HJ	*Historical Journal*
JBS	*Journal of British Studies*
ODNB	*Oxford dictionary of national biography* , ed. H. C. G. Mathew and B. Harrison, Oxford 2004
P&P	*Past and Present*
SRP	*Stuart Royal Proclamations*, I: *Royal proclamations of King James I, 1603–1625*; II: *Royal proclamations of King Charles I, 1625–1646*, ed. J. F. Larkin and P. L. Hughes, Oxford 1973, 1983

Introduction: Interpreting the Royal Touch

'Saturday being appointed by his Majesty to touch such as were trou-
bled with the *Evil*, a great company of poor afflicted Creatures were met
together, many brought in Chairs and Flaskets, and being appointed by his
Majesty to repair to the Banqueting house, his Majesty sat in a Chair of
State, where he strok'd all that were brought to him, and then put about
each of their Necks a white Ribbin with an Angel of Gold on it. In this
manner his Majesty strok'd about 600, and such was his princely patience
and tenderness to the poor afflicted Creatures that though it took up a
very long time, his Majesty being never weary of wel-doing, was pleased to
make enquiry whether there were any more that had not yet been touch'd.
After Prayers were ended, the Duke of *Buckingham* brought a towel and
the Earl of *Pembrook* a Basin and Ewer, who after they had made their
obeisance to his majesty, kneeled down till his Majesty had washed'
                                   Mercurius Publicus, 21–28 June 1660

As soon as Charles II was restored to the throne at the end of May 1660 he
began to hold public ceremonies at least twice a week in London at which
he touched between 200 and 600 people who were ill with scrofula. This
disease was also known as struma, or the king's evil ('evil' as in malady, the
king's as he was thought to be able to cure it) or, as in the newspaper extract,
it was sometimes just called 'the evil'. It is an infection of the lymph nodes
by the tubercular bacillus, known in the modern world as tubercular adenitis;
its symptoms include painful and disfiguring abscesses and suppurations on
the face and neck.[1]

The ceremonies performed by Charles II were structured around prayers
and passages from the New Testament, following a practice that had existed
in different forms in England and France since the early Middle Ages. The
purpose of these services was to cure the sick in an imitation of Christ,
whom the Gospels recorded as having healed numerous people by his touch,
including those who were blind or had leprosy, or were physically infirm. Just
as Christ's cures were described as miraculous, so were those attributed to the
royal touch. Each person touched by the king was given a commemorative
gold medal known then as an Angel and today as a touch-piece; records kept
by staff at the Chapel Royal, who were responsible for supplying the correct
number of medals for each service, reveal that by the end of his reign in 1685
Charles had touched some 96,000 people.[2] This staggering figure is especially

---

[1]   Scrofula is discussed in more detail at pp. 17–19 below.

[2]   J. Browne, *Adenochoiradelogia*, London 1684, 79, 197–207. Unless otherwise stated
all references to this work are to book III, *Charisma basilicon*. The book and its author
are discussed at pp. 157–60 below.

intriguing when compared to the Tudor data: between 1530 and 1532 Henry VIII touched just sixty-five people.[3] Greater numbers of people were touched for scrofula during the Restoration by both Charles II and James II, and with greater regularity, than at any other time in English history.

The royal touch ceremonies at which Charles II officiated in 1660 were the largest that early modern England had yet known. London had experienced an influx of sick people who wanted the new king to cure them of their scrofula by his sacred touch, possibly as many as 2,000, with more arriving every day.[4] Charles had made no official announcement that people with scrofula should come to him to be touched but the practice was so central to English culture that it was expected that the restoration of the monarchy included the reinstatement of royal therapeutics, which had ceased during the Interregnum. Charles had already made clear his willingness to undertake his therapeutic duties by touching the sick throughout his exile on the continent, thus continuing a royal custom that was thought to date back to Edward the Confessor. Just before Charles embarked for England from The Hague he held three ceremonies on three consecutive days, the first two of which were private, for people with connections at court, whereas the third was a public ceremony at which he touched forty-eight people. Before this he had touched 260 people at Breda at a number of services, and his ceremonies at Brussels were equally popular: his 'patients' there included the two daughters of the marquis of Caracena, governor of the Spanish Netherlands, both of whom he apparently cured.[5] All of these ceremonies were attended by people from various parts of Europe: belief in the English king's ability to heal scrofula was not limited by national boundaries.

The restoration of the monarchy was met with much popular joy and celebration as well as sermonising that reflected on its rapid, peaceful and largely unpredicted nature, to the extent that it was often referred to as 'miraculous'.[6] The fervour for the royal touch was part of this tide of popular royalism, and the description of it from *Mercurius Publicus* reflects this enthusiasm, as well as informing the public of the ceremonial proceedings. It contrasts vividly the supplicants, many so unwell that they had to be carried in chairs or long basket-like stretchers known as flaskets, with the king sitting on his throne, an implicitly healthy state of affairs. It also records Charles's generosity and patience: each of the 600 people was touched and given a gold coin in a rite that lasted 'a very long time'.

---

[3] See p. 45 below.

[4] *Mercurius Publicus*, 21–28 June 1660; *Parliamentary Intelligencer*, 18–25 June 1660.

[5] A. van Wicquefort, *A relation in form of a journal, of the voyage and residence which the most excellent and most mighty Prince Charles the II of Great Britain, &c. hath made in Holland, from the 25 of May, to the 2 of June, 1660*, trans. W. Lower, The Hague 1660, 76, 78; Browne, *Adenochoiradelogia*, 157–8.

[6] N. H. Keeble, *The Restoration: England in the 1660s*, Oxford 2002, 32–5. See pp. 102–3, 106–9 below.

People who were sick with scrofula accessed the king's therapeutic touch through a ritual process. The supplicants first had to acquire a certificate from the minister of their parish stating that they had scrofula and had not been touched before; then they had to travel to London, some journeying great distances. On arrival they were examined by the king's personal surgeons, known as serjeant surgeons, to ensure that they did have scrofula, the only disease thought to be curable by the royal hand. Those who passed the medical assessment were given an admission token to the next ceremony, which in the first weeks of the Restoration would be held very soon. The ceremony was performed in the morning, so people had to arrive early at the correct venue, which was often the Banqueting House at Whitehall. Prior to attending, the king would have taken communion and heard a sermon, and he might have fasted; these rituals suggested that he needed to be purified in order to heal the sick by acting as a conduit for God's grace. The king took his place in the designated room, seated on a throne but not wearing formal robes, surrounded by courtiers. The ceremony began with two royal chaplains reciting a liturgy which comprised prayers and passages from the New Testament. The surgeon then led the first ill person to the monarch; both knelt together in obedience in front of the sovereign and then one of the chaplains read out Christ's words to his disciples after his resurrection: 'They shall lay their hands on the sick and they shall recover' (Mark xvi.18). At this moment the king used both hands to touch and stroke the scrofulous sores on the ill person's face and neck. The sick person was then led away to wait at one side, and this process continued until everyone had been individually touched. Once this had happened, the sufferers were each presented to the monarch for a second time in order to receive their commemorative gold medal, the Angel or touch-piece. Each of these had been threaded onto a white ribbon and was hung around each person's neck by the king as a passage was read from the Gospel of St John: 'It was the true light that lighteth every man which cometh into this world' (John i.9). Once everyone had received their Angel the king's hands were ritually cleansed in public by the Lord Chamberlain or other high-ranking nobles and the ceremony was closed with further prayers.[7]

During the initial weeks of the Restoration the government found that the demand for the royal touch exceeded its supply. In July scrofulous people were still arriving in droves, with the press reporting that 1,000 people from all over England and further afield were still waiting to be touched. Added to this problem was the convention that the royal touch was not practised in the capital during the summer due to the heat and the fear of the plague. Trying to find a middle road, the government announced in the newspapers that henceforth the ceremony would occur weekly on Fridays, in the Banqueting House, with the crowd limited to 200 people until everyone

---

[7] Browne, *Adenochoiradelogia*, 83–103; van Wiquefort, *Relation*, 74–8.

waiting in London had been touched.[8] This proved too stringent though, and shortly afterwards it was announced that healings would occur on Wednesdays and Fridays.[9] This was the new administration's first taste of trying to control the demand for royal therapeutics, an issue that would preoccupy the crown until the royal touch ceased to be practised in 1714 with the death of Queen Anne.

The royal touch was a remarkable phenomenon. Although it does not often feature in modern accounts of early modern England it was a central aspect of English culture. The kings and queens regnant who performed it were political leaders who took on the role of religious healers, something that can be difficult for modern minds to accommodate. For secular-minded people in modern democracies, politics and religion are meant to be separate from each other, although in practice this is not always the case: for example, there are still bishops in the British House of Lords. It might also seem alien that political or religious leaders should claim to heal the sick by touch. Today, in the West, medical science dominates the treatments available for those who are unwell, religious or spiritual healing practices occupying a more marginal position. Whatever form of therapy is undertaken, today it is likely to be administered privately, whereas crowds of people who had scrofula were treated together in public by the monarch. On the other hand, the royal touch was available for no cost; in today's world, any form of free medical care is an increasingly scarce and precious commodity.

The realisation that it was during the Restoration that the highest numbers of scrofulous people were touched by the crown is also not without its problems. It might be assumed that the trial and execution of Charles I in 1649 had ended belief in the mystical aspects of kingship. The Restoration was the time when the new science was emerging and the Enlightenment dawned, both of which can seem incompatible with thaumaturgic monarchy. It can also appear strange that Charles II touched the sick on such a large scale: was not his sacral role at odds with his great appetite for sexual conquest? At first glance it would seem to make more sense if the royal touch had been in greatest demand during the Middle Ages, given the cult of saints, healers and relics associated with Christendom at that time; more specifically, the numbers might be expected to have peaked during the reign of a medieval saintly king such as Edward the Confessor or Henry VI.

These problems are all addressed in this book. The royal touch originated in medieval France, and so the process by which it came to be practised in England must be examined. The ceremony was originally Roman Catholic: whereas numerous Catholic practices did not survive the Reformation, the royal touch did, and it went on to flourish in the seventeenth century, an age characterised by its virulent anti-popery. The royal touch survived these

---

8   *Mercurius Publicus*, 28 June–5 July 1660; CSPV xxxii. 182.
9   *Parliamentary Intelligencer*, 16–23 July 1660; *Mercurius Publicus*, 19–26 July 1660.

vicissitudes because at various junctures it was reformed in order to make it more Protestant. A key preoccupation of this book is therefore change over time. This is why a chronological approach has been chosen – a more thematic one would obscure this important and revealing theme.

The survival of the royal touch after the Reformation, and the resources that were required to make it more Protestant, are testament to its importance. The significance of the ceremony was three-fold: it projected monarchical authority, it sought to heal people who were ill with scrofula, and it was an imitation of Christ. Thus it will be argued that the royal touch was a place at which politics, medicine, and religion intersected. Hitherto within the scholarly literature it is the political value of the ceremony to the crown that has been privileged, and so before discussing the aims of the current book in more detail an examination of the historiography is in order.

The historiography of the royal touch

In 1911 the first of the two twentieth-century books on the royal touch, *The king's evil*, was published by the physician and historian of medicine, Sir Raymond Crawfurd. He shone much light on how doctors understood scrofula in pre-modern Europe and was sensitive to how the royal touch ceremony changed over time. Between 1916 and 1919 the numismatist Helen Farquhar published four articles in which she provided a meticulous history of the production and significance of the touch-pieces.[10] Then, in 1924, Marc Bloch published *Les Rois thaumaturges*, which was later translated and published as *The royal touch* (1973).[11] His book superseded earlier studies and

---

[10] R. Crawfurd, *The king's evil*, Oxford 1911; H. Farquhar, 'Royal charities, I: Angels as healing-pieces for the king's evil', *BNJ* xii (1916), 39–135; 'Royal charities, II: Touch-pieces for the king's evil', *BNJ* xiii (1917), 95–163; 'Royal charities, III: Continuation of touch-pieces for the king's evil: James II to William III', *BNJ* xiv (1918), 88–120; 'Royal charities, IV: Conclusion of touch-pieces for the king's evil: Anne and the Stuart princes', *BNJ* xv (1919), 141–84. A number of nineteenth-century antiquarians wrote about the royal touch: the three most useful articles are J. Pettigrew, 'The royal gift of healing', in his *On superstitions connected with the history and practice of medicine and surgery*, London 1844, 117–54; W. Sparrow Simpson, 'On the forms of prayer recited "At the healing" or touching for the king's evil', *Journal of the Archaeological Association* xxvii (1871), 282–307; and E. Law Hussey, 'On the cure of scrofulous diseases attributed to the royal touch', *Archaeological Journal* x (1883), 187–211. The full historiography is discussed in S. Brogan, 'The royal touch in early modern England: its changing rationale and practice', unpubl. PhD diss London 2011, 13–30.

[11] M. Bloch, *Les Rois thaumaturges: étude sur le caractère surnaturel attribué a la puissance royale particulièrement en France et en Angleterre*, Strasburg–Paris 1924, trans. J. E. Anderson as *The royal touch: sacred monarchy and scrofula in England and France*, London 1973; trans. into Italian as *Il re taumaturghi*, Turin 1973. All citations in this book are from the English edition of 1973, with corresponding French page references from the 1983 reprint in parentheses. The reasons for commissioning the English translation remain speculative as

remains very influential to this day.[12] Bloch (1886–1944) himself is one of the twentieth century's most important historians, a co-founder, with Lucien Febvre, of the Annales School.[13]

Bloch's impulse for working on the royal touch derived from his doctoral work on kings and serfs which fostered his interest in ritual. *The royal touch* was pioneering for a number of reasons. It broke away from the dominant positivist tradition of political history of the day, instead offering a comparative and interdisciplinary study of the healing practices of the French and English monarchies. It was a *longue durée* political narrative that incorporated insights from anthropology, medicine, psychology and sociology. Bloch sought to unearth the 'collective mentality' that allowed for belief in royal thaumaturgy; his historical method was influenced by the French sociologist Emile Durkheim, who privileged the importance of human societies and collective norms over individual agency.[14] This marked out Bloch's book from earlier treatments of the royal touch that tended to assume that belief in it was 'superstitious'. The result of Bloch's sensitivity to disciplines other than history is that his highly perceptive book used a wide variety of sources including texts, images and coins.

Bloch's concern with 'collective mentalities' led him to contextualise the royal touch by discussing other magical beliefs and practices that were associated with the English and French monarchies, such as the case of St Marcoul,

neither publisher has kept their relevant file, but by 1973 all of Bloch's books had been translated into English so English publishers were aware that his books sold well. At that time the recent discovery of anthropology by historians had opened up new areas of study such as magic and witchcraft, making royal thaumaturgy more topical than it had been. The English translation is unusual in that it lacks an introduction by a modern scholar, thus differing from both the Italian translation, also of 1973, that has one by Carlo Ginzburg, and the French reprint of 1983 that has one by Jacques Le Goff.

[12] I have been greatly helped by treatments of the royal touch published since that of Bloch. These include Keith Thomas, *Religion and the decline of magic*, London 1971, repr. 1997, 192–211; F. Barlow, 'The king's evil', *EHR* xcv (1980), 3–27; N. Woolf, 'The sovereign remedy: touch-pieces and the king's evil', *BNJ* xlix (1980 for 1979), 99–121, and 'The sovereign remedy: touch-pieces and the king's evil, II', *BNJ* l (1981 for 1980), 91–116; D. J. Sturdy, 'The royal touch in England', in H. Duchhardt, R. A. Jackson and D. J. Sturdy (eds), *European monarchy: its evolution and practice from antiquity to modern times*, Stuttgart 1992, 171–84; H. Weber, 'The monarch's sacred body', in his *Paper bullets: print and kingship under Charles II*, Lexington, KY 1996, 50–87; S. Clark, *Thinking with demons*, Oxford 1997, ch. xliii; J. F. Turrell, 'The ritual of royal healing in early modern England', *Anglican and Episcopal History* lxviii/1 (1999), 3–36; S. Werrett, 'Healing the nation's wounds: royal ritual and experimental philosophy in Restoration England', *History of Science* xxxviii/4 (2000), 377–99; J. Shaw, *Miracles in Enlightenment England*, New Haven 2006, 64–73; and A. Keay, *The magnificent monarch: Charles II and the ceremonies of power*, London 2008, 112–19.

[13] C. Fink, *Marc Bloch, a life in history*, Cambridge 1989.

[14] Ibid. 109; R. Colbert-Rhodes, 'Emile Durkheim and the historical thought of Marc Bloch', *Theory and Society* v/1 (1978), 45–73; Bloch, *Les Rois thaumaturges*, 28–30 (52–4).

a French saint born about 540 whose relics were said to heal scrofula.[15] For Bloch, the royal touch came into being because people already had a magical outlook on life, the origins of which he found in primitive cultures in which people believed that kings were special and often possessed magical powers. This partly explained the Judeo-Christian practices of anointing kings, which, as Bloch noted, some commentators said was prerequisite for the royal touch.[16] Central to Bloch's treatment was the idea that the royal touch was used by the monarchy to assert its authority and proclaim its divine right to rule; and this has become the prevailing historiographical view.[17] He stated that the 'physician princes' did not cure scrofula but that they were not deceiving the populace as, just like them, the sovereigns believed in mystical or sacral monarchy.[18]

However, like many early twentieth-century intellectuals Bloch rejected magic and 'superstition' and concluded that belief in the efficacy of the royal touch was due to 'mass belief and collective error'.[19] He discussed two possible explanations for this. He initially postulated that the close proximity of the sovereign to sick people might stimulate their imaginations and bring about a psychosomatic cure, but when he discussed this with medical doctors they were hostile, so he dismissed it. Instead, Bloch favoured science over psychology: he stated that modern science maintains that scrofula can sometimes go into remission of its own accord, giving the appearance of a cure.[20] Because of the widespread belief that monarchs possessed mystical powers people were predisposed to expect wondrous things from them, Bloch suggested, so if someone's scrofula went into remission after they were touched then it could be attributed to the royal hand. Since Bloch other scholars have speculated that belief in the royal touch can be explained either by the power of suggestion or by the sometimes-episodic nature of scrofula, the implication being that early modern people were not aware of these possibilities.[21] In fact both topics were debated in early modern England which means that explaining belief in the royal touch is more complex than is sometimes thought.

When Bloch's book was published some historians praised it for its innovative qualities, but the sociologist Maurice Halbwachs – a colleague of Bloch's at Strasbourg University – objected that Bloch could have shed more light on why people believed in the ritual if he had concentrated on the period

---

[15] Bloch, *The royal touch*, 151–76 (261–308).

[16] Ibid. 3, 28–48 (18, 51–86).

[17] It is explicit or implicit in the works mentioned at n. 12 above.

[18] Bloch, *The royal touch*, 238 (420).

[19] Ibid. 238, 243 (420, 429); Fink, *Bloch*, 129.

[20] Bloch, *The royal touch*, 237–8, 242 (419–20, 428).

[21] See pp. 167–73 below.

when those beliefs were most fully developed rather than by taking his *longue durée* approach.[22] This is one of the aims of this study.

The scope of Bloch's book was weighted towards France, which as he explained was because he was only able to make one trip of three month's duration to England at the beginning of his research.[23] While his book examined the royal touch over many centuries it was the medieval period that dominated the book: the early modern period occupied a mere fifty-one pages.[24] As Bloch was a medievalist this may not be surprising, but paradoxically the bulk of the evidence concerning the royal touch dates from the early modern period. This is partly because it was during that period that the ritual was practised on a greater scale in both England and France. Bloch engaged closely with the relatively sparse medieval evidence, using it to construct a daring history that placed the royal touch at the heart of French and English culture. He paid less attention to the more plentiful early modern sources because the closer he got to the Enlightenment, and the 'birth of modernity', the more difficult it was for him to explain the persistence of the royal touch, let alone its increasing popularity. The early modern texts that discuss the healing rite were given only very brief mention, as was pre-eighteenth-century scepticism about it, referred to as 'the first awkward steps of childhood'.[25] This was because neither fits his thesis. In other words, according to Bloch, a society whose mind-set allowed for belief in miraculous healings would not have been able to analyse the royal touch or discuss it critically. His emphasis on mass belief did not allow much room for scepticism, so Bloch overstated the degree to which people believed in the royal touch in England and France. He said that 'as for the crowds, they believed in miracles with whole-hearted passion' and he claimed that doubt was only expressed by people in other countries, as in England and France the 'sceptics were reduced to a policy of silence'.[26] Bloch's tendency to homogenise belief was true of his own times too: he said that 'nowadays' no one believed in things like the 'physiological influence of the stars'.[27]

Bloch's book is an insightful and ground-breaking study that offers a provocative thesis concerning belief in the ritual. It is pioneering, and like many such books it is compelling because it covers new ground while at the same time leaving many unanswered questions. Bloch himself was aware of

[22] S. Friedman, *Marc Bloch, sociology and geography: encountering changing disciplines,* Cambridge 1996, 118.

[23] Bloch, *The royal touch,* 293 n. 6 (21).

[24] Ibid. 177–228 (309–405).

[25] Ibid. 235 (414).

[26] Ibid. 232, 233 (410–11).

[27] Ibid. 236 (417).

this, stating that he made 'no claim at all to completeness' but rather hoped he would stimulate further research.[28]

This book endorses Bloch's argument and also the prevailing historiographical tradition that the royal touch could project monarchical authority. However, this could only be the case if people believed in the possibility of thaumaturgic monarchy. The belief system that allowed for this was composed of three parts – politics, medicine and religion – each of which will be considered in turn. These often overlap, but for the sake of clarity they will initially be discussed separately, concentrating on the Stuart Restoration, when the ceremony reached its apogee in England.

The political interpretation can be subdivided. The first aspect is, of course, Bloch's view concerning monarchical authority and is 'top down'. By administering to thousands of people with scrofula as soon as he was restored, Charles II asserted that he was the legitimate king, appointed by God. Charles touched the sick in imitation of Christ, thus uniting throne and altar, while those who flocked to him as healer paid allegiance to the crown. In exile the ceremony had played a similar role, albeit on a smaller scale. The only other country in which sovereigns touched for scrofula was France; Charles's therapeutic practices therefore aligned him with his cousin Louis XIV. The French king also touched on a large scale and he too was involved in re-building monarchical authority after civil wars, in his case The Fronde, something that cannot have been lost on contemporaries.

The great demand for Charles II's touch much be acknowledged. This leads to the second political aspect of the practice, which is 'bottom up'. Charles and his government responded sensitively to the great demand for royal therapeutics, organising ceremonies that took up a lot of time and resources, not least the great sums spent on minting the touch-pieces. This sensitivity partly reflects the fact that the king was administering to people who had been unable to access the royal touch in London since Charles I fled the capital in 1642. Since then Charles I had been defeated in two civil wars, and in 1649 tried as a war criminal and executed. The House of Lords had been abolished, as had the episcopate, and the country ruled by Oliver Cromwell and his major-generals, none of whom touched the sick despite their desire to create a Godly commonwealth. Yet this acute turmoil and strife, sometimes said to have desacralised the monarchy,[29] had done nothing to undermine belief in the royal touch. In fact, it had greatly increased the demand for it. It is worth reiterating that between 1530 and 1532 Henry VIII had touched sixty-five people,[30] whereas Charles II touched an average

---

[28] Ibid. 7 (23)

[29] See especially R. Zaller, 'Breaking the vessels: the desacralisation of monarchy in early modern England', *Sixteenth-Century Journal* xxix/3 (1998), 757–78.

[30] See p. 45 below.

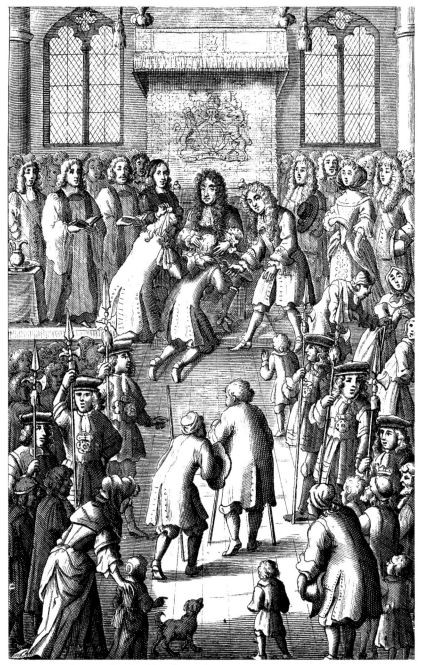

Figure 1. 'The royal gift of healing', frontispiece to Browne, *Adenochoiradelogia*.

of 4,000 each year until 1680 when the figure rose to 6,000; the total for Charles's reign was some 96,000.

The 'bottom up' political reading of the royal touch leads to the second part of the analysis, which is medical. Even though the royal touch could project monarchical authority and allow others to bow down to it, it was not just a metaphor. People really were ill and wanted to be cured, not least because scrofula was often very difficult to treat. Sometimes they travelled great distances to get to Charles II, despite being severely unwell, journeying from all over Britain and even from as far away as Russia and the New World. This means that there is a medical interpretation of the royal touch. Indeed, the king had no monopoly on curing scrofula. Doctors prescribed medicine and recommended the royal touch to their patients and they wrote tracts on scrofula in which they discussed their patients being touched by the king; surgeons operated on scrofulous tumours; and a range of healers administered medicinal remedies and charms, some even offering tactile therapy. Sometimes the royal touch was the last resort for especially hard-to-treat cases of scrofula when all other options had failed.

The third interpretation is religious. The rationale for healing by touch was that it was a continuation of Christ's ministry. This was particularly evident in the verse that was read aloud each time the king stroked someone's scrofulous sores: 'They shall lay their hands on the sick and they shall recover.' Apologists for the practice stressed that the king's hands acted as a conduit for God's healing powers and that when someone's scrofula was cured it was a miraculous event. The ceremony was structured around passages from the New Testament and prayers; these were recited by two royal chaplains; the rite was often performed in chapels or cathedrals. Furthermore, religion and health were very closely linked in pre-modern Europe: disease was associated with sin, recovery with God's blessing, forgiveness and redemption. Prayer was usually thought to supplement medicine, or might even be a remedy on its own.

One of the central arguments of this book is that the royal touch lends itself to political, medical and religious interpretations and that, given the belief systems, structures and practices of early modern England, these have a great tendency to overlap. Indeed, the royal touch could act as an intersection where politics, medicine and religion met. This is evident in the extract from *Mercurius Politicus*, and in Robert White's striking engraving of Charles II touching for scrofula in John Browne's *Adenochoiradelogia* (*see* Figure 1).[31] To begin with the king himself: in the text he is the authority figure, sitting on the chair of state and attended by a duke and an earl; in the image Charles sits under a canopy bearing the royal coat-of-arms, flanked by courtiers and guarded by armed yeomen. This all bears out the 'top down' political reading. Yet in pre-modern Europe authority was usually thought

---

[31] This image will be introduced and examined in detail in chapter 5 below.

to be ordained by God, so politics was underpinned by religion. Charles's role in the ceremony was that of healer, which combines the religious with the medical. As far as the supplicants are concerned, the text informs us that some were so ill that they had to be carried; in the image there are in the foreground two people waiting to be touched, one stooping, the other walking with crutches, while to the right someone waits with a bandaged head. These people were sick and they had been assessed twice to ensure that they did have scrofula, once in their place of residence and again at the royal court: this is indicative of the medical interpretation as well as the 'bottom up' political one that reflects the demand for the royal touch. The supplicants turned to their king in the hope of a cure, an action that embodies politics, medicine and religion. In the image the medical reading is further evident in that the man being touched by the king is flanked by two surgeons who officiate at the ceremony. The religious aspect of the ceremony includes mention in the text that it was structured around prayers, while in the image two chaplains stand to the left of the king, reading the liturgy from prayer books.

By broadening out the analysis from 'top down' politics to include medicine, religion and the demand for the royal touch, this study interprets the unprecedented enthusiasm for the ceremony during the Restoration in new ways. It allows us to think about the reassertion of royal authority in 1660 as well as the great appetite for it. It draws attention to the relationship between medicine and religion, and to the link of both to politics. But what expectations did people have of the ceremony: exactly how efficacious was it? If the ceremony were to have a significant role in the projection of monarchical authority then surely it must have been important that the king did heal people. And yet, not surprisingly, there is no evidence that during Charles II's reign some 96,000 people were completely cured of their scrofula at the very moment that he touched them. But if the ceremony did not work in the way that the Bible recounts Christ's miracles, why were so many people determined to access it? As people believed that the monarch could cure by touch one wonders if the healing power was only available during the ceremony, or whether sovereigns could touch the sick at any time, in the way that Christ had. We must also ask why the thaumaturgic rulers only touched for scrofula, and why people with other ailments sometimes tried to gain admission to the ceremonies. The particularity of the royal touch in connection with scrofula highlights the need to examine the origins of the ceremony and its early history. This must then be compared with how the early modern apologists presented the ritual's history. Did the ceremony remain unchanged over the years? If not, when and why did it change and how popular were these innovations? During the Restoration the new science emerged, which rejected ancient orthodoxies in favour of observation and experimentation, and yet at the same time as this crucial intellectual change the appeal of thaumaturgic monarchy escalated as never before. It might seem counter-intuitive that the numbers touched by the king should increase at a time when belief in royal therapeutics might be expected to have declined with the emergence of science and Enlightenment. How can this be explained? How did people elucidate their belief in the healing powers of the monarch's hands? Did everyone believe in the royal touch? Or was belief in it limited to people who were uneducated, or to royalists and High Church Tories, some of whom might not have understood or welcomed intellectual and social advances? Did anyone doubt the efficacy of the ceremony? If so, who, and on what grounds, and how was their scepticism articulated?

These are some of the questions that this book seeks to answer. Understanding of the early modern period has changed immensely since the publication of Bloch's book in 1923. Consequently this study asks new questions about the royal touch, finds new evidence to answer them, and sometimes offers revised interpretations of evidence that is already known to scholars. This new treatment of the royal touch is therefore both timely and interdisciplinary. Understanding of the construction and projection of monarchical authority has greatly increased in recent decades, by works including Kevin Sharpe's trilogy on the Tudor and Stuart sovereigns.[32] This book furthers knowledge in this area; but it also examines how that authority was received and debated. As well as power, this study is interested in the benevolent and charitable aspects of kingship, and the imperatives and belief systems that underpinned them.

The place of religion in early modern England is hotly debated, with the effects of the Reformation occupying a central position in the discourse. The royal touch survived the Reformation, which supports the recent historiographical turn that emphasises that not all the old beliefs and practices were swept away in the 1530s and 1540s, as was once believed to be the case.[33] On the other hand, the royal touch was reformed during the Tudor and Stuart age, in order to 'Protestantise' it and bring it into line with new ideas concerning the relationship between humankind and God. The present study should therefore be of interest to scholars of early modern religion who are interested in continuity, as well as those who are concerned with theological and ceremonial innovation.

Another important advance in our understanding of early modern England is the key role of the supernatural in people's lives. The royal touch was predicated on belief that the physical world was influenced by the supernatural

[32] K. Sharpe, *Selling the Tudor monarchy: authority and image in sixteenth-century England*, London 2009; *Image wars: promoting kings and commonwealths in England, 1603–1660*, London 2010; and *Rebranding rule: the Restoration and revolution monarchy, 1660–1714*, London 2013. See also S. Anglo, *Images of Tudor kingship*, London 1992; Keay, *Magnificent monarch*; and R. G. Asch, *Sacral kingship between disenchantment and re-enchantment: the French and English monarchies, 1587–1688*, New York–Oxford 2014.

[33] For example, E. Duffy, *The stripping of the altars: traditional religion in England, 1400–1580*, London 1992.

realm, that God was omnipotent and interventionist. It was usual to think that the world was a Manichean battle ground in which God and his angels fought the devil, his demons and his witches; not surprisingly, salvation and damnation were chief preoccupations of many early modern people. Again, recent scholarship stresses the continuity of supernatural belief throughout the early modern period which has led to a re-thinking of the Reformation and the Enlightenment.[34] Similarly, historians of science and intellectual change are aware that eminent natural philosophers such as Robert Boyle and Isaac Newton were preoccupied with magical investigation as well as scientific activities.[35] All of this makes more difficult the task of explaining the 'disenchantment' and secularisation that would eventually characterise the eighteenth century. This book should be of interest to scholars working on witchcraft and the occult because it has much to say about the supernatural; it should also interest those preoccupied with how and why such beliefs and practices were abandoned, and by whom.[36] Not all early modern people were devout, of course, the age being characterised by an increasing fear of atheism and irreligion. The wits, libertines and free thinkers associated with the later Stuart age demonstrate that this was not mere paranoia. This book pays attention to those who doubted the efficacy of the royal touch, critics who were castigated as atheists by the rite's apologists. We will see who was ambivalent and sceptical and on what grounds, which will further understanding of marginal and heterodox ideas in early modern England.[37]

The history of medicine has also revolutionised thinking about pre-modern England and Europe. Not only is more known about medical theory and practice, but recent scholarship has privileged the importance of the medical market place, the negotiations between doctors and patients, and the expectations that both had of therapies. The huge variety of practitioners, from doctors to quacks to cunning men and women, is a feature of much recent work.[38] This book addresses how people understood scrofula, and the

[34] A. Walsham, *The reformation of the landscape: religion, identity and memory in early modern Britain and Ireland*, Oxford 2011; P. Monod, *Solomon's secret arts: the occult in the age of Enlightenment*, London 2013.

[35] M. Hunter, *Boyle: between God and science*, New Haven 2009; R. S. Westfall, *Never at rest: a biography of Isaac Newton*, Cambridge 1980. For definitions of occult and science see J. Henry, *The scientific revolution and the origins of modern science*, Basingstoke 2008, esp. ch. iv.

[36] M. Hunter, 'The Royal Society and the decline of magic', *Notes and Records of the Royal Society* lxv (2011), 103–19.

[37] J. Champion, *The pillars of priestcraft shaken: the Church of England and its enemies, 1660–1730*, Cambridge 1992; S. Ellenzweig, *The fringes of belief: English literature, ancient heresy, and the politics of freethinking, 1660–1760*, Stanford, CA 2008.

[38] R. Porter, *Mind forg'd manacles: a history of madness in England from the Restoration to the Regency*, London 1987, and *Bodies politic: disease, death and doctors in Britain, 1650–1900*, London 2001, 101–17; A. Wear, *Knowledge and practice in English medicine, 1550–1680*, Cambridge 2000, and (ed.), *Medicine in society: historical essays*, Cambridge 1992;

role of the surgeons at the royal court who diagnosed it and then participated in the royal touch ceremony. It also furthers understanding of how
religion underpinned medicine. However, it avoids the positivist question
of whether or not people really were cured by the laying on of royal hands.
To dismiss the royal touch as working by psychosomatics or to explain away
cures by the coincidence of scrofula going into remission of its own accord
soon after someone was touched seems disrespectful and reductionist. Early
modern people differed in their opinions of how efficacious the ceremony
was, and this debate will be analysed objectively. Historians of witchcraft
discuss witches, spells and magic rather than 'witches' 'spells' and 'magic' and
this book engages with royal therapeutics in a similarly impartial manner.

The present study concentrates on the royal touch in early modern
England because, although the ceremony originated in the Middle Ages, in
terms of its vitality it was an early modern phenomenon, reaching its zenith
during the Restoration. A wide range of sources has been utilised, including
manuscripts, printed texts and images, touch-pieces, liturgies, ballads, and
playing cards. No source is 'innocent' of course; all contain bias and subjectivity whether or not those who produced them were aware of it. Many of the
sources used in this book were produced by royal touch apologists, meaning
that at times one has to tread carefully in order to avoid hyperbole and flat-
tery. Yet the apologists were also capable of candid objectivity and sometimes
they were even critical of aspects of their subject, while knowledge of doubt
concerning royal therapeutics owes much to their refutation of it. This study
has learned much from historians of witchcraft and popular culture, who
are used to negotiating evidence at one remove through archival sources
that comment on their subject, rather than first-hand testimonies.[39] Most
of the sceptical comments concerning the royal touch were expressed orally
before the eighteenth century, and so the importance of the oral tradition
is acknowledged. Beyond the word, coins and images can also be analysed,
often yielding as much useful information as textual sources.[40]

D. Harley, 'Spiritual physic, providence and English medicine, 1560–1740', in P. O. Grell
and A. Cunningham (eds), *Medicine and the Reformation*, London 1993, 101–17; P. O.
Grell and A. Cunningham (eds), *Religio medici: medicine and religion in seventeenth-century
England*, Aldershot 1996.

[39] Thomas, *Religion and the decline of magic*; P. Burke, *Popular culture in early modern
Europe*, London 1978; T. Harris (ed.), *Popular culture in England*, c. 1500–1850. London
1995; M. Gaskill, *Crime and mentalities in early modern England*, Cambridge 2000.

[40] A. Griffiths, *The print in Stuart Britain*, London 1998; Sheila O'Connell, *The popular
print in England*, London 1999; H. Pierce, *Unseemly pictures: graphic satire and politics
in early modern England*, London 2008; M. Hunter (ed.), *Printed images in early modern
Britain: essays in interpretation*, Farnham 2010; M. Jones, *The print in early modern England*,
London 2010.

Structure

The royal touch originated in medieval France so that although this book is concerned with early modern England it is necessary trace the French origins of the ceremony and its assimilation into English culture. This is the concern of chapter 1. The context for this will be seen to be royal benevolence and charity, and the relationship between the English and French monarchies. The example of royal thaumaturgy that was unique to the English crown, the blessing and distribution of medicinal cramp rings will also be considered.

The royal touch was practised only intermittently in England during the Middle Ages but was revived by the Tudors. The reasons for this are examined in chapter 2, as are the reforms that enabled the ceremony to survive the Reformation. Gender is an issue, given that the rite was performed by two queens regnant, Mary Tudor and Elizabeth I. The first two books published in England on the royal touch date from the end of Elizabeth's reign and these are used to tease out the rationale of the Tudor cult. New light is also shone on the reforms of the ceremony that date from Elizabeth's reign.

Chapter 3 surveys the royal touch during the seventeenth century, from the accession of James VI and I in 1603 until the Glorious Revolution of 1688. It explains the increasing popularity of the ceremony during the reigns of the first two Stuart kings of England and the effects that this had on its practice, and then clarifies why the disruptions of the Civil War did not diminish demand for royal therapeutics. During the Republic the royal touch ceased to be practised but the Restoration experienced a huge reaction in favour of thaumaturgic monarchy, which is explained by reference to contemporary beliefs concerning the body politic and sin. Alongside this will be considered the case of Valentine Greatrakes, the Irish 'stroker' who came to England in 1666, and who is sometimes described as a rival healer to Charles II. Chapter 4 then teases out the ritual process during its Restoration heyday, from prior announcements to the ceremony itself to retrospective assessments of it, utilising written, visual and numismatic sources. We will see that at times the great demand for the royal touch led to problems in managing the crowds, meaning that the rite was not always as dignified as the official accounts of it maintained. Chapter 5 turns to the Restoration debate on the efficacy of the royal touch: vews on it ranged from belief to ambivalence to scepticism, all of which were expressed by a wide range of people from across the different ranks of society.

Chapter 6 is concerned with William III who did not touch for scrofula, and Anne who did, as well as the debate concerning the efficacy of the practice that raged well after its cessation in 1714, until the middle of the eighteenth century. The extent to which the debate was party-political is scrutinised, as is the effect on it of the intellectual revolution of the period.

The medical context

It makes sense to end the introduction to this book by returning to the medical context and examining it in more detail, because the theory and practice of medicine remained fairly static during the medieval and early modern periods. More specifically, the treatments available to someone who had scrofula remained the same. The medical context is an important component of our study that illuminates some of the interpretative problems within it.

Plate 1 and Figure 2 are nineteenth-century depictions of young men with scrofula. The lymph nodes of the neck were especially vulnerable to infection by the tubercular bacillus, as is evident in both images, and when scrofula is untreated suppurations occur which can affect the face and eyes. The bovine strand of the bacillus was particularly robust, so scrofula was transmitted largely by the consumption of unpasteurised milk. Airborne transmission was also possible, though this would result in a tubercular infection of the respiratory system rather than scrofula. The disease has almost disappeared from the developed world today, largely due to the pasteurisation of milk that began in the mid-nineteenth century, though it is found in some minority ethnic communities in the West, especially among immigrants, and is still prevalent in parts of Africa and Asia.[41]

Scrofula was rife in pre-modern Europe. The London Bills of Mortality record that 6,353 people died from scrofula, between 1629 and 1758.[42] However, the bills only record burials in Church of England churchyards, and so do not include dissenters, Roman Catholics or non-Christians. The disease could manifest itself in a number of ways: it might be acute, whereby the sufferer had periods when scrofula was visibly present and other times when it went into remission; it might be a chronic, long term condition; or it might even be fatal. Doctors were very familiar with it and so usually

41 B. Phillips, 'The prevalence and alleged increase of scrofula', Journal of the Statistical Society of London ix/2 (1846), 152–7; B. Bramwell, Atlas of clinical medicine, Edinburgh 1892–6, ii. 1–5; Bloch, The royal touch, 11–12 (27–8); R. K. French, 'Scrofula', in K. F. Kiple (ed.), Cambridge historical dictionary of disease, Cambridge 1993, 292–4; S. Grzybowski and E. A. Allen, 'The history and importance of scrofula', The Lancet, 2 Dec 1995, 1472–4; K. F. Kiple, 'Scrofula: the king's evil and struma Africana', in K. F. Kiple (ed.), Plague, pox and pestilence in London, London 1997, 44–9.
42 John Graunt records 656 deaths between 1629 and 1636 and 1647 and 1659, in his Natural and political observations made upon the Bills of Mortality, London 1663. A further 5,697 are recorded in the Bills between 1660 and 1758: J. Postlethwayt, J. Graunt, W. Petty, C. Morris and W. Heberden, A collection of the yearly Bills of Mortality, from 1657 to 1758 inclusive, London 1759. In the parish of St Botolph without Aldgate, London, 4,253 deaths were recorded between 1583 and 1599, of which five were attributed to scrofula: T. Rogers Forbes, Chronicle from Aldgate: life and death in Shakespere's London, New Haven 1971, 101. I am grateful to Phil Baker for this reference. See also pp. 207–8 below.

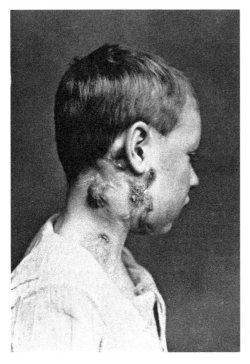

Figure 2. 'A young man with scrofula', from B. Bramwell, *Atlas of clinical medicine*, Edinburgh 1892–6, ii, plate 31.

diagnosed it correctly, even though the boundaries of the diagnosis could be porous, with other similar infections of the eyes, glands, face and neck sometimes being loosely diagnosed as scrofula.[43]

The millenarian mood of sixteenth- and seventeenth-century Europe meant that for many people scrofula was analogous to leprosy, which reinforced the Christ-like aspect of the thaumaturgic sovereigns.[44] Indeed, that no English or French monarch ever caught scrofula must have added to the mystique of royalty (although Edward VI probably died of a tubercular respiratory infection).[45] However, great care was taken with royal hygiene. In France the royal touch was practiced outdoors to minimise the amount of bad odours that the king would smell, and to guard against miasma. In England the ceremony appears to have been performed indoors, in cathedrals, chapels and palaces, though the designated room was fumigated for the same reasons. In both countries the ceremony closed with the sovereign's

---

[43] Bloch, *The royal touch*, 11 (27); Thomas, *Religion and the decline of magic*, 272–8, 242–3; Barlow, 'King's evil', 4.

[44] Barlow, 'King's evil', 4.

[45] Also noteworthy is the Spanish queen Maria Luisa of Savoy, the wife of Philip V and the niece of Louis XIV, who died of scrofula in 1714: Louis de Rouvroy, duc de Saint-Simon, *Memoirs of duc de Saint-Simon, 1710–1715: the bastards triumphant*, ed. and trans. L. Norton, Warwick, NY 2007, 200, 319.

hands being thoroughly washed in a public, an act of ritual cleansing that signified that the healing role was now over.

In pre-modern Europe there was no scientific rationale for life. It was usual to believe that the primary cause of disease and misfortune was sin, meaning that medicine and religion were inextricably linked together. It followed from this that recovery depended on acknowledging one's sins to God, praying for forgiveness, and having faith, all of which were believed to be essential if medicine and other therapies were to be effective.[46] When the sovereign laid hands on the sick with the intention of curing them, the royal touch signified the potential triumph of health over disease, of good over evil (this rationale was made clear in the inscriptions and depictions on the gold Angels given to supplicants).[47] As such, there is a striking resemblance between the ceremony and another early modern healing rite, exorcism.

Both the royal touch and exorcism began as Roman Catholic curative practices that connected the physical world to the spiritual. Contracting scrofula and demonic possession could both be explained by sin, a point of view that assumed that health was vulnerable to supernatural forces. Demonic possession produced visible symptoms such as physical contortions, writhing, talking in tongues, vomiting foreign objects and revulsion at sacred things; scrofula was especially noticeable as it attacked the glands of the neck and often affected the eyes. Both sets of symptoms could be episodic, the capriciousness of which could reinforce belief in their mysterious or spiritual origins. The royal touch and exorcism both relied on intermediary figures to act as a conduit for God's curative powers, the king and the priest; both rites were structured around prayers and liturgies that attested to the power of sacred language. Indeed, in the eighteenth century it was suggested that Henry VII codified the royal touch liturgy out of the service for dispossession.[48]

During the English Reformation exorcism was initially rejected as idolatrous as it had no biblical sanction, a criterion that reformers argued was required for religious practices; although Christ had cast out demons he had not used the Roman formula to do so. Counter-Reformation Catholics continued to exorcise demons, which enabled them to claim superior spiritual power: they successfully exorcised possessed people in England, a sign, they argued, that theirs was the true faith. By way of response, reformers reintroduced exorcism by giving it scriptural authority which in turn reframed the practice so that it centred on prayer and fasting. The scriptural mandate came from Mark ix.14–29, in which Jesus exorcised a youth possessed by a

---

[46] R. Porter, *The greatest benefit to mankind: a medical history of humanity from antiquity to the present*, London 1997, chs iv–v; C. Rawcliffe, *Medicine and society in later medieval England*, Stroud 1999, ch. i.

[47] See pp. 142–5 below.

[48] W. Becket, *A free and impartial enquiry into the antiquity and efficacy of touching for the cure of the king's evil*, London 1722, 52; pt III, 14.

deaf and dumb spirit whom his disciples had been unable to help. When asked by his Apostles why they had failed, Jesus replied that 'This kind can come forth by nothing, but by prayer and fasting.' Faith, scriptural authority and a strong desire to quash Catholic propaganda led to Protestants dispossessing people by means of marathon sessions of prayer and fasting.[49] In a similar fashion the royal touch survived the Reformation partly because Protestants emphasised the curative potential of the prayers involved.[50]

The supernatural interpretation of the royal touch was accompanied by medical theories of secondary causation that concentrated on the physical body and its environment. The spread of disease was explained by miasma theory, as opposed to the modern germ theory. Miasma theory maintained that decaying matter in the air caused a poisonous vapour or miasma which then infected people.[51] Contemporaries described the putrid sores that characterised scrofula as foul smelling, which can only have reinforced this theory of infection.

Since antiquity one of the key ways in which people understood their health was humoralism, whereby the body was composed of four liquids or humours – blood, yellow bile, black bile and phlegm. Good health, it was believed, depended upon all four humours being in balance with each other, whereas a surplus or deficit of one or more humour caused disease. The four humours related to the theory of four elements (blood with air, yellow bile with fire, black bile with earth, and phlegm with water), as well as to the four seasons (spring, summer, autumn, winter, respectively).[52] People with scrofula were thought to have an excess of bile and phlegm trapped in their glands. This could be attributed to a number of factors: corrupt air, inappropriate food, too much sleep, insufficient exercise, or a change of temper. It was also thought that cold climates were responsible for scrofula, which partly explained why it was so prevalent in Britain. Whether or not scrofula could be hereditary was debated, as sometimes both parents and their children suffered with it, but not always.[53]

Theories of causation influenced treatments. Aside from the royal touch, there were three main strands: medication, surgery and diet and lifestyle. People who were ill often tried a range of treatments, not least because scrofula was often difficult to cure no matter which option was tried. Doctors, quacks, apothecaries and cunning folk offered medication that could be consumed, purges and 'cathartics' that were meant to cleanse the blocked glands of trapped matter and re-balance humours. They also applied emollients to the

---

49 M. MacDonald, *Witchcraft and hysteria in Elizabethan London: Edward Jorden and the Mary Glover case*, London 1991, pp. xix–xx.

50 See pp. 62–3, 72–3, 152, 162–3, 169 below.

51 Porter, *Greatest benefit*, 79.

52 Ibid. 9, 56–8.

53 Browne, *Adenochoiradelogia*, bk II, 4, 104.

sores, the hope being that they would draw out the excess humours and dry the infected areas. Bleeding was not used to treat scrofula as blood was not thought to play a role in its causation. Surgeons made incisions and cut away scrofulous tumours. Diet and lifestyle factors included avoiding a 'flatulent, vaporous and windy Dyet', with beans, pork, cheese, leeks and onions best avoided. A diet that enabled good digestion was recommended, including veal, capon, mutton, lamb and small birds; corn bread; and broth with mint and marjoram. It was also important not to sleep for too long, and to guard against melancholy.[54]

Not surprisingly, patients in pre-modern Europe had very different expectations to their modern counterparts. In the modern developed world medical science is expected to cure ailments because of the incredible recent advances in science and healthcare; it is true that some diseases remain incurable, but nevertheless we tend to believe that in the future science will triumph over them. By contrast, in pre-modern Europe people had different expectations of doctors and medicine because so many diseases were difficult or impossible to treat: they were therefore much less cure-fixated. Furthermore, Christian doctrine taught that salvation came through suffering. The role of the doctor was primarily to provide pain management, to fortify the body and to adjust the whole constitution by rebalancing the humours. Treatment went beyond drugs and involved psychological consolation and rituals of comfort and condolence; if someone's disease was also cured, this was an additional benefit. Life was far more precarious then than now, which helps to explain why it was usual to believe that one's existence lay in the hands of God rather than those of the doctors.[55]

Bearing this in mind, what motivated ill people to seek the royal touch? This is complex, but three imperatives can be identified. First, faith: people hoped that God would intervene during the royal touch service and cure or alleviate their ailment. Second, opportunism: no doubt small numbers of people were attracted by the gift of the gold coin, or the prospect of a day out and the chance to see the monarch. Third, pragmatism: others might not have placed much faith in the royal hand at all, but attended the ceremony as their scrofula had proved resistant to other treatment.[56] But the expectations that sick people had of health care were completely different to ours

[54] Ibid. bk II, 99–103; R. Wiseman, *Several chiurgical treatises*, London 1676, pt IV. For recipes and household medicine see A. Stobart, ' "Lett her refrain from all hott spices": medicinal recipes and advice in the treatment of the king's evil in seventeenth-century south-west England', in M. DiMeo and S. Pennell (eds), *Reading and writing recipe books, 1550–1800*, Manchester 2013, 203–24.

[55] R. Porter, 'The patient's view: doing medical history from below', *Theory and Society* xiv/2 (1985), 175–98 at p. 193; H. J. Cook, 'Good advice and little medicine: the professional authority of early modern English physicians', *JBS* xxxiii (1994), 1–31 at pp. 13–14.

[56] For opportunism see pp. 81, 86–7, 125, 147 below; for pragmatism see pp. 92, 160, 161, 179.

today. Contemporaries must have appreciated that the royal touch did not miraculously heal people's scrofula in the immediate way that the Gospels recounted Christ's miracles. People with scrofula approached the sovereign hoping to be cured, but also seeking psychological consolation from being in close proximity to God's representative on earth, which allowed them the opportunity to act out in public their humility and obedience to the crown. The hope surely was that this would please God, who might alleviate their condition. Even a small incremental improvement in someone's condition soon after the ceremony signified the effectiveness of the royal touch.

1

The Origins and Medieval History of the Royal Touch, 1000–1485

The royal touch originated in France during the eleventh century and was practised intermittently until it became a regal prerogative in the thirteenth century. In England the origins are less certain, but by the thirteenth century the ceremony had been assimilated into English royal custom by the Plantagenet kings. Touching for scrofula was the key aspect of sacral monarchy, whereby the sovereign was anointed and performed religious duties. This chapter therefore argues that although the royal touch could enhance the political authority of the English and French crowns, it was a key component of the religious aspects of both monarchies during the Middle Ages. The religious duties of both crowns were of great importance to the theory and practice of kingship, and were closely interwoven with civil power. During the thirteenth century these religious observations were increased in number and performed more often due to the piety of Louis IX and his English counterpart Henry III. Some of these duties, such as alms-giving, were already established but others, such as the royal touch, were new or revived. Beyond this, a number of the dominant Christian values of medieval Europe provide further insight into the rationale and context of the royal touch, while the close relationship between England and France helps to explain why the English monarchs imitated their French kinsmen. It is worth noting, though, that the evidence concerning the origins and early history of the royal touch in both countries is fragmentary, meaning that sometimes questions can only be answered with speculation or left open.

This chapter will first consider the context of the royal touch, namely sacral monarchy and alms-giving, before turning to an analysis of its origins in France, and its early history in England. From Edward II to Mary Tudor English monarchs also performed a second thaumaturgic duty, the blessing and distributing of cramp rings – finger rings that were worn to ward off epileptic seizures – and so this practice too will be analysed.

Sacral monarchy and alms-giving

Kings needed to set themselves apart from the nobility, and, from the conversion of Constantine onwards, the Christian Church provided justification and sanction for temporal rulers. They were said to rule 'by the grace of God', meaning that they were chosen as God's representatives on earth.

Further endorsement from the Church came during the coronation, as in some countries kings were anointed by an archbishop with holy oil, on the head, chest and hands, in imitation of Old Testament kings. The model for this was Charlemagne, crowned and anointed in 800 as the first Holy Roman Emperor. Anointing consecrated the sovereign: it made their body holy, and, like the clergy, it separated them from the laity. It also raised the sovereign above their un-anointed counterparts in the hierarchy of European rulers. In theory unction gave the king his sacral character, turning him into a quasi-divine being; by contrast, in ancient Rome, some emperors had actually been made into Gods. Yet in reality kings were mortal and fallible, which partly explains the development of the political theory of the king's two bodies that also strengthened the monarchy. This maintained that each king had a physical, human body that was mortal, and a mystical body – the office of king – that was immortal. Again, the Church played an important role because it had already conceptualised itself in a similar manner. Christ, it was said, had two bodies. One was divine, but also human, physical, male and finite; the other was the Church, which was universal, perpetual and often represented as female.[1]

Sacral monarchy reached its apogee in France and England. From the ninth century the kings in both countries were anointed;[2] they each received communion in both kinds, the bread and the wine, as did the clergy but not the laity; both royal houses boasted a saint (Edward the Confessor in England, as well as a number of earlier Anglo-Saxon kings, and Louis IX in France); in both countries the crown was strengthened by primogeniture, whereas in countries such as Poland the king was elected. The annual cycle of the royal court centred on holy days, while the royal day itself was religious in character. Mass was heard each morning, ceremonies and prayers accompanied dining, as well as the *lever* and *coucher*, and on special occasions such as Twelfth Night the king's clothes were blessed.[3]

These were the preconditions for the ultimate expression of sacral monarchy, touching the sick in imitation of Christ. This was the most prolific example of royal thaumaturgy, but it was not the only one. In the ancient world Vespasian and Hadrian were each recorded as having healed a blind person by touch, while in medieval Europe the kings of Castile performed exorcisms. The counts of Hapsburg were said to be able to cure scrofula by handing their supplicants a liquid remedy to drink, and to cure by an embrace anyone who stammered. The kings of Hungary were reputed to be able to

---

[1]   P. Monod, *The power of kings: monarchy and religion in Europe, 1589–1715*, New Haven 1999, 36–42; J. Adamson, 'The making of the *ancien régime* court, 1500–1700', in J. Adamson, *The princely courts of Europe, 1500–1700*, London 2000, 7–42 at pp. 27–33; E. H. Kantorowicz, *The king's two bodies: a study in medieval political theology*, Princeton 1957.

[2]   Bloch, *The royal touch*, 38 (70).

[3]   C. M. Woolgar, *The senses in late medieval England*, New Haven 2006, 47–8.

cure jaundice.[4] These practices – real or imagined – could give a sacred aura to the rulers concerned. Thus myths could also arise concerning earlier sovereigns: in early modern France it was thought that Clovis (481–511) had healed by touch the sores on his favourite, Lanicet, though this seems very doubtful. The point was that it was usual to think that kings stood above their subjects but below the Almighty in the divinely-ordained hierarchy, so in theory sovereigns could act as intercessors between this world and God, channelling his grace, as did the clergy.[5]

Touching for scrofula obviously affirmed the God-given authority of kings, even if the apologists were divided as to whether this healing gift resulted from being anointed on the hands, or was hereditary. Whilst it was not until the early modern period that beliefs concerning the scriptural basis for royal authority became codified as the divine right of kings, its four components were well known in the medieval world. Monarchy was divinely ordained; hereditary right was indefeasible and regulated by primogeniture; kings were accountable to God alone; and non-resistance and passive obedience were enjoined by God.[6] If a king were personally devout, this enhanced the sacral aura of monarchy.[7]

While subjects owed obedience to their king, similarly the king was accountable to God. Christian kings therefore needed to be conspicuously devout and benevolent, or at least needed to act so in public on certain occasions, just as they were meant to rule within the law, dispense patronage fairly, protect the Church, provide for the succession and be victorious in battle. Medieval kings were peripatetic charismatic leaders and they came into contact with large numbers of destitute and ill people because it was a royal duty to make regular, charitable donations. Like provincial nobles, it was important that the king was a good lord.[8]

Poor and sick people journeyed to wherever the royal court resided to receive alms and to be fed. The records for Edward I's reign are particularly useful in this regard, revealing that the king usually fed at least 200

4   Bloch, *The royal touch*, 84–91 (146–57).

5   J. G. Frazer, *The golden bough: a study in magic and religion* (1922), abridged edn, London 1929, 9–11, 83–91; J. N. Figgis, *The divine right of kings*, Gloucester, MA 1970, 17–38; Crawfurd, *The king's evil*, 15; Bloch, *The royal touch*, 34 (63–4); J. M. Bak (ed.), *Coronations: medieval and early modern monarchic ritual*, Berkeley 1990; T. F. Ruiz, 'Unsacred monarchy: the kings of Castile in the late Middle Ages', in S. Wilentz (ed.), *Rites of power: symbolism, ritual and politics since the Middle Ages*, Philadelphia 1999, 109–44; S. Bertelli, *The king's body: sacred rituals of power in mediaeval and early modern Europe*, trans. R. Burr Litchfield, University Park, PA 2001.

6   Figgis, *Divine right*, 5–6.

7   Obviously the sacral aspects of monarchy were debated and sometimes even pious kings had doubts concerning the exact nature of their role and powers: N. Vincent, *The holy blood: King Henry III and the Westminster blood relic*, Cambridge 2006, 192.

8   H. Johnstone, 'Poor-relief in the royal households of thirteenth-century England', *Speculum* iv/2 (1929), 149–67; Barlow, 'King's evil', 14.

poor people every week. Special provision was also made for the poor and sick during Easter, Whitsun, Pentecost and Christmas, and on certain saint's days: at Christmas 1283, Edward gave 500 paupers one and half pence each. Charity was also dispensed by the royal family to commemorate joyous occasions, such as the birth of a son, or sad ones such as a death.[9]

After a king's demise it was customary for alms to be distributed lavishly at his funeral and then at his tomb, and in England a number of tenth- and eleventh-century Anglo-Saxon kings were said to have wrought miraculous cures posthumously at their tombs. Thus the line between caring for the sick and healing them could sometimes be very blurred, which reinforced the unique status of kings.[10] This was especially pertinent given that at this time disease and misfortune were usually understood providentially, and healing was associated as much with prayer and relics as with medicine.[11]

Alms-giving was a Christian duty. According to Thomas Aquinas, it was an act of mercy 'whereby something is given to the needy out of compassion and for God's sake'. Since man could be needy both spiritually and physically there were two forms of gift. The seven kinds of spiritual alms were listed as: 'instructing the ignorant, giving advice to those in doubt, consoling the sorrowful, reproving sinners, forgiving offences, putting up with people who are burdensome and hard to get on with and finally, praying for all'. The forms of material alms, also called the seven corporal works of mercy, were: 'feeding the hungry, giving drink to the thirsty, clothing the naked, giving hospitality to strangers, visiting the sick, ransoming prisoners, and burying the dead'.[12]

At the heart of the rationale for alms-giving and charity was the medieval theology of Christ's mystical presence within crowds of poor people, which allowed the better off to encounter Jesus, serve him, and be saved. This belief came directly from Christ's discourse on the Last Judgement.[13] Matthew's Gospel records that Christ addressed the righteous, who are to receive the Kingdom of Heaven as their inheritance, saying, 'For I was hungry and you gave me food, I was thirsty and you gave me drink, I was a stranger and you welcomed me, I was naked and you clothed me, I was sick and you visited me, I was in prison and you came to me.' The righteous asked him when it was that they saw him and did these things, and he replied 'Truly, I say

9   M. Prestwich, 'The piety of Edward I', in W. M. Ormrod (ed.), *England in the thirteenth century: proceedings of the 1984 Harlaxton Symposium*, Woodbridge 1985, 120–8 at pp. 120–3.

10   Barlow, 'King's evil', 14.

11   Rawcliffe, *Medicine and society*, 21–4, 70, 95–6, 98–9, 200, 218; Thomas, *Religion and the decline of magic*, 26, 41, 192, 194, 273, 275, 478, 489, 491.

12   T. Aquinas, *Summa theologiae*, ed. R. J. Batten, XXXIV: *Charity* (2a 2ae), London 1975, 239, 241.

13   S. Dixon-Smith, 'Feeding the poor to commemorate the dead: the *pro anima* almsgiving of King Henry III of England, 1227–72' , unpubl. PhD diss. London 2002, 68–77.

to you, as you did it to one of the least of these my brothers, you did it to me.' Jesus then spoke to those who were damned, saying that they had not responded to his needs in the way that the righteous had; the damned asked when this had happened and he replied that whenever they had failed to help anyone in need they had failed him (Matt. xxv.31–46). Given that the royal touch was practised until 1714 and that the New Testament exerted a great influence on English culture throughout the medieval and early modern periods, it seems very likely that the idea of Christ's mystical presence amongst the poor continued to underpin the royal touch during the sixteenth and seventeenth centuries.

From a humanitarian viewpoint people who are vulnerable always need help. From a theological perspective the giving of alms was also intended to allow the more affluent to atone for sins, or to develop a spiritually healthy attitude towards their wealth, as cupidity could bar entry to Heaven. Neglect of alms-giving risked damnation. Thus it was important that a king dispensed alms and cared for the destitute and ill. The *quid pro quo* was that the poor people who received charity were expected to pray for their king and to be loyal subjects.[14]

The French origins

When the royal touch was first practised in eleventh-century France it was associated with individual kings as opposed to the office of king. This was because the ritual was new, and because monarchs were expected to be in a state of grace if they were to cure the sick: they were meant to have confessed beforehand and to be free from sin. The first monarch to touch the sick was the French king Robert II, 'the Pious' (996–1031). The 'sick' was a general category that we know to have included lepers and the blind and it must have taken account of scrofulous people, given the prevalence of the disease and the eventual specialisation of the French crown. Robert touched lepers as he believed that 'Christ was often entertained under the guise of a leper';[15] the French king prayed and made the sign of the cross over each sick person that he touched, as did doctors and others who treated and attended ill people, in accordance with the religious underpinnings of medicine.[16] Those who had leprosy and scrofula were disfigured and so touching the 'untouchable' with the intention of curing them was both benevolent and brave because of the fear of contagion. Crucially, it was an imitation of Christ, whose touch had healed the blind on four separate occasions,

---

[14] Ibid. 73–4.

[15] Helgald the monk wrote a life of Robert soon after the king's death: Crawfurd, *King's evil*, 12.

[16] Bloch, *The royal touch*, 18–21 (36–40); Barlow, 'King's evil', 14–15.

and lepers on two others.[17] As an especially devout king, presumably Robert the Pious was thought to be very suitable for the role of healing, while at the same time his ceremonies were said to be effective, which must have increased his aura of holiness.

Nothing is known about Robert's successor Henri I (1031–60) in relation to therapeutic practices, but Henri's son Philip I (1060–1108) and his successor Louis VI (1108–37) both touched for scrofula alone, as opposed to a wider range of conditions. The reason why the French kings began to specialise just in scrofula was that the disease was especially widespread and there were many reported cases of it being healed by the monarch's hand. In other words, the royal touch was thought to be most efficacious when treating scrofula. This pattern of beginning with a number of illnesses and then narrowing down to scrofula followed the precedent of the French saint St Marcoul, whose healings in the sixth century had followed this course. It is interesting that Philip I was said to have lost his thaumaturgic powers as a result of committing adultery and being excommunicated.[18] This is noteworthy because it questions the traditional 'top down' interpretation of the royal touch that privileges its political role, rather than its moral element.

There is very little evidence that the royal touch was practised from 1137 until the reign of Louis IX (1226–70), suggesting that it declined or ceased during this time.[19] Louis IX revived the royal touch, touching large numbers of ill people with great regularity; consequently, it was during the thirteenth century that the rite became a fully established part of French royal ceremonial. At the same time the rite began to be performed regularly by the kings of England. Louis IX therefore occupies a central place in the history of the royal touch on both sides of the Channel; his practice of royal therapeutics is hence highly significant.

Humility and piety were important motivating factors for Louis IX's practice of the royal touch. Thirteenth-century French chronicles state that he touched more people with scrofula than had any of his predecessors and that this was consolidated after his return from the Seventh Crusade in 1254.[20] This venture had lasted for six years and was a dismal failure for the Christians. Louis was captured, imprisoned and ransomed, events that were thought to indicate God's anger at the king because he had financed his crusade by plundering the French Church. This was a usual interpretation for

---

[17] For the blind see Mark x.46–52; Matt. xx.29–34; Luke xviii.35–43; Matt. ix.27–31; John ix.1–12. For lepers see Matt. viii.1–4; Mark i.40–5; Luke v.12–16; Luke xvii.11–19.

[18] Bloch, *The royal touch*, 12–21 (29–41); Barlow, 'King's evil', 17–24.

[19] Bloch, *The royal touch*, 18–21 (37–41); Barlow, 'King's evil', 26; P. Buc, 'David's adultery with Bathsheba and the healing power of Capetian kings', *Viator* xxiv (1993), 101–20.

[20] A. D. Hedeman, *The royal image: illustrations of the Grandes Chroniques de France, 1274–1422*, Berkeley 1991, 2; Barlow, 'King's evil', 24.

the time, and it was very powerful. The experience of defeat changed Louis profoundly, and, beginning in Palestine during his captivity, his religious practices became more intense, even obsessional: he lived a life of penance, seeking both punishment and absolution. His punishments included flagellation, the wearing of a hair shirt, and touching the sick, the ugly and the filthy. He buried fallen crusaders with his own hands and was renowned for not holding his nose despite the odour of putrefaction; and he visited leper houses where he held lepers and fed them with his own hands. Louis's friends were disgusted by these actions, sensory aberrations that marked his self-punishment. Nevertheless, the king found a new empathy for the sick and the poor. He ensured that he came into regular, sometimes daily, contact with both groups, feeding the poor at his own table with his own hands, and touching the sick with the hope of curing them.[21]

Louis acted out his piety, humility and benevolence in the Holy Land at a time when he was politically disempowered. He sought atonement. Yet because he was a king, these public acts displayed his own charisma as well as his imitation of Christ. It was on this foundation that Louis created a new cult of kingship when he returned to France, continuing his penitential lifestyle and touching large numbers of people who had scrofula. Alongside this public religiosity, Louis facilitated a successful programme of governmental reforms in order to improve the health of the body politic.[22]

Louis's drive to create a new cult of kingship was expressed further in ways connected to ceremony. He collected prestigious relics that were displayed in his architectural masterpiece, La Sainte Chapelle.[23] He established the cathedral at St Denis as the royal mausoleum, thus ending the practice of kings choosing to be buried in religious houses that they had patronised. From Louis's reign onwards royal funerals became state occasions, whereas previously they had been relatively small, private affairs.[24] He changed the coronation *ordo* and incorporated into it the claim that the oil used at every French anointing had originally been given by the Holy Dove to King Clovis.

---

[21] W. C. Jordan, *Louis IX and the challenge of the crusade: a study in rulership*, Princeton 1979, 127–8.

[22] E. M. Hallam, 'Royal burial and the cult of kingship in France and England, 1060–1330', *Journal of Medieval History* viii (1982), 359–80; W. M. Ormrod, 'The personal religion of Edward III', *Speculum* lxiv (1989), 849–77 at p. 853; J. Richard, *Saint Louis: crusader king of France*, trans. J. Birrell, Cambridge 1992, 155–83; E. M. Hallam and J. Everard, *Capetian France, 987–1328*, Harlow 2001, ch. v.

[23] Richard, *Saint Louis*, 80, 239–40.

[24] Hallam, 'Royal burial', 367, 372–4; B. Schneidmüller, 'Constructing identities in medieval France', in M. Bull (ed.), *France in the central Middle Ages*, Oxford 2002, 15–42 at p. 41.

Although the papacy had given the title 'Most Christian King' to the French crown in the Carolingian period, it was Louis who personified this ideal.[25]

Thaumaturgic kingship epitomised Louis's cult of sovereignty and was proclaimed in the manuscript that he commissioned which was widely copied and distributed, Les Grandes Chroniques de France. In it is a striking image of Louis touching for scrofula (see Plate 2) as well as other images that show him being baptised and crowned, at confession and leading the Seventh Crusade. The text states that during the royal touch ceremony there were customary words spoken, although no detail is given as to what they were, and that Louis made the sign of the cross over each person whom he touched. The king attributed the healing power to this gesture.[26] He also fed those whom he touched and gave each of them a piece of silver.[27] The image shows the king in a central position, wearing a crown and a robe decorated with fleur de lis; he extends his right arm to touch the chin of a man to the right of him, whose legs are bent at the knee, suggesting deference. Louis's left hand is raised up almost to the level of his face: this gesture signified piety and was found in other important Christian images such as the baptism of Christ.[28] Both of Louis's hands are depicted as larger than life, no doubt in order to emphasise their healing qualities. To the right of the man being touched stands another similar-looking male who might be waiting to be touched, while to the left of Louis stands another man who could also be waiting or could be an attendant. The healing dominates the scene which is closely framed, enclosed within an architectural motif comprising two columns to the left and right joined by a crenelated arch. Although it is an arresting image, it was probably meant to record Louis's thaumaturgic practices rather than to convince people that he was a healer king. This is because images from illuminated manuscripts were only seen by relatively small numbers of people as compared to those that were printed from the late fifteenth century onwards.

Louis died in 1270 and was canonised in 1297. After his death the royal touch was practised by every French king for the next five hundred years, until the outbreak of the Revolution in 1789. This is testament to the cult of the royal saint.

---

[25] Schneidmüller, 'Constructing identities', 36–41.

[26] Hedeman, Royal image, 2; Les Grandes Chroniques de France, BL, MS Royal 16 G VI, fo. 424v; Les Grandes Chroniques de France, ed. J. Viard, Paris 1920–53.

[27] Richard, Saint Louis, 241.

[28] L. Twining, Symbols and emblems of early and medieval Christian art, London 1885, 134.

The English origins

The sparse evidence means that a number of candidates have been proposed as the first English king to heal by touch, namely Edward the Confessor (1042–66),[29] Henry II (1154–89)[30] and Henry III (1216–72).[31]

Edward the Confessor did not perform the ceremony of the royal touch, but he was the first English sovereign recorded as having cured a single person of scrofula. A young woman who was married but childless had scrofula which disfigured her face and was 'evil smelling'. She dreamt that if Edward washed her sores she would be cured. She went to the royal court and Edward obliged; he also made the sign of the cross over her suppurations. At that moment, the scrofula that he touched came away from the woman's face and the king then drained her sores of pus. He gave orders that the woman should be fed daily until her disease had gone, after which she conceived and bore twins.[32] The suggestion is that the touch of the pious king and the sign of the cross brought about divine intervention which precipitated the young woman's recovery, the fulfilment of which was her ability to produce children. Thus this episode contains some elements pertinent to the later royal touch ceremony. Edward was recorded as having cured a total of five sick people during his lifetime, all of whom were anointed with water with which he had washed his hands, while miracles were said to have been wrought posthumously at his tomb. Yet three of the five postulants were instructed in a dream to approach Edward, and there is no suggestion that he took the initiative as a thaumaturgic healer – indeed, he may well have been a reluctant one.[33] Despite this, medieval and early modern royal touch apologists claimed that the ceremony originated with Edward the Confessor, whom they said had regularly performed it.

The earliest evidence hinting that an English king touched for scrofula as a royal duty is anecdotal, concerning Henry II. Philip of Blois, a French cleric at Henry's court, wrote that kings were sacred because they healed scrofula as well as a certain plague that affects the groin, although he did not mention any English monarchs by name.[34] Stronger evidence came to light in 1995 when Geoffrey Koziol drew attention to a brief, hitherto unknown reference to Henry II touching a girl for scrofula who was cured but then developed

---

[29] Crawfurd, The king's evil, 20–3; Thomas, *Religion and the decline of magic*, 193; Turrell, 'Ritual of royal healing', 6; Shaw, *Miracles*, 64.

[30] Bloch proposed both kings: *The royal touch*, 22–7 (41–9).

[31] Barlow, 'King's evil', 25. However, Barlow did allow (p. 20) that Henry II might have touched for scrofula.

[32] *The Life of King Edward: who rests at Westminster*, ed. and trans. F. Barlow, London 1962, 61–2 and pp. 122–3.

[33] F. Barlow, *Edward the Confessor*, London 1970, ch. xii, esp pp. 260–1.

[34] Bloch, *The royal touch*, 22–7 (41–9).

paralysis.[35] Nothing is known of the scale or method of Henry's therapeutic activities, or his motivation for undertaking them; but the close connections between England and France at this time provide some context. The French kings ruled what is now the Ile de France and some of Flanders, but the kings of England from Henry II to Edward III were also the dukes of Aquitaine: for two hundred years English monarchs ruled a third of what is now France, and the two nations shared many social, cultural, intellectual, political and religious ideas and practices.[36]

After Henry II there is no evidence of royal therapeutics for nearly a century, until the reign of Edward I (1272–1307). The administrative records from Edward's reign reveal that, from early in his reign, he touched the sick regularly and on a large scale. In light of this, it has been suggested that the rite must have been revived by Edward's predecessor Henry III but left no archival trace.[37] This is certainly plausible given that Henry's almoners' records have not survived, and given his close relationship with Louis IX. The devotional aspects of Henry III's reign therefore merit examination.

The context for the devotional practices of Henry III and Louis IX is revealing. During the thirteenth century the religious practices of both crowns rose in importance. The royal touch was not the only imitation of Christ that was incorporated into the panoply of both monarchies at this time: both also began to wash the feet of the poor, a re-enactment of one of Jesus' acts during the Last Supper. The kings performed this ceremony on Maundy Thursday and other occasions, having adopted it from senior clergymen amongst whom it had been a regular act of humility for a number of centuries.[38] For the monarchy, both foot washing and touching for scrofula could be perceived in at least two ways. Monarchs could wield immense political power, and their public appearances included the majesty of coronations, royal entries and processions; yet the two re-enactments of Christ provided a communal display of humility and benevolence, a reminder that kings were mortal and answerable to God. But the self-effacement involved in both practices also reinforced the unique status of sovereigns and could enhance the charisma or allure of office and office-holder.

If Henry III did touch for scrofula this was probably done in emulation of Louis IX and out of devotion to Edward the Confessor. The relationship between Henry and Louis is revealing. Henry was less powerful than his kinsman due to the political instability of the reigns of Henry's father John

---

[35] G. Koziol, 'England, France, and the problem of sacrality in twelfth-century ritual', in T. N. Bisson (ed.), *Cultures of power: lordship, status, and process in twelfth-century Europe*, Philadelphia 1995, 124–48 at pp. 139–40.

[36] J. Arnold, *What is medieval history?*, Cambridge 2008, 17.

[37] Barlow, 'King's evil', 25. It is also possible that Henry III did not touch for scrofula and that Edward I revived a moribund practice, as suggested by Nicholas Vincent: *The holy blood,*, 194.

[38] Dixon-Smith, 'Feeding the poor', 93–6.

and his uncle Richard I, which meant that Henry might have sought to strengthen his authority by incorporating thaumaturgic practices into his kingship. Henry probably witnessed Louis touch the sick as he visited the French king on five occasions, the first being in November and December 1254, soon after Louis's return from the crusade.[39] The two men were personally close and both were devout, though Louis was more austere than Henry, with his preference for flagellation, fasts and hair shirts; Henry exceeded Louis in the scale of his public piety, giving alms and food on a bigger scale, and washing the feet of the poor more often.[40] This suggests that the royal touch would have appealed to Henry, who also held religious ceremonies in great esteem; indeed, at times there was even a sense of competitiveness between him and Louis with regard to their religious observances.[41] Henry would have been aware that Louis had revived the royal touch and so might have thought that he too could rejuvenate the practice in England.

Whilst Henry III and Louis IX undoubtedly shared many sacred practices, unlike Louis, Henry was devoted to a saintly predecessor, Edward the Confessor, whose cult had been developing since his death. Henry's veneration for the Confessor is evident in that he named his sons Edward and Edmund after the Confessor and his brother, and that he rebuilt Westminster Abbey and had his saintly predecessor's remains transferred to a new shrine there.[42]

Reverence for the Confessor during the thirteenth century explains the production of the manuscript *La Estoire de Seint Ædward le Roi* that dates from c.1245, and was written for Henry III's wife Eleanor of Provence.[43] In it is a depiction of the Confessor touching a young woman for scrofula (*see* Figure 3).[44] Entitled 'Miracle of the scrofulous woman', *La Estoire* states that:

[U]ne fem[m]e jofne e bele	[A young and pretty girl
Suz la goue out escrouele,	Affected on the cheek with scrofula
Ne pout avec gareisun	Could not eat, despite being treated
Par art d'umme, se Deu nun,	By art of man, nor by God,
Ke purrir li fait la buche;	That made her mouth rot;
Le rois la garist ki la tuche.[45]	The king healed it by touch.][46]

---

[39] D. Carpenter, 'The meetings of kings Henry III and Louis IX', in M. Prestwich, R. Britnell and R. Frame (eds), *Thirteenth Century England*, X: *Proceedings of the Durham Conference, 2003*, Woodbridge 2005, 1–30 at p. 3.

[40] Ibid. 17–19, 27.

[41] Hallam and Everard, *Capetian France*, 264.

[42] D. A. Carpenter, 'King Henry III and Saint Edward the Confessor: the origin of the cult', *EHR* cxxii (2007), 865–91.

[43] *La Estoire de Seint Ædward le roi*, CUL, MS Ee.3.59.

[44] The image is described in *Lives of Edward the Confessor*, ed. H. R. Luard, London 1858, 12. See also Farquhar, 'Royal charities, I', 5, 44 n. 1, and Bloch, *The royal touch*, 24, 181, 254 (45, 319, 450).

[45] *Lives of Edward the Confessor*, 12.

[46] I am grateful to John Arnold for help with translating this from the medieval French.

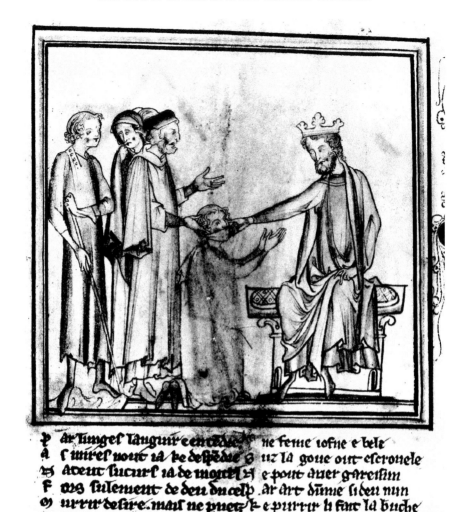

P ar lunges languir e en oedie ne feme tofue e bele
A f mires nout ra be desp̃edue o uz la goue out escrouele
o Adeut lucurs ra de morel u e pout auer garesiш
F oes fulement de deu du celp ar art dume si deu nun
o urrur desire. mais ne puet k e purrir li fat la buche
p ar murrir. kar deuf uel ueut li rois la garst. k la ruche

Figure 3. 'Edward the Confessor touches a scrofulous woman', from *La Estoire de Seint Ædward le roi.*

The king is shown to the right of the image, wearing a crown and sitting on a carved stool; he extends his right hand to touch the kneeling woman's left cheek. His left hand rests on his knee and the index and second finger are shown curved and separate from the other digits: were these raised, it would signify a blessing or benediction.[47] The woman being touched kneels to the left of the king and occupies the centre of the image; she wears a piece of fabric around her mouth which might contain herbs or other medicines, or might be intended to hide her unsightly swellings, which are just visible on her right cheek. Not surprisingly, people with scrofula on their faces sometimes hid their sores with fabric.[48] The king and the woman are making eye contact, and she echoes his outstretched arm by holding her arms up to him. This gesture, along with her cupped hands, suggest that she is submitting to him and receiving his healing powers. To the left of her stand three people – a younger man supporting himself with a crutch, an older man who also touches the kneeling woman's face, and behind them a figure that could be male or female. Close up it can be seen that all three have scrofula on their faces so they might be waiting to be touched as well. Unlike early modern depictions of the royal touch, no clergymen are present and no one is reading from a text: this is because the ceremony had not yet been given liturgical expression. The depiction provides a sense of intimacy between the people in it, noticeably by touch and eye contact between king and supplicant. At the same time attention is drawn to the monarch's power by the crown, his decorated seat and his kingly distance from the other characters within the frame. It is a quintessentially thirteenth-century English image, and as such it is revealing with regard to how the Confessor was viewed at that time. If Henry III did touch for scrofula, this image could be based on his practice.

Turning to Edward I: by good fortune his almoners' accounts have survived. These constitute the strongest of the medieval evidence for the English royal touch, revealing that Edward touched on a large scale – some 9,896 persons during thirty years – giving one penny to each scrofulous person (*see* Table 1).[49] The extant data demonstrates high and consistent totals: not until the seventeenth century will a similar level be reached. A number of issues arise from these figures. Although Edward succeeded in 1272 his earliest extant alms accounts date from 1276: the figures for the royal touch suggest that it was well established by this time. A further point is that, given the great popularity of Edward's royal touch, it is strange that

---

[47] J. Hall, *Illustrated dictionary of symbols in eastern and western art*, London 1994, 122.

[48] Browne tells of a man whose face 'was so monstrous to view, and accompanied with many deplorable and fetid Ulcers, that he was forced to cover them with green silk': *Adenochoiradelogia*, 157. In the eighteenth century the Spanish queen Maria Luisa of Savoy, whose scrofula would be fatal, wore a hood that covered 'her head and her throat and also part of her face': *Memoirs of duc de Saint–Simon*, 200.

[49] Barlow, 'King's evil', 24; Prestwich, 'Piety of Edward I', 125. For Edward I, II and III see Bloch, *The royal touch*, 56–60 (97–105).

Table 1 The number of people touched for scrofula
by Edward I, 1276–1306

Year	Total
1276–7	627
1277–8	928
1283–4	237
1284–5	888
1288–9	519
1289–90	1736
1296–7	757
1299–1300	983
1300–1	0
1303–4	1219
1305–6	2002

Table 2 The number of people touched for scrofula
by Edward II, 1316–21

Period	Total
27 July–30 Nov. 1316	214
20 Mar.–7 July 1320	93
8 July 1320–7 July 1321	79

Table 3 The number of people touched for scrofula
by Edward III, 1336–44

Period	Total
25 Jan. 1336–30 Aug. 1337	108
12 July 1338–28 May 1340	885
Nov. 1341 –Apr. 1344	396

no commentaries or images relating to it have surfaced from his reign. The low total for 1283 was due to poor accounting, while the total of zero for the years 1300–1 was due to Edward being in Wales, where he was preoccupied with military conquest, and so was unlikely to attract native supplicants. Yet Edward's thaumaturgic practices were not limited to England, and not necessarily rejected by those with whom he was in conflict: between 1303 and 1304 he touched 995 people when in Scotland, a country that he was trying to subjugate, suggesting that sometimes the desire for a cure could override the king's unpopularity. The high numbers for 1289–90 were due to the king's absence from England since 1286, meaning that he had a 'backlog' to deal with, while in 1305–6 Edward was not on campaign, so that he was available to his sick subjects.[50]

A smaller amount of similar evidence reveals that both Edward II (1307–27)[51] and Edward III (1327–77)[52] touched for scrofula, although its fragmentary nature means that no firm conclusions can be drawn about the frequency or scale of the ritual during either reign (*see* tables 2, 3). Yet the figures are fairly impressive and suggest that the ritual remained an established custom. The low totals or incomplete records from Edward II's reign may reflect his unpopularity. Yet he held provincial healings. On 26 July 1316 he left London to begin his journey to York, before going to fight the Scots. On 27 July he touched twenty-two people at St Albans Abbey; on 1 August he touched seventeen at Kingscliff; the next day he touched eleven at Clipsham and fifteen at Wilsford; between 2 and 10 August he resided at Lincoln, where he touched a total of twenty-six. He crossed the Trent, touching twenty-seven at Bentley and seventeen at Todcaster. Between 16 August and the end of November he stayed at York, where he touched a total of seventy-nine people on various occasions.[53] As for Edward III, between 12 July 1338 and 28 May 1340 he was campaigning in Flanders and only resided in England for four months, which means that he touched for scrofula on the continent, which is interesting in itself. During this conflict which became known as the Hundred Years' War, Edward claimed suzerainty over France through his mother, Isabella. In 1340 Edward challenged Philip VI (1328–1350) to prove his right to rule France. He suggested that this might be done by personal combat, or by braving ravenous lions (legend had it that they would not harm a true king), or by a contest in which both kings would touch for scrofula in order to see who had the greatest thaumaturgic powers.[54] The French king declined, but the use of the royal touch to assert royal legitimacy speaks volumes about the power of the ritual and its use to the crown at this time.

A further piece of evidence from Edward III's reign is the commentary of Thomas Bradwardine (c.1290–1349), the king's chaplain and archbishop of

[50] Prestwich, 'Piety of Edward I', 125–6.

[51] For Edward II see Edward II treasury records, BL, MS Add. 9951, fo. 3, and T. Stapleton, 'A brief summary of the wardrobe accounts of the tenth, eleventh and fourteenth years of King Edward II', *Archaeologia* xxvi (1836), 318–45 at pp. 319–20.

[52] TNA, Exchequer accounts 388, 5; Royal Society, London, Treasury of receipt, miscellaneous books, 203, fo. 177; BL, MS Cotton Nero C VIII, fo. 208; Ormrod, 'Personal religion of Edward III', 862–5.

[53] Stapleton, 'A brief summary', 319–20.

[54] *CSPV 1, 1202–1509*, 8–9; Bloch, *The royal touch*, 1–2, 60 (15–17, 104–5); Ormrod, 'Personal religion of Edward III', 862.

Canterbury, which testifies to the popularity of the rite as well as providing a brief description of the ritual. He wrote that Edward would cure those who were ill with scrofula

> in the name of Jesus Christ, with prayer poured out, with laying on of hands, and with a blessing given along with the sign of the Cross. For this he does continually, and very often did it to the foulest of men and women, who flocked to him in crowds, in England, in Germany, and in all parts of France … And this is a thing that all Christian kings of the English have been accustomed to do by gift of God, and French kings too, as the books of ancient records and the unanimous tradition of these kingdoms testify.[55]

After the reign of Edward III the administrative records are silent until Henry VII, which could be due to the book-keeping reforms of Edward III that began in 1344 and sought to provide better budgeting and cut down on scribal work. Hitherto the penny given to each person touched was recorded as special alms given from the Wardrobe Account at the king's personal instructions. This then had to be copied into the Household Accounts. The new system was that payments by the almoner were made from the statutory 4s. allocated each day for almsgiving, recorded under general household expenses without specific detail concerning the nature of the charity.[56]

It is strange that Richard II appears not to have touched for scrofula, given his exalted view of kingship; however, anecdotal evidence reveals that the saintly Henry VI touched for scrofula and that Henry IV and Henry V might have done so. The Lancastrian apologist and political theorist Sir John Fortescue (c. 1397–1479) wrote a number of tracts in defence of Henry VI whilst exiled in Scotland between 1461 and 1463. In one of these he stated that Henry VI healed people: 'at the touch of his most pure hands … you can see even today sufferers from the King's Evil, including those despaired of by physicians, recovering their longed-for health by divine intervention'.[57] The records of Henry VI's posthumous miracles include two women cured of scrofula as a result of praying at his tomb, which is suggestive of his practising royal therapeutics whilst alive.[58]

In another of Fortescue's tracts he gave a vague hint that might refer to Henry IV and Henry V. He wrote that legitimate English kings healed scrofula by their sacred touch, having been anointed on their hands, but frustratingly he provided no details of which kings did so.[59] Fortescue had been

---

55 Crawfurd, *The king's evil*, 39; Bloch, *The royal touch*, 310 n. 20 (99).

56 Ormrod, 'Edward III', 863–4.

57 Bloch, *The royal touch*, 65 (111–12).

58 R. Knox and S. Leslie (eds), *The miracles of Henry VI*, London 1923, 109–10, 124–5; J. M. Theilmann, 'The miracles of king Henry VI of England', *Historian* xlii/3 (1980), 456–71 at pp. 465–6.

59 Crawfurd, *The king's evil*, 45–6; Bloch, *The royal touch*, 65 (111–12).

Lord Chief Justice of the King's Bench, and he would have had memories of Henry IV and Henry V so it is just possible that his reference to legitimate kings implied that these kings touched for scrofula.

The paucity of evidence concerning the royal touch from the mid-fourteenth to the late fifteenth century means that it might have been practised only intermittently during this time. This could be connected to the Black Death that raged from 1348 to 1350, which would have reduced the numbers of people who had scrofula and lessened the appeal of assembling those who remained; while the political instability of the Wars of the Roses could have undermined the notion of hereditary healing powers.

Epilepsy and the English crown

If English kings did not touch for scrofula consistently from the middle of the fourteenth century to the end of the fifteenth, they did practise another healing rite throughout this period. From Edward II to Mary Tudor all but two English sovereigns distributed gold (and occasionally silver) medicinal finger rings known as cramp rings on Good Friday or soon after; these were intended primarily to ward off epileptic seizures. The rings were made from coins presented on an altar by the sovereign, which were then blessed before being distributed: just as the monarch was thought to act as an intermediary for God's healing powers when touching for scrofula, so too they were thought to be able to channel divine grace into cramp rings.

As well as epilepsy, cramp sometimes referred more generally to muscular pains and spasms, rheumatism, convulsions or paralysed limbs.[60] Cramp rings were thought to be able to ward off such seizures because they resembled ligatures, which since antiquity had been recommended as medical treatments for epileptic attacks and similar problems.[61]

The earliest record concerning cramp rings dates from 1318, its language suggesting that the custom was already established:

---

[60] In Shakespeare's *The Tempest* I.2, Prospero says, 'For this be sure, to-night thou shalt have cramps, Side-stitches that shall pen thy breath up'; and later, 'Go, charge my goblins that they grind their joints, With dry convulsions; shorten up their sinews, With aged cramps.' See also E. Waterton, 'On a remarkable incident in the life of St Edward the Confessor, with notices of royal cramp rings', *Archaeological Journal* xxi (1864), 103–13; R. Crawfurd, 'The blessing of cramp-rings: a chapter in the history of the treatment of epilepsy', in C. Singer (ed.), *Studies in the history and method of science*, i, Oxford 1917, 165–87 at pp. 180–2; C. J. S. Thompson, *Royal cramp and other medycinable rings*, London 1921; Bloch, *The royal touch*, 92–107 (159–83); Thomas, *Religion and the decline of magic*, 198–9; J. Cherry, 'Healing through faith: the continuation of medieval attitudes to jewellery into the Renaissance', *Renaissance Studies* xv/2 (2001), 154–71.

[61] Crawfurd, 'Blessing of cramp-rings', 182.

Item, likewise the King must for certain offer on Good Friday five shillings which he is accustomed to receive in person from the hand of the chaplain to make rings of them to give for medicine to divers persons.[62]

Cramp rings were very popular and were often bequeathed in wills, and, like the royal touch, there is also evidence that they were sought in Europe: Anne Boleyn sent some cramp rings to Stephen Gardiner when he was in Rome in 1529 trying to secure Henry VIII's divorce, to distribute as he thought best.[63]

Cramp was supposed to have supernatural causes because its key symptoms were unpredictable pain and seizures: the ceremony occurred on Good Friday because these symptoms were said to be a reminder of Christ's passion. The cramp ring service formed part of the intense religious practices of that day. Good Friday began with the Creeping to the Cross ceremony at which the monarch, queen consort and nobility prostrated themselves on their chapel floors and crept along the floor to the crucifix on the altar in order to physically and emotionally submit themselves to Christ's passion. The Plantagenets did this in front of the Welsh Neith Cross, believed to be a relic of the true cross.[64] An offering of new gold coins was then made by the king and sometimes the queen consort at the altar; these were taken away to be made into cramp rings and distributed sometime afterwards by the monarch, having first been consecrated on the altar.[65]

From 1442 onwards a significant change in the ceremony occurred in that the rings were made before Good Friday and then distributed straight away, which made the ceremony more self-contained.[66] Descriptions of this new practice include the manner in which the rings were blessed: they were placed on the altar, the monarch prayed over them and held them and rubbed them, and then sprinkled them with holy water.[67] It has been suggested that

---

[62] 'Household ordinance of York, June 1323', in T. F. Tout (ed.), *The place of the reign of Edward II in English history*, Manchester 1914, 317, and trans. in Thompson, *Royal cramp and other medycinable rings*, 6.

[63] For the popularity of cramp rings see Crawfurd, 'Blessing of cramp-rings', 171–7; *Letters and papers, foreign and domestic, of the reign of Henry VIII*, ed. J. S. Brewer and others, London 1862–1932, iv. 5422.

[64] Crawfurd, 'Blessing of cramp-rings', 168; Ormrod, 'Personal religion of Edward III', 864; E. Owen, 'The Croes Nawdd', *Y Cymmrodor* xliii (1932), 13–17; W. C. Tennant, 'Croes Naid', *National Library of Wales Journal* (1951–2), 102–15.

[65] For queen consorts see Bloch, *The royal touch*, 102–3 (176–8). The evidence relates to Philippa, wife of Edward III.

[66] Ibid. 104, 251 (178–80, 446–8). The key records are, for Henry VI: TNA, exchequer acccounts 409, 9, fo. 32 [30 Mar. 1442]; for Henry VII: EA 413, 9, fo. 31 [5 Apr. 1493]; for Henry VIII: BL, MS Add. 35182, fo. 31 V [11 Apr., 1533]; for Edward VI: TNA E101/426/1, fo. 19 [8 Apr. 1547] and BL, MS Add. 35184, fo. 31 V [31 Mar. 1553].

[67] John Fortescue, *Defensio iuris domus Lancastriae*, trans. in Crawfurd, 'Blessing of cramp–rings', 171, and *King's evil*, 45; Marco Antonio Faitto to Ippolito Chizzola, Doctor in Divinity, 3 May, 1556, in *CSPV*, vi/1, 434–7; Mary Tudor's missal, Westminster Cathedral

this emphasised that the healing properties of the rings resulted from contact with the anointed hands of the monarch as opposed to their consecration, which represented an increase in the sacral nature of English monarchy.[68] This might be so, but the problem is that there is no description of how the rings were distributed before the changes made in 1442, and so it seems safer to suggest that both before and after 1442 the ceremony emphasised that the rings' healing properties were given by God via the intermediary figure of the monarch.

This is evident from an examination of Mary Tudor's missal. This remarkable manuscript owned by Westminster Cathedral, is held in the Library and Muniment Room of Westminster Abbey. It contains Mary's liturgy for the cramp ring ceremony as well as for the royal touch, and it was intended for Mary's personal use at both ceremonies.[69] It has a number of illustrations attributed to the female artist Levina Teerlinc (1510/20–76), daughter of Simon Bennink, one of the chief exponents of the Ghent-Bruges school of illuminators.[70] One illumination is of the cramp ring ceremony which depicts Mary praying alone in an oratory, facing an elaborate altar and a crucifix (*see* Plate 3). She stands at a table draped with cloth, reading a prayer book that rests on a cushion; next to her on the table are two bowls of cramp rings. This probably represents the practice that was first described during her reign, namely that two bowls of rings were blessed, one containing rings made in the usual manner, the other rings that were sent in by their owners to be blessed.[71] The accompanying liturgy made continuous reference to the power of God and his ability to bless the rings and his people with his grace.

Treasury, London, MS 7; *Liber regie capelle: a manuscript in the Biblioteca Publica, Evora*, ed. Walter Ullmann, London 1961, 62–3.

[68] Bloch, *The royal touch*, 105–7 (180–3).

[69] Mary Tudor's missal. The liturgy was transcribed three times in the seventeenth century: 'The Patrick papers', CUL, MS Add. 44, item 9; MS Mm. 1.51; St John's College, Cambridge, MS Cam. L. 13. Crawfurd transcribed the Latin liturgy in 'Blessing of cramp-rings', 182–4, and Bloch translated much of it in *The royal touch* at pp. 105–6 (182–3). It can be compared to *The office of consecrating cramp rings, used by the Catholick kings of England*, London 1694.

[70] Sparrow Simpson, 'On the forms of prayer recited "At the healing"', 295; R. Strong, *Artists of the Tudor court: the portrait miniature rediscovered, 1520–1620*, London 1983, 52; cf. J. Backhouse, 'Queen Mary's manual for blessing cramp rings and touching for the evil: the rituals of the royal healing ceremonies, written and illuminated for Mary I (1553–58)', in J. Browne and T. Dean, *Westminster Cathedral: building of faith*, London 1995, 200–2 at p. 202. Backhouse insists that the attribution must remain open because 'no miniature can as yet be associated with her beyond doubt. Furthermore the manuscript work of the mid 16th century has still to be exhaustively investigated'. For biographical details of Teerlinc see Strong, *Artists of the Tudor court*, 52. Teerlinc produced images of the ritual year, including (probably) the image of the Elizabethan Maundy Thursday ceremony, reproduced in Strong, *Artists of the Tudor court*, 55.

[71] CSPV vi/1, 436.

The cramp ring ceremony and the royal touch had much in common. Both were performed by the sovereign acting as an intermediary for the Almighty, although Philippa, wife of Edward III, is recorded as also distributing cramp rings; both practices sought to alleviate illness by means of a religious ceremony; both cramp and scrofula can manifest themselves episodically, without warning, and so were thought to have supernatural causes, meaning a supernatural remedy seemed to be appropriate; both were available free of charge; yet neither ceremony had a monopoly, as sick people could also turn to doctors, surgeons and other healers in the hope of a cure. However, there is a significant difference between the ceremonies, which may help to explain why cramp rings flourished at a time when the royal touch declined, the context for which is the Black Death. The cramp ring ceremony happened only once a year and did not involve the monarch having physical contact with hundreds of ill people, meaning that sovereign and supplicants were not exposed to infectious diseases as they could be during the royal touch ceremony.

One further issue that connects cramp rings to the royal touch is that the rings were meant to be worn if they were to ward off seizures; likewise when Henry VII revived the royal touch he almost certainly instigated the practice of giving each sick person a gold Angel coin to wear until their scrofula was healed. Both practices related to a whole culture connected to the curative properties of amulets, rings, stones and jewels.

A number of beliefs and customs surrounded the wearing of rings in pre-modern Europe. They were worn for a variety of purposes. They could be worn as beautiful ornaments that signified status, wealth and power; or as commemorative mementoes, that recalled the death of a loved one, for example, or a legally binding contract; they were useful as seals; they proclaimed allegiance, friendship or love, especially if the ring were a gift; they could be worn as a talisman; or as any combination of these. Since antiquity rings had been widely worn as talismans that were valued for their magical, prophylactic or healing properties, protecting travellers, providing a good night's sleep, or preventing or alleviating sickness.[72]

Rings could acquire their supposed magical or healing properties in a number of ways, one of which was via contact with a special source. The Roman naturalist Pliny the Elder (AD 23–79) described putting rings into a jar with temporarily blinded lizards: when they regained their sight, the rings were worn to help restore poor eyesight in humans.[73] Alternatively, special words or images could be engraved onto a ring: these were often astrological, as the stars were thought to influence human affairs. During the medieval period rings were often engraved with the names of the three Magi – Casper,

---

[72] T. Blaen, *Medicinal jewels, magical gems: precious stones in early modern Britain*, Crediton 2012, 33; G. F. Kunz, *Rings for the finger*, London 1917, 32–50, 340.

[73] Pliny the Elder, *Natural history* XXIX.38.

Melchior and Balthazar – in order to ward off diseases. Copper rings, especially if engraved with a lion, crescent moon and star were believed to ward
off or cure the stone.[74]

Two further ways in which a ring could acquire properties were due to the
substance from which it was made, or to having a precious stone set within
it. Horn rings were believed to treat cramp and so the royal cramp rings were
not the only medicinal jewellery used to alleviate this ailment.[75] Precious
stones could acquire a mystical quality as they were an important component of medieval art and religion, encrusting reliquaries, crucifixes and book
covers.[76] Henry VIII wore a ruby ring to protect himself from scrofula whilst
touching the sick,[77] while priests used stones to promote health or heal sickness. Sapphires such as the one kept at St Paul's Cathedral in London were
used to treat sore eyes, garnets to ward off flies and insects.[78]

In relation to cramp rings, it was usual to think that coins received as a gift
by the church were ideal for making healing rings.[79] Apart from resembling
ligatures the therapeutic qualities of cramp rings were also thought to derive
from their consecration on the altar, and their contact with the monarch's
anointed hands. A further mythical explanation associated a special ring
with English royalty. Just as it was widely thought that Edward the Confessor
had touched for scrofula, so it was said that he had given a ring to a beggar
who later revealed himself to be St John the Evangelist; subsequently the
ring was returned to the king via intermediaries.[80]

Thus cramp rings belonged to a culture in which health and disease
were connected to the spiritual world. Religion, natural magic and medicine provided remedies for sickness, while certain people and objects were
thought to be able to connect the natural and supernatural spheres, thus
having the potential to cure illness.

To conclude, the royal touch originated in the medieval period. Its practice by the French and English kings demonstrates the close relationship
between political power and Christian doctrine. The thaumaturgic kings
re-enacted aspects of Christ's healing ministry and passion as a way of
appealing to God for redemption for the sick and poor. It was thought that
Christ himself might be present within the crowds of impoverished and
unwell people, which helps to explain the enthusiasm for royal therapeu-

---

[74] Blaen, *Medicinal jewels*, 25–6; Thompson, *Royal cramp*, 2, 3.

[75] Thompson, *Royal cramp*, 3.

[76] Blaen, *Medicinal jewels*, 6, 71.

[77] *The inventory of King Henry VIII: Society of Antiquaries MS 127 and British Library MS
Harley 1419*, ed. D. Starkey, London 1998, 75.

[78] Thompson, *Royal cramp*, 3.

[79] Bloch, *The royal touch*, 97 (169).

[80] Crawfurd, 'Blessing of cramp-rings', 165–7, 171, 182.

tics as well as the regular charitable donations made by royalty to the poor. Although kings could wield great political power it was important that at times they humbled themselves in public and acknowledged the sovereignty of the Almighty. Failure to do this could lead to excessive pride, which like avarice and selfishness could prevent someone from entering heaven. The recipients of royal charity and benevolence were meant to be obedient to the king, just as the sovereign complied with the will of God. The Almighty was therefore thought to be omni-present and to intervene in human affairs. Thaumaturgic kings acted as intercessionary figures for God's healing powers, the royal touch and cramp rings both acting as conduits for divine grace.

2

The Tudors: Revival and Reform of Royal Therapeutics, 1485–1603

Henry VII revived the royal touch after which it was practised by all the Tudors, although the evidence for Edward VI is weaker than for the others. The numbers touched by the Tudors are small though, when compared to Edward I, Edward II or Edward III, or to the Stuarts. Yet the continuity with which the Tudors touched the sick meant that the ceremony became an established part of English royal ritual during the sixteenth century, whereas it might have been practised intermittently towards the end of the Middle Ages.

The fragmentary evidence reveals that the scale of Tudor thaumaturgy was initially very small, although an increase can be detected by the end of the sixteenth century. Between December 1491 and June 1505 Henry VII may have held fourteen ceremonies at which he touched a total of thirty-four people, averaging between two and three people per ceremony.[1] Between January 1530 and December 1532 Henry VIII is recorded as having touched a total of sixty-five people on twenty-six occasions: although the number of ceremonies is greater, the average is still between two and three people. The records reveal that Henry VIII touched in London, as well as when he was on progress, and even in France. He held ceremonies at York Place, Westminster, Greenwich, Windsor, Woodstock, Grafton, The More, Havering and King's Langley, and at Calais when he visited François I in November 1532.[2] The records are silent for Edward VI's reign and sparse for the reigns of Mary Tudor and Elizabeth I. Yet it is known that at Easter 1556 Mary touched a crowd of people who had scrofula that numbered 'not above 20'.[3] Elizabeth touched nine people when staying at Kenilworth in 1575, but towards the end of her reign she touched thirty-eight at Easter 1596. Easter was the most popular time to be touched,[4] so this figure is probably indicative of the largest

[1] Household-book of Henry VII, as kept by John Heron, Treasurer of the Chamber, 1499–1505, BL, MS Add. 21480, fos 20–1; account book of John Heron, TNA, E 101/415/3; W. Bentley, *Excerpta historica*, London 1833, 87; Farquhar, 'Royal charities, I', 74–6; Crawford, *The king's evil*, 50.

[2] N. H. Nicolas, *The privy purse expences of king Henry VIII from November 1520 to December 1532*, London 1827, 16, 20, 37, 40, 46, 135, 145, 150, 156, 160, 161, 163, 164, 170, 203, 213, 217, 221, 225, 237, 243, 249, 253, 264, 272, 278.

[3] *CSPV* vi. 436.

[4] See pp. 165–6 below.

of Tudor ceremonies. In November 1596 she touched another ten people.[5] The next year her chaplain boasted that she performed the ceremony every Sunday and feast day.[6]

If it was usual for Henry VII to touch only two people at each ceremony, whereas by 1596 thirty-eight were touched at Easter, evidently the rite had become more popular during the intervening period. This was due in part to the constancy with which the Tudors practised it. Yet this chapter will stress that the Tudor ritual was characterised by change, the motor for which was political, religious and medicinal. Particularly important is Henry VII's revival of royal thaumaturgy, especially the liturgy which almost certainly dates from his reign and includes departures from the medieval practice. Then in the 1530s the royal touch survived the Reformation: the reforms that enabled this demonstrate that the rationale and practice of the rite was altered in accordance with religious and political change. These modifications reveal the priorities of different sovereigns, while also confirming that ceremonies were not static. A further change during the sixteenth century was that for the first time the royal touch was practised by women: Mary and Elizabeth performed the rite for a total of fifty years. The effect of gender on the rite is therefore an issue. The first two books on the royal touch published in England date from the end of Elizabeth's reign and these will enable an assessment of the ceremony which by then had been continually performed by the Tudors for more than a century. The numbers touched suggest that all these innovations were popular.

Reviving the royal touch

The earliest Tudor commentary on the royal touch is in the Italian historian Polydore Vergil's *English history*, written between 1506 and 1513. He said that English kings had healed 'loathesom swellings' by their touch since Edward the Confessor, and that 'presentlie' the ritual involved hymns and 'ceremonies'.[7] Although Vergil was wrong concerning the chronology of royal therapeutics, his comment on hymns and ceremonies was accurate. The ceremony had recently undergone a major innovation: it had been given liturgical expression, which included the new practice of giving each sick person a prestigious gold Angel coin instead of one penny. These changes probably date from Henry VII's reign and lasted until royal therapeutics ceased with the death of Queen Anne in 1714. If, as seems likely, the royal touch had

---

[5] Crawfurd, *The king's evil*; 78, W. Tooker, *Charisma sive donum sanationis*, London 1597, 100; *CSPV* ix. 238.

[6] See p. 65 below.

[7] *Polydore Vergil's English history*, ed. H. Ellis, London 1846, i, bk VIII, p. 294.

46

declined in the 150 years before Henry VII became king, he must have revived it. Why did he do so? And why did he introduce these changes?

The most apparent reason for his revival of royal therapeutics was that it could project monarchical authority and thus aid him in establishing the Tudors as rightful sovereigns. With hindsight we know that the succession of the Tudors would end the Wars of Roses and that they would rule England for more than a century, but this was far from certain in the early years of Henry VII's reign. Henry's supporters argued for a providential reading of his assumption of power, claiming that although he acquired his crown by conquest rather than primogeniture he was chosen by God to rescue England from the tyranny of Richard III. The royal touch could fit into this pairing of politics and religion; indeed, the earliest record of Henry touching for scrofula dates from 24 December 1491,[8] the year in which the pretender Perkin Warbeck first landed in Ireland hoping to rally support against Henry. The royal touch bolstered Tudor authority as it signified God's blessing on the royal house while at the same time it marked continuity with the medieval kings who had practised it, whether real or imagined. Consequently, it is not surprising that Vergil, whose history was written at the instigation of Henry VII, stressed that the ceremony had been performed by all English kings since Edward the Confessor.

In pre-modern Europe political authority was thought to be ordained by God, and this needs to be borne in mind when assessing Henry's motives for touching the sick. Henry was devout. By practising the royal touch he associated the Tudors with Edward the Confessor. Like Edward, Henry was an orthodox medieval king who continued the royal custom of giving large sums to the poor, often on a daily basis. Henry commissioned the Savoy Hospital as well as alms houses at Westminster, both of which signify his Christian compassion. More ostentatiously, he blended piety and monarchical authority in a number of magnificent building projects, including continuing the building of the chapel at King's College, Cambridge, founded by Henry VI, and his own burial chapel at Westminster Abbey.[9]

A further way in which monarchical power and religious faith could be jointly expressed was royal ceremony. Henry was skilled at projecting majesty and he had a great regard for ceremony, sometimes introducing ceremonial innovations: as soon as he became king he reformed the annual protocol of the Chapels Royal expressed in the *Liber Regie Capelle*.[10] In light of this it has been suggested that Henry VII was the first king to codify a liturgy for

---

8   Bentley, *Excerpta historica*, 87. Henry VII minted Angels from 4 November 1485, I am grateful to Barrie Cook, curator of medieval and early modern coinage at the British Museum, for this information.

9   F. Bacon, *The history of the reign of Henry VII*, ed. R. Lockyer, London 1971, 228; S. B. Chrimes, *Henry VII*, London 1972, 240–4; S. J. Gunn, 'Henry VII (1457–1509)', ODNB.

10   *Vergil's English history*, 145–6; Chrimes, *Henry VII*, 298–324; *Liber regie capelle*, 5, 62–3.

the royal touch.[11] This is very plausible, especially given Vergil's comments: specifically his use of 'presentlie' which could be taken to imply that the ceremonies were new. But the situation is not quite straightforward. No liturgy that dates from Henry's reign has come to light, the evidence used being the documents published by James II in 1686, one in English, the other in Latin, entitled *The ceremonies for the healing of them that be diseased with the kings evil, used in the time of king Henry VII*.[12] The most that can be said about these is that they were attributed by James II to Henry VII.[13] The earliest royal touch liturgy is to found in Mary Tudor's missal, which refers to 'the king' rather than 'the queen'. This might be a scribal error, or, more likely, it implies that the liturgy dates from the reign of Henry VII or Henry VIII.[14]

On balance it is probable that Henry VII was the first monarch to provide the royal touch with its own liturgy. Written and spoken in Latin, it was structured around prayers that included mention of the saints and the Virgin Mary and passages from the New Testament, and it might have codified earlier practices. Both the chaplain and the king recited various parts of the liturgy, though the supplicants and others present remained silent. Each sick person was presented individually to the king, who touched the sores on their head and neck as the chaplain recited 'Ac super aegrotos manus inponent et bene habebunt' ('They shall lay their hands on the sick and they shall recover') (Mark xvi.18). After more prayers, each ill person was presented again to the king, who, holding the gold Angel in his hand, made the sign of the cross with it over the sores. The coin was then put around the neck of the supplicant, having been threaded onto a white ribbon (whether at that time or prior to the ceremony is not stated). While this happened the chaplain recited 'It was the true light that lighteth every man which cometh into this world' (John i.9). The ceremony closed with further prayers and the sick people departed. The king and the chaplain then 'prayed in secret', asking God to grant that those just touched be healed and their souls saved from sin.[15] While some of the ceremony originated in France around 1100

---

[11] Sparrow Simpson, 'Forms of prayer', 284; Crawfurd, *The king's evil*, 51–2; Farquhar, 'Royal charities, I', 46; Bloch, *The royal touch*, 54 (93); Thomas, *Religion and the decline of magic*, 193; G. MacDonald Ross, 'The royal touch and the Book of Common Prayer', *Notes and Queries* n.s. xxx (1983), 433–5 at p. 434; C. Levin, '"Would that I could give you help and succor": Elizabeth I and the politics of touch', *Albion* xxi/2 (1989), 191–205; Shaw, *Miracles*, 65.

[12] *The ceremonies us'd in the time of King Henry VII for the healing of them that be diseas'd with the kings evil*, London 1686; Crawfurd, *The king's evil*, 52–6, Sparrow Simpson, 'Forms of prayer', 301–3.

[13] Bloch, *The royal touch*, 54, 219, 381–2 n. 31 (93, 389). As a Catholic monarch, James had his own good reasons for publishing what he said was the original Catholic royal touch liturgy in 1686: see ch. 3 below.

[14] Westminster Cathedral Treasury, MS 7; Crawfurd, *The king's evil*, 60–3.

[15] *The ceremonies … used in the time of king Henry VII*.

(the touch, the sign of the cross) some of it had evolved later (the prayers, the gift of gold).

It seems likely that Henry introduced the liturgy and the gift of the gold Angel (*see* Plate 4) to supplicants in order to make the ceremony more effi-cacious, possibly because he was aware that it did not always cure people of their scrofula. In part, this showed his concern for his ill subjects, but at the same time a more effective ceremony could strengthen his authority as king, given that his accession disrupted the direct line of succession.[16] One way of enhancing the power of the royal touch was evidently to standardise the ritual; the other concerns the Angels.

The Angel was the most commonly used gold coin of its day, so in one respect it was an obvious choice to include in the ceremony. Angels were first minted in 1465 by Edward IV – who does not appear to have touched for scrofula – in emulation of the French Angelot coin that was first produced in 1340. Angels were a standard part of English currency until the 1590s, after which their primary use began to be ceremonial (this explains why Tudor Angels are not always pierced, whereas later ones usually are).[17] The Angel was the standard fee charged by a reputable doctor for a consultation.[18] This meant that people who were not well off tended to consult apothecaries, whose fees were lower; indeed the apothecary Nicholas Culpeper quipped that physicians were like Balaam's ass – they would only speak when they saw an Angel.[19]

Yet the addition of the Angel to the royal touch ceremony was signifi-cant. The gold coin increased the prestige of the ritual as Angels were made from 22 carat gold and contained more of this metal than any other English coin.[20] During the reign of Henry VII the Angel was worth 6s. 8d.: medieval kings had given each person whom they touched one penny, so the gift of the Angel marked a very substantial increase in value.[21] Although Henry VII

---

[16] Becket, *A free and impartial enquiry*, 51. The author and his book are discussed at pp. 206–12 below.

[17] I am grateful to Barrie Cook for clarification of these points.

[18] J. Maxwell, *A poem shewing the excellencie of our soveraigne king James his hand*, in *The laudable life and deplorable death of ... prince Henry*, London 1612, D3; W. S. C. Copeman, *Doctors and disease in Tudor times*, London 1960, 51. Maxwell says that doctors took an Angel from their patients 'yet oftentimes give them noe health for their gold', whereas the kings gives his patients both gold and health.

[19] A.W. Sloan, *English medicine in the seventeenth century*, Durham 1996, 4.

[20] For Angels see Farquhar, 'Royal charities, I, II, III, IV', and Woolf, 'The sovereign remedy', and 'The sovereign remedy, II'; R. L. Kenyon, *The gold coins of England*, London 1884, esp. pp. 18–20, 52; and C. E. Challis, *The Tudor coinage*, Manchester 1978, esp. p. 213.

[21] Marc Bloch suggested that the Angel might have been intended to encourage ill people to seek recourse from their king (*The royal touchs*, 66 [114]); but he did not examine the numbers touched, which were low.

became notoriously parsimonious as his reign progressed, he remained generous to the poor and sick.[22]

The coin played a key role in the ceremony, contributing to the restoration of health alongside the king's touch, which is why both have equally prominent places in the liturgy. Supplicants were presented twice to the monarch, first to be touched, and then to be blessed with an Angel with which they were then presented, each occasion having its own passage from the New Testament recited aloud. The liturgy states that people were to wear their Angels until they were fully restored to health, meaning that they both commemorated the ceremony and aided recovery.

The thaumaturgic properties of the Angel related to the depictions and inscriptions engraved upon it (see Plate 4). They were named thus because each had on its obverse a portrayal of the Archangel Michael slaying the devil in the form of a two-legged dragon or wyvern. The Archangel Michael was the warrior who led the fight against God's enemies (Revelation xii.7), as well as the guardian of souls.[23] His image on the coin was an allusion to the triumph of good over evil and hence of health over disease, given the contemporary belief that illness related to sin. On the coin's reverse appeared the ship of state, the central mast of which had a cross beam to make it look like Christ's cross. This image symbolised the godly body politic.

Some of Henry VII's Angels bore the legend 'Per Crucem Tuam Salva Nos Christie Redemptor' ('Through Thy Cross Save Us, Christ Redeemer'), thus retaining Edward IV's inscription, whilst others read 'Jesus Autem Transiens Per Medium Illorum Ibat' ('But Jesus Passing Through Their Midst Went His Way'). These words, from Luke iv.30, tell of Christ's rejection by the people of his own town of Nazareth: they drove him to the brow of a hill and were going to throw him over it, but he walked through them unhurt. The second Latin verse had appeared on some of Edward III's Nobles, a different coin from the Angel. Henry VII's return to Edward III's inscription associated him with his Plantagenet predecessor, which was desirable because Henry's claim to the throne was through his mother, Margaret of Beaufort, who descended from Edward III. Since in pre-Reformation Europe it was usual to believe in the therapeutic properties of sacred language, verses from the Bible, holy words or even spells could be written out and worn by a person to aid wellbeing.[24] Edward III's Nobles had sometimes been worn as protective amulets in battle – the legend is suggestive of this – so Henry VII probably wanted to emphasise that his Angels were equally special.[25] Indeed, in the

[22] Farquhar, 'Royal charities, I', 68, 72–6.

[23] L. J. Taylor and others (eds), Encyclopedia of medieval pilgrimage, Leiden–Boston 2010, 420–1; R. Johnson, Saint Michael the archangel in medieval English legend, Woodbridge 2005.

[24] Thomas, Religion and the decline of magic, 180–1; Becket, A free and impartial enquiry, 47.

[25] Becket, A free and impartial enquiry, 46; Farquhar, 'Royal charities, I', 70–1.

early eighteenth century William Becket, who conducted thorough archival work on the royal touch, said that Henry VII specifically chose the inscriptions for the Angels as they were thought to aid recovery.[26] The practice of wearing an Angel to aid recovery was evidently popular because it continued throughout the seventeenth century, despite the fact that Protestants were supposed to shun thaumaturgic objects.

The exalted status of the Angel also had the effect of bringing the ceremony in line with pilgrimages made by the sick to healing shrines. Of course it had always been the case that people with scrofula had to travel to the royal court, and pilgrims to a shrine, and that both healing rituals required faith and involved prayer, but the Angel added a new aspect to the royal touch in the way that badges and souvenirs did for pilgrimages. Just as pilgrims could buy badges at shrines to honour their petition to a saint, or souvenirs such as phials of holy oil, so people who had been touched were meant to wear their Angel around their neck afterwards. The badges and souvenirs were sometimes said to have thaumaturgic properties, just like the Angels, as were other Christian amulets such as the Agnus Dei, a wax disc stamped with an image of Jesus as the lamb of God bearing a cross, that was blessed by the pope and worn on a chain. The inscriptions on these objects were crucial to their perceived therapeutic properties because, whereas a prayer lasted for as long as it was spoken, wearing the text meant that it was with someone all the time, and so would hopefully be more efficacious.

Angels and other Christian tokens can be thought of as part of a gift economy, material objects that marked the process whereby supplicants offered allegiance to an intercessionary figure who could act as a conduit for God's grace which could cure their ailments, or ward off misfortune.[27] For Henry Tudor and those who supported him or wanted peace, this allegiance was important given the recent turmoil of the Wars of the Roses, while the ability of the king to cure scrofula marked God's blessing on the nation.

Reforming the royal touch

The royal touch survived the Henrician and Edwardian Reformations. The reformers were hostile to 'popish' doctrines and practices such as the real presence of the eucharist and its associated ceremonies; they were opposed

---

[26] Becket, A free and impartial enquiry, 47. The supposed thaumaturgic properties of Angels, including the occult properties of gold, are further discussed at pp. 142–5, 163–5 below.

[27] Thomas, Religion and the decline of magic, 30–2; A. M. Koldeweij, 'Lifting the veil on pilgrim badges', in J. Stopford (ed.), Pilgrimage explored, York 1999, 161–88; D. Webb, Pilgrims and pilgrimage in the medieval west, London 1999, 124–32; Sarah Hopper, To be a pilgrim: the medieval pilgrimage experience, Stroud 2002, 120–34; D. Webb, Medieval European pilgrimage, c. 700–c. 1500, Basingstoke 2002, 163–6; Walsham, The reformation of the landscape, 49–66.

to healing shrines, relics and thaumaturgic objects because they denied their authenticity and curative powers. But both reformers and Roman Catholics agreed that sickness could result from sin, and that recovery depended on divine will and should involve prayer and repentance.

The earliest extant reformed royal touch liturgy dates from Elizabeth's reign and is changed in a number of ways in keeping with the new doctrine. The date of these innovations is uncertain, however, as there is no definitive liturgy from the reigns of Henry VIII or Edward VI (the earliest liturgy is from Mary Tudor's reign and refers to the king, so could possibly date from the reigns of Henry VII or Henry VIII). The changes in the reformed Elizabethan liturgy are revealing: it is shorn of the references to saints and the Virgin Mary; it is still spoken by the chaplain but no longer the monarch, and there are communal prayers for all to speak; the statement that supplicants must wear their Angels until they were fully recovered is deleted; and there is no final prayer said by the chaplain and king after everyone has left. The rest of the ceremony remained intact, and surprisingly the queen still made the sign of the cross with the Angel over the sores, an issue which needs further discussion. The survival of reverence for the cross is also evident in Henry VIII and Edward VI's Angels which kept the legend 'Per Crucem Tuam Salva Nos Christie Redemptor' ('Through Thy Cross Save Us, Christ Redeemer').[28]

The liturgical reform of the royal touch highlights the attitude of the reformers to ritual.[29] Although evangelical theologians such as Jean Calvin and Huldrych Zwingli idealised a pure, intellectualised faith, many reformers had a selective attitude to ritual and were not hostile to it *per se*. This was partly because religious and secular rituals proliferated in pre-modern Europe, and helped to maintain order.[30] It was also because people could be very attached to the old ways. This meant that it was often difficult to decide exactly what to keep, reform or abolish, creating a highly complex state of affairs. The legislation of the Henrician Reformation reveals that the radicalism of some of the reformers who led the initial changes was tempered by more conservative forces that reflected the king's position. Thus, initially, the legislation revoked many traditional religious rituals because they were thought to be 'superstitious' and 'idolatrous', and so offend God and 'diminish His honour and glory'.[31] But later legislation reintroduced many

---

[28] For Mary and Elizabeth's legends see p. 62 below.

[29] For ritual and the Reformation see R. Hutton, *The rise and fall of merry England: the ritual year, 1400–1700*, Oxford 1994; E. Muir, *Ritual in early modern Europe*, 2nd edn, Cambridge 2005; and J. Bossy, 'The mass as a social institution, 1200–1700', *P&P* c (Aug. 1983), 29–61, and *Christianity in the West, 1400–1700*, Oxford 1985, esp. pp. 153–61.

[30] N. Z. Davis, 'The sacred and the body social in sixteenth-century Lyon', *P&P* xc (1981), 40–70 at p. 59.

[31] 'The second royal injunction of Henry VIII, AD 1538', in *Documents illustrative of the history of the English Church*, ed. H. Gee and W. J. Harvey, London 1896, 277.

rituals, although their intrinsic efficacy was downplayed and emphasis placed upon their symbolism:

> [The King's loving subjects are commanded] to observe and keep the ceremonies of holy bread, holy water, procession, kneeling, and Creeping on Good Friday to the Cross, and on Easter day setting up of lights before the Corpus Christi, bearing of candles upon the day of the Purification of our Lady, ceremonies used at the purification of women, delivered of child, and offering of their chrisoms ... and all other laudable ceremonies heretofore used in the Church of England ... so as they shall use without superstition.[32]

This last point was emphasised:

> And so it shall be well understood and known that neither holy bread nor holy water, candles, bows nor ashes hallowed, or creeping or kissing the cross be the workers or works of our salvation, but only as outward signs and tokens whereby we remember Christ and his doctrine, his works and his passion, from whence all good Christian men receive salvation.[33]

Attachment to pre-Reformation ritual is evident even at the royal court. Archbishop Thomas Cranmer had to write to Thomas Cromwell in 1537 to express his dismay that the saints' days and ceremonies that had been abolished were nevertheless still being celebrated and performed at court.[34] At a more popular level, Christopher Haigh has found evidence that parishioners sometimes put pressure on their clergy to reintroduce banned rituals such as the wearing of the surplice, and the signing of the cross at baptism.[35]

Reform of ritual was clearly a delicate subject, but a key criterion underlay it. In theory a true rite had to be found in the Bible, and so the seven sacraments of baptism, confirmation, the eucharist, extreme unction and anointing the sick, marriage, ordination and penance were reduced to two: baptism and the eucharist. The royal touch survived the Reformation partly because its apologists claimed that its origins lay in Christ's healing ministry and the continuation of this by his disciples after the resurrection. However, the reformers knew that in reality rituals had often developed as the result of centuries of lay and clerical pious practices and so rather than abolishing

---

[32] '[Proclamation] Prescribing rites and ceremonies, pardoning Anabaptists', Westminster, 26 Feb. 1539, 30 Henry VIII, in *Tudor royal proclamations*, ed. P. L. Hughes and J. F. Larkin, New Haven, 1964–9, i. 278.

[33] Ibid. i. 279.

[34] F. Kisby, ' "When the king goeth a procession": chapel ceremonies and services, the ritual year, and religious reforms at the early Tudor court, 1485–1547', *JBS* xl (2001), 44–75 at pp. 71–2.

[35] C. Haigh, 'The taming of the Reformation: preachers, pastors and parishioners in Elizabethan and early Stuart England', *History* lxxxv (2000), 572–88 at p. 585.

them because they had no biblical origin, they reformed them. This usually involved the removal of anything to do with intercessionary figures such as the saints and the Virgin Mary.[36]

The liturgical reforms of the royal touch were popular as is clear from the fact that the scale of the practice evidently increased after the Reformation. There are two points to be made in this connection. First, the Reformation swept away many other religious healing practices, such as those associated with shrines and relics. The suppression of other forms of spiritual healing could be unpopular, not surprisingly. This might explain why after the Reformation it is reported for the first time that the royal surgeons examined people who had come to court to be touched, as not all of them had scrofula: people who were ill with other diseases sometimes tried to access the royal touch.[37]

The second effect of the Reformation on the royal touch was that it enhanced the sacral nature of the English monarchy.[38] Most obviously, the sovereign was now Supreme Head of the English Church. The reformed pattern of devotion changed from a eucharist-centred liturgy to one of preaching and reading, while leaving intact all the ceremony attached to the exalted nature of the monarchy. Thus processions in which the eucharist was carried under a canopy were discarded, as were the canopies and tabernacles for the host and altar; bowing to the altar also ceased. Yet all these objects and practices remained in connection with royal ritual, while other aspects of royal ceremony also enhanced the monarch's sacral role. The king heard service in the Chapel Royal in a closet elevated above the courtiers below. He dined publicly in the Presence Chamber in a ceremony that was full of ecclesiastical references. The table at which he ate was placed to the east and was covered with a fine cloth, just like an altar; grace was said by the highest ranking prelate at court; the king washed his hands before and after eating, with the towel carried by the gentleman usher above his head like a holy relic. The monarch also washed the feet of the poor on Maundy Thursday in imitation of Christ and dispensed cramp rings on Good Friday, until this ceased in 1558. More broadly, the entire court calendar was structured around the Church's ritual year, a situation that continued after the Reformation, although a small number of 'popish' feast days were removed such as Corpus Christi. In sum, the Reformation removed 'the real presence of the eucharist while leaving intact the royal presence of the monarch'.[39]

---

[36] Muir, *Ritual*, 79,163–4.

[37] Tooker, *Charisma*, 93.

[38] J. Adamson, 'The Tudor and Stuart courts, 1509–1714', in Adamson, *Princely courts*, 104–5.

[39] Ibid. 104.

Edward VI and the royal touch

It seems likely that England's most feverently Protestant king did touch for scrofula even though the Edwardian Reformation was more radical than the Henrician and there is no direct evidence that Edward touched the sick.[40] Indeed, this lack of evidence is not unusual for Edward's reign given that much material was destroyed by the reformers themselves when Mary Tudor defeated Northumberland's coup, and then by the subsequent, more systematic Marian annihilation of documents concerning her brother's reign.[41] However, there are convincing hints of Edward touching for scrofula.

First, a record from the last ten months of Edward's reign details the gold that he distributed at the traditional festivals of the Church during that period, totalling £10 3s., revealing that he spent another 25s. on cramp rings on Good Friday 'according to the ancient order and custom'.[42] This surely means that Edward distributed cramp rings throughout his reign, which is surprising given the hostility of radical reformers towards thaumaturgic objects. Yet this hostility was due to wonder-working objects being said to be fraudulent, whereas cramp rings could not be described as false since they were made at the behest of the king, who then blessed them. It is almost inconceivable that Edward should dispense cramp rings and not touch for scrofula, especially given the taste for exalted monarchy that was characteristic of Edward's court.[43]

Next, Elizabeth I's chaplain William Tooker (1553/4–1621) commented in his book on the royal touch that the queen's thaumaturgic abilities exceeded her 'brother, sister, father, and grandfather'.[44] The point here is that Tooker was correct in noting that Henry VII, Henry VIII and Mary Tudor all practised the royal touch, implying that he was right about Edward VI as well. Although Tooker could not himself have witnessed Edward VI touching for scrofula, many of his contemporaries such as Elizabeth could have done so. He was unlikely to have made a mistake in this regard, and so his explicit reference to Edward is important.

---

[40] Crawfurd leaves the question open: *The king's evil*, 65–6. See also Farquhar, 'Royal charities, I', 92; Bloch, *The royal touch* 188 (330); Brogan, 'Royal touch' (dissertation), 63. For the Edwardian Reformation see W. K. Jordan, *Edward VI: the young king: the protectorship of the duke of Somerset*, London 1968, 125–225, 305–38; J. Loach, *Edward VI*, ed. George Bernard and P. Williams, New Haven 1999, 116–35; and D. MacCulloch, *Tudor Church militant: Edward VI and the Protestant Reformation*, London 1999.

[41] I am grateful to Professor Diarmaid MacCulloch for this pointt.

[42] BL, MS Add. 35183, fo. 31v, 31 Mar. 1553; account book of Sir William Paget, controller of the household 1547–8, TNA, E 101/426/1.

[43] For exalted sovereignty see W. K. Jordan, *Edward VI: the threshold of power: the dominance of the duke of Northumberland*, London 1970, 420–6; Loach, *Edward VI*, ch. xi, esp. pp. 143–4.

[44] Tooker, *Charisma*, 87–8.

A further piece of evidence that suggests that Edward touched for scrofula is a commentary by the physician and cleric Andrew Boorde (1490–1549). He wrote in his *Breviary of health* (1547) that people with scrofula should 'make frendes to the kynges maiesty for it doth pertaine to a kynge to helpe this infyrmyte … by the grace the which is geven to a kynge anornted'.[45] Boorde worked at the royal court and was a noted medical practitioner;[46] his *Breviary* was the first medical manual written in English and was aimed primarily at practitioners who needed a handbook and at patients from the upper ranks of society.[47] Though Boorde wrote his *Breviary* in 1542, implying that his comment relates to Henry VIII rather than to his successor, it was not published until July 1547. Henry died in January of that year and Edward VI would have been expected to touch the sick at Easter: had he not done so Boorde would surely have amended his text. Boorde died in 1549 and his *Breviary* was re-issued in 1552 due to high demand; the second edition contains the same reference to scrofula, which reinforces the view that Edward touched for scrofula.[48] Furthermore, in Borde's companion volume *The fyrst boke of the introduction of knowledge* (also written in 1542 and published in 1547), he stated that the kings of England healed scrofula and distributed cramp rings at Easter.[49]

Lastly, the clergyman Hamon L'Estrange (1605–60) wrote in *The alliance of divine offices* (1659) that, 'All along King Edward the six'th, and Queen Elizabeth her Reign, when the strumosi, such as had the king's Evil, came to be touched, the manner was for her to apply the sign of the Cross to the tumour.'[50] L'Estrange was a royalist apologist who published his book more than a century after Edward's death, which might seem to undermine his comments. Yet L'Estrange was correct with regard to Elizabeth and the sign of the cross, so notwithstanding his awkward phraseology, his comments provide a further hint that Edward touched the sick.

Such evidence that might imply that Edward did not touch for scrofula is weak and unconvincing. The king's diary contains no mention of the ceremony but this is not significant as the journal is primarily concerned with court politics, foreign affairs and administrative matters; it also contains

---

[45] A. Boorde, *Breviary of health*, London 1547; 2nd edn, 1552, fo. lxxxxvi.

[46] E. Furdell, 'Boorde, Andrew (*c.* 1496–1549)', *ODNB*.

[47] P. Slack, 'Mirrors of health and treasures of poor men: the uses of the vernacular medical literature of Tudor England', in C. Webster (ed.), *Health, medicine and mortality in the sixteenth century*, Cambridge 1979, 237–73 at pp. 256, 260.

[48] Boorde, *Breviary*, fo. lxxx.

[49] Idem, *The fyrst boke of the introduction of knowledge*, London 1547, ch i, pp. B.i.–B.ii.

[50] H. L'Estrange, *The alliance of divine offices*, London 1659, 250. For a fourth, less significant, suggestion that Edward VI touched for scrofula see R. Holinshed, *Chronicles of England, Scotlande, and Irelande*, London 1577, 279. In the 1587 edition it is at bk VIII, p. 195.

no mention of cramp rings – which were distributed.[51] It has been suggested that Edward was too sickly to have touched ill people, but in fact he was a healthy young man until the last year of his life.[52] Edward's accounts contain no information germane to him distributing Angels to people whom he had touched, but they were minted during his reign. The numismatist Christopher Challis has argued convincingly that this must mean that Edwardian Angels were produced for use in the royal touch ceremony, mainly because the coins were beginning to be replaced within the currency by the half-sovereign.[53] Although no Edwardian royal touch liturgy survives, that of Elizabeth I does, reformed of its Roman Catholic elements: just as Elizabeth adopted Edward VI's prayer book perhaps her liturgy for the royal touch might also derive from her brother's.[54]

The royal touch and two queens regnant

Mary Tudor's accession in 1553 meant that the royal touch was practised for the first time by a woman, a situation that continued for fifty years until the death of her successor Elizabeth I in 1603. By contrast to Edward VI, there is concrete evidence that Mary and Elizabeth touched for scrofula. Did it matter that they were women? The answer appears to be no, not least because the numbers of people touched by both queens were seemingly higher than those regarding their male Tudor predecessors. Like kings but unlike queen consorts, queens regnant were anointed on their hands as part of the coronation ritual, thus giving them full thaumaturgic powers.[55] However, there appear to have been two changes connected to the royal touch in light of it being practised by a woman. The first point is that during the reign of a queen regnant scrofula was sometimes referred to as the 'queen's evil' rather than the 'king's evil'.[56] The second is to do with hygiene and sensitivity, and is only germane to Elizabeth. If she were to touch

---

[51] *The chronicle and political papers of king Edward VI,* ed. W. K. Jordan, London 1966.

[52] Farquhar, 'Royal charities, I', 92. I am grateful to Professor Diarmaid MacCulloch for information concerning the king's health.

[53] Challis, *Tudor coinage,* 213.

[54] Crawfurd, *The king's evil,* 65; Bloch, *The royal touch,* 385 n. 65 (330–1).

[55] C. G. Bayne, 'The coronation of queen Elizabeth', *EHR* xxii (1907), 650–73 at p. 668 n. 80; Bloch, *The royal touch,* 103, 331 n. 36; A. L. Rowse, 'The coronation of queen Elizabeth I', *History Today* (May 1953), 301–10 at p. 310; D. Starkey, *Elizabeth: apprenticeship,* London 2000, 272; A. Hunt, *The drama of coronation,* Cambridge 2008, 210 n. 18. For the primary sources see *The accession, coronation, and marriage of Mary Tudor as related in four manuscripts of the Escorial,* ed. and trans. C.V. Malfatti, Barcelona 1956, 33; *The accession of Queen Mary: being the contemporary narrative of Antonio de Guaras, a Spanish merchant resident in London,* ed. and trans. R. Garnett, London 1892, 121; and *English coronation records,* ed. L. G. Wickham Legg, London 1901.

[56] R. Scot, *The discoverie of witchcraft,* London 1584, bk XII, ch. xiv, pp. 4, 137; bk XIII, ch. ix, pp. 303–4.

someone who had open sores her surgeons sometimes bandaged them so that she did not have to make physical contact with the abscesses.[57] Elizabeth was noted for her fine-looking hands, which must have contrasted greatly with the sores that she touched. William Tooker stated:

> how often have I seen her, with her very beautiful hands, radiant as white-washed snow, courageously free of all squeamishness, touching their abscesses not with her finger tips, but pressing hard and repeatedly, with wholesome results, and how often did I see her handling ulcers as if they were her own?[58]

The fact that English queens regnant touched for scrofula can be placed within the polemical debate concerning female rulers. This 'problem' was exemplified by the works of the Calvinist John Knox, an especially polemical and patriarchal theorist who abhorred the rule of females; and yet queens regnant were expected to marry a man, produce a male heir and take counsel from noblemen.[59] Thus a female prince was expected to practise as much kingcraft as possible.

A good evocation of female sacral monarchy can be found in Mary Tudor's missal. As well as the miniature of her blessing cramp rings at an altar in an oratory, another image depicts her touching for scrofula within an architectural setting (see Plate 5). This corroborates the description by the Venetian observer Marco Antonio Faitto of the ritual at Greyfriars Church in Greenwich in May 1556. The queen is shown in the centre of the image in her characteristic dress and headdress. She kneels behind a reading desk that has an open book on it, presumably the Bible, and is shown in the act of touching the neck of a young man who has scrofula whilst the clergyman on the right reads from a prayer book. Mary has a hand on either side of the young man's neck, which she is holding or pressing: it does not look like a brief moment of contact. Faitto recorded that when the infirm were brought to the queen one by one, Mary 'kneeling the whole time … commenced pressing, with her hands in the form

---

57 Tooker, *Charisma*, 94.

58 Ibid. 99–100.

59 J. Knox, *First blast of the trumpet against the monstrous regiment of women* (Geneva 1558), in *The works of John Knox*, ed. L. David (1895), New York 1966. For a defence of female rulers see J. Aylmer, *An harborrowe for faithful and trewe subiectes, agaynst the late blowne blast, concerning the government of wemmen*, London 1559. For early modern female rulers see (as well as Levin's work) M. Mendle, *Dangerous positions: mixed government, the estates of the realm, and the answer to the XIX propositions*, Tuscaloosa, AL 1985; P. L. Scalingi, 'The sceptre or the distaff: the question of female sovereignty, 1516–1607', *The Historian* xli (1978), 59–75; and J. E. Phillips, Jr, 'The background of Spencer's attitude toward women rulers', *Huntington Library Quarterly* v (1941), 5–32. For women more generally see N. Z. Davis 'Women on top', in N. Z. Davis, *Society and culture in early modern France*, Stanford, CA 1975, 124–51; M. Weisner, *Women and gender in early modern Europe*, Cambridge 1993; and M. Sommerville, *Sex and subjection: attitudes to women in early modern society*, London 1995.

of a cross, on the spot where the sore was, with such compassion and devotion as to be a marvel'.[60]

The young man kneels partly on a rug, partly on a tiled floor, and has his hands clasped in prayer. He wears a tunic (or possibly rolled up britches), while the neck of his garment has been fully opened to expose his shoulders and the glands of his neck. Unfortunately the position of Mary's hand means that we cannot see his scrofulous swellings. To his left kneels a clergyman, probably Mary's clerk of the closet John Ricorde, who is holding down the young man's clothing.[61] In the image there is no sight of the Angels, but further details of the ceremony are given by the Venetian observer who said that after Mary had touched each person they were again presented individually to her. The queen then touched their scrofula with an Angel and made the sign of the cross over it, threading the coin onto a ribbon and giving it to them. Mary made them promise 'never to part with it' unless they were in 'extreme need' because it was 'hallowed'. The queen then washed her hands in public to signify that the ceremony had finished. This is the earliest eyewitness description of the ceremony, and the reference to the sick person possibly selling their Angel is intriguing because in the seventeenth century a royal touch apologist complained that the coins could be bought second-hand in London in goldsmith's shops.[62]

The Tudor cult

At the end of Elizabeth's reign the first two books devoted to the royal touch were published. Both of these greatly increase understanding of the ceremony, especially its underlying principles, not least because both authors assisted in the ceremony and so provide first-hand evidence of it. The first was by the theologian William Tooker, Elizabeth's chaplain and later dean of Lichfield. His Latin text *Charisma sive donum sanationis*, translated as *The royal gift of healing* (1597), was aimed at a learned audience and seems always to have been a rare book.[63] Tooker wrote his book because he was an ardent royalist and he used his text to refute the excommunication of Elizabeth I by Pope Pius V in 1570.[64] The pope claimed that the Protestant Elizabeth was a usurper. Tooker replied that as Elizabeth had touched so many people for scrofula, often with apparent success, this demonstrated that she was the rightful sovereign. Tooker strengthened his rebuttal by including mention of a Roman Catholic Englishman who had been a prisoner but who was

---

[60] CSPV vi. 434–7 at p. 436.

[61] J. Bickersteth and R. W. Dunning, *Clerks of the Closet in the royal households*, Stroud 1991, facing p. 66.

[62] See p. 165 below.

[63] Becket, *Free and impartial enquiry*, 60; Crawfurd, *The king's evil*, 69.

[64] J. A. Löwe, 'Tooker, William (1553/4–1621)', ODNB; Tooker, *Charisma*, 90–2.

touched by Elizabeth, and healed. This showed the queen's great benevolence as she did not withhold her curative powers from religious minorities, and by implication her enemies. The man then realised that the papal bull had no authority over Elizabeth and that she was the rightful queen of England.

The second book, *A right fruitful and approved treatise for the artificial cure of that malady called in Latin struma* (1602), was written by the surgeon William Clowes (1543/4–1604).[65] This is a medical treatise written in English, as were all Clowes's publications: he wanted to reach as broad an audience as possible, so as to benefit his countrymen.[66] Clowes was serjeant-surgeon to Elizabeth and his book concentrated on the symptoms and treatment of scrofula, probably so that people would not approach the queen to be healed before they had sought medical help. This was in the interests of the queen, who was elderly, and it reflected the contemporary notion that the royal touch should be a last resort for especially hard-to-treat cases of scrofula.[67] Indeed, Clowes provided a vivid case to illustrate this last point. He described a Dutchman, the scrofula on whose neck was so bad that it was not safe to operate on him. Medicine that Clowes and others had prescribed had made the man's condition worse rather than better, and Clowes feared that the man would develop gangrene. The Dutchman was subsequently touched by Elizabeth and was cured within five months. He told Clowes that that after he was touched he 'never applyed any Medicine at all' but kept himself clean 'with sweet and fresh clean clothes, and now and then washed the sore with White Wine'.[68] He also wore his gold touch-piece at all times. The suggestion here is that the royal touch was not always expected to work on its own, nor was it expected to provide an immediate cure.[69] The man mentions that he did not use medicine afterwards, implying that other people did; he emphasises the need for good hygiene; and he wore his Angel constantly in keeping with the pre-Reformation rationale that this was essential for the cure.

Both Tooker and Clowes explained that the ability to heal scrofula by touch was an important component of sacral monarchy, with the ultimate source of thaumaturgic power being God. It was important to stress this because the apologists maintained that the monarch acted as a conduit for God's healing powers during the royal touch ceremony; there was no suggestion that the sovereign had innate healings powers, such as those of Christ.

---

[65] For Tooker see Löwe, 'Tooker'; for Clowes see I. G. Murray, 'Clowes, William (1543/4–1604)', *ODNB*, and *Selected writings of William Clowes*, ed. F. N. L. Poynter, London 1948.

[66] Murray, 'Clowes'.

[67] W. Clowes, *A right fruitful and approved treatise for the artificial cure of that malady called in Latin struma*, London 1602, 'Epistle to the reader', pp. A2r, 48–50. See also Tooker, *Charisma*, 93, 104.

[68] Clowes, *Treatise*, 50.

[69] The effectiveness and timescale of cures is discussed at chapter 6 below.

It appears that sometimes this distinction could be blurred and so apologists and successive governments continued to reiterate this message until royal therapeutics ceased.

Tooker stated that all English monarchs since Edward the Confessor had healed by touch – his source for this was Polydore Vergil – and he voiced the orthodox view that the gift of healing was hereditary and solemnised when sovereigns were anointed. Yet Tooker prioritised God over heredity, writing that English monarchs 'rely not so much on some innate power from their ancestors … rather they are granted a particular divine gift'.[70] Tooker dealt only briefly with the anointing, probably reflecting his reformist view that sacramental acts had no intrinsic value. Despite this, it is worth noting that sacral monarchy was given ritual expression at the coronation, whether Protestant or Roman Catholic.[71] The royal vestments were similar in appearance to the sacerdotal clothing of the clergy; the monarchs were anointed with oil said to have come down from heaven, in a tradition that was traced back to Old Testament kings; and the English monarch was said to descend from a royal saint, Edward the Confessor.[72] Healing by touch demonstrated that the sovereign was separate from the laity and that they were blessed with a divine charisma. The fact that no English monarch caught scrofula can only have added to the mystique of the monarchy.

Tooker further explained the royal touch by reference to Christ's healing ministry, maintaining that the Messiah was the first person to heal by touch diseases that were otherwise incurable, such as epilepsy, dropsy and dysentery. This work was continued by the Apostles, their pupils and the early Church Fathers, and then the English monarchs. The reference to incurable diseases is pertinent given that doctors like Clowes recommended the royal touch to patients whose scrofula was especially resistant to treatment. Tooker quoted St Paul who explained that the ability to heal by touch was a gift given to certain individuals by God for the greater benefit of humankind (1 Corinthians xii.7). As the head of state was chosen by God, Tooker explained that it was only natural that they outshone others in terms of heavenly gifts; thus the ability of the English monarchs to heal by touch proved the favour in which God held them. Tooker stressed the importance of faith, not just for the sick people but for the royal healer as well. He cited the instance of when Christ's disciples had been unable to exorcise a demon from a possessed man; they took the man to Jesus who healed him and said

[70] Tooker, Charisma, 85, 89; Clowes, Treatise, 49–50.

[71] Bloch, The royal touch, 128, (221).

[72] P. E. Schramm, A history of the English coronation, trans. L. G. Wickham Legg, Oxford 1937, 116. See also Bayne, 'Coronation of Queen Elizabeth'; H. Wilson, 'The coronation of Queen Elizabeth', EHR xxiii (1908), 87–91; Bak, Coronations; and R. Strong, Coronation: a history of kingship and the British monarchy, London 2005.

to the disciples 'For verily I say unto you, if ye have faith … nothing shall be impossible unto you' (Matt. xvii.20).[73]

Elizabeth I was aware of the need for faith when practising the royal touch, and of the great responsibility incurred by being a conduit for God's grace. When preparing to touch the sick the queen galvanised herself psychologically: she 'visualized God about to restore physical and spiritual health … so that by touch alone … with the assistance of divine power' she could perform the ritual.[74] Prayer was also very important during her preparations, sometimes producing dramatic results. Tooker wrote 'how often have I seen her most serene Majesty down on her knees, worshipping with her whole body and mind, calling upon the true God, humbly beseeching Christ the Savior on behalf of such people?'[75]

Elizabeth herself explained that royal healing powers were a gift from God and advocated prayer as a remedy for disease when she was approached by people with scrofula whilst on progress in Gloucestershire, although the exact place and date are not recorded. She said to them that she was merely God's conduit: 'If only I could bring you benefit and help; God, God is the best and greatest doctor of them all. He is Jehovah wise and holy, who will bring relief to your ills, you should pray to him.'[76] After the Restoration it was sometimes claimed that Elizabeth's response indicated that she stopped touching for scrofula for a while 'in a Fitt of Puritanisme'.[77] Puritans did sometimes object that the royal touch was 'superstitious', but this interpretation of Elizabeth's words is mistaken. It tells us more about Restoration anti-Catholicism and the way that Elizabeth was seen at this time as being more Protestant than she really had been than it does about the queen herself. There is no evidence that Elizabeth ceased practising the royal touch at any point and her words merely voiced the inscription on the Marian and Elizabethan Angels that was changed to 'A Domino Factum Est Istud, Et Est Mirabile in Oculis Nostris' ('This is the Lord's Doing, And It Is Marvellous In Our Eyes', Psalm cxviii.23). More recently, it has been suggested that Elizabeth might have refused to carry out the royal touch when petitioned because she was menstruating. In pre-modern Europe the touch of a menstruating woman was thought to pollute the recipient.[78] This interpretation is certainly plausible. But the key to understanding the Gloucestershire incident lies in Tooker's overlooked introductory passage in which he explained

---

73 Tooker, *Charisma*, 1, 3.

74 Ibid. 106.

75 Ibid. 99.

76 Ibid. 105.

77 H. Stubbe, *The miraculous conformist*, London 1666, 9; Becket, *Free and impartial enquiry*, 48. See also Turrell, 'Ritual of royal healing', 3, 9–10. In 1684 Browne explained that Elizabeth's words merely meant that God was the source of her thaumaturgic powers: *Adenochoiradelogia*, 124.

78 Levin, 'Help and succour', 200.

that in fact the queen gave in to demand and touched the petitioners, albeit reluctantly. Tooker revealed that this episode was not unique. Elizabeth was sometimes approached by crowds of scrofulous people who hoped that she would touch them, which itself is enlightening in terms of the demand for royal therapeutics. On occasion she gave in to pressure and appeared to perform the ceremony somewhat unenthusiastically.[79] When Elizabeth told the people in Gloucestershire that only God could cure them, she presumably meant that, unlike Christ, she did not have an innate ability to heal, and advised them to pray because she did not intend to perform the royal touch ceremony, but to no avail. She then touched the people half-heartedly, whether immediately or later is not recorded. Her reluctance could have been due to a number of reasons: she had no opportunity to prepare herself for the ceremony; her itinerary was probably interrupted; she might have been menstruating; her surgeons and chaplains might not have been with her. This is the earliest of many examples when the public demanded the royal touch, and the sovereign acquiesced.

The emphasis on prayer helped the apologists in another way, namely in answering criticisms of the ceremony. Although it was usual to believe in the efficacy of the royal touch, not least due to the religious underpinnings of medicine, not everyone believed that the monarch could cure by touch. In responding to these arguments, Tooker reveals their content. The main objections were that prayer had no intrinsic efficacy; cures might be wrought by wearing the gold Angel rather than the royal touch, which was problematic for Protestants as it was suggestive of magic; or that they might be caused by the power of suggestion. This debate continued into the Stuart age and there is far more evidence of it from the Restoration. Suffice it to say here that in relation to prayer Tooker maintained that reading the word of God could not be condemned because it was an 'antidote to poison' and by implication disease. The thaumaturgic properties of the Angels represented a survival of pre-Reformation belief as Henry VII's liturgy had explicitly stated that they must be worn to effect a cure. By contrast Tooker said that the Angel was only an example of royal alms-giving but he allowed that doctors sometimes thought that wearing one aided recovery though it did not bring it about on its own. And he castigated the power of suggestion as bringing about cures as, in his view, it was not strong enough to do so.[80]

One key criticism levied at Elizabeth herself was that she made the sign of the cross over the sores that she had touched.[81] Presumably this objection was made by Puritans, the issue dying out in 1603 when James VI and I

---

[79] Tooker also mentions (*Charisma*, 93) scrofulous people asking the queen to touch them.

[80] Ibid. 109–10, 117. Although unidentified the objections probably came from Puritans: see chapter 6 below.

[81] Tooker, *Charisma*, 96.

removed the gesture from the ceremony.[82] Elizabeth's continued use of this pre-Reformation sign is telling in terms of her traditional views on religion: the context for this is the queen's liturgical conservativism, one example being her retention of crucifixes in the Chapel Royal.[83] These practices were controversial for 'hotter' Protestants who maintained that they were 'superstitious' and hence Roman Catholic. All that Tooker could reply was that 'the most powerful respect ... should be rendered to the cross'.[84] He then reminded his readers that the sign of the cross was still used in the Church of England during the ceremony of baptism. His views on the royal touch are summarised thus:

> The liturgy is entirely holy, the simplicity and purity of the rituals is praiseworthy, the person performing them is sacrosanct; there is no superstition; magic, bad taste and swearing are completely absent. The author of the whole activity is the Holy Spirit. There is nothing here that is not beneficial: prayer, laying on of hands (a healthy form of touch), making the sign of the cross, which is the same ritual as in baptism ... there is nothing here but God worshipped, veneration of Christ, the care and health of the Christian.[85]

Tooker obviously needed to refute the arguments of those who were sceptical of the royal touch: the stakes were high because the ritual was theorised as an act of Christian healing. To deny it was therefore to question whether God did intervene in the world in the manner that the orthodox maintained.

The Elizabethan reform of the ceremony

During Elizabeth's reign the royal touch underwent two changes: the liturgy was reformed and the ceremony became grander. Beginning with the liturgy, this had its residual Roman Catholic prayers removed and was almost certainly translated into English. Transcribed by Tooker, although he translated it back into Latin which was the language in which he wrote, this is the earliest extant Church of England royal touch liturgy.[86] No copy of the Elizabethan liturgy survives in English but it was almost certainly translated into the vernacular in accordance with the priorities of the reformers.[87]

These liturgical changes increased the popularity of the royal touch. This is evident in Tooker's comments that, whereas Elizabeth washed the feet of the poor annually on Maundy Thursday, by contrast no special day was set aside for

[82] See pp. 73, 76 below.
[83] M. Aston, *England's iconoclasts*, I: *Laws against images*, Oxford 1988, 306–14.
[84] Tooker, *Charisma*, 109.
[85] Ibid. 97–8.
[86] Ibid. 92–7, cf. Crawfurd, *The king's evil*, 72–4, who provides it in English.
[87] Crawfurd, *The king's evil*, 71.

the royal touch because she practised this so regularly, on Sundays and feast days, sometimes even on a daily basis.[88] Although Tooker does not mention a healing calendar, evidence from James I's reign reveals that Elizabeth touched seasonally during the spring and autumn so as to avoid the heat of the summer and the risk of plague.[89]

As for those who sought Elizabeth's sacred touch, it is frustrating that so little is known about them. However, two categories of people were thought to be especially suitable: the poor, who could not afford a doctor, and those whose scrofula was so bad that medicine could not alleviate it. These two types of people emphasised the benevolent aspect of the royal touch and are suggestive of the belief in Christ's mystical presence within the crowds of poor and ill people.[90]

By the end of the sixteenth century Tooker could boast that Elizabeth's touch was sought by people of every age, sex and rank, and that they came from all over England, including the north and both universities.[91] Hence by the 1590s the royal touch had become more current than ever before, which also helps to explain the appearance of the two books devoted to it at that time, as well as the debate concerning its efficacy. Indeed, Tooker tells us that other books and pamphlets also discussed the royal touch, and that it was debated in sermons. He even mentions an image of Elizabeth I touching the scrofulous that was engraved by the mapmaker Joos de Hondt. Unfortunately the books, pamphlets and image do not seem to be extant, while the only sermon reference to have been traced is a brief, orthodox comment on royal therapeutics.[92] On the other hand, even Tooker acknowledged that not everyone believed in the royal touch and he admitted that although Elizabeth had cured 'many thousands' not everyone was healed, castigating those who remained ill as being 'unworthy of such healing assistance'.[93]

The other change to the Elizabethan ceremony is that it became grander. In 1596 it was reported that after the queen had touched ten people, she closed the ceremony by washing her hands in public. During this act of hygiene she was

> served by the Lord Treasurer, the Lord Chancellor and the Earl of Essex, all three on their knees, the Treasurer in the middle, opposite the Queen, holding a basin, the Chancellor to the right with a ewer of warm water, and

---

[88] Tooker, *Charisma*, 94, 113.

[89] See p. 77 below.

[90] See pp. 26–8 above.

[91] Tooker, *Charisma*, 94.

[92] Ibid. 10, 89, 107, 122. For an Elizabethan sermon that mentions the royal touch see J. Howson, *A sermon preached at St. Maries Oxford the 17 day of November, 1602, in defence of the festivities of the Church of England and namely that of her Majesties coronation*, Oxford 1603, D2.

[93] Tooker, *Charisma*, 106.

on the left the Earl of Essex with a napkin, which the Queen used to wipe her hands.[94]

The only earlier account of the Tudor ceremony is that from Mary Tudor's reign. This mentions the cleansing ritual but says that her towel was passed to her by Cardinal Reginald Pole rather than three of the most prominent of the nobility.[95] As Mary was a traditionalist it is likely that she followed the precedent of the first two Tudor kings; this means that by the end of Elizabeth's reign a change had occurred, with the nobility participating in the ceremony as well as the monarch and the clergy. The Lord Chancellor was responsible for the organisation of all court ceremonies, and the holder of that office handed the monarch his or her towel to clean their hands throughout the Stuart period. The Treasurer was responsible for ordering the Angels, which explains his presence (but in subsequent reigns he was not mentioned as a participant in the ritual). Although it might be thought that a clergyman was more appropriate to wash the royal hands at the end of the ceremony, these innovations reflected the inventiveness of those who organised the royal touch, as well as the exalted nature of the Tudor monarchy.[96]

The royal touch was practised throughout the Tudor age regardless of whether the official faith was Roman Catholic or that of the English Church, or whether the sovereign was male or female. It survived the Reformation because it was purged of some of its Roman Catholic elements, and it may have increased in popularity in part because other healing practices were swept away. On the one hand the royal touch projected monarchical authority during a century of great religious and political upheaval and so provided a sense of constancy and legitimacy to a ruling house whose claim to sovereignty was sometimes disputed; on the other, the rite was subjected to many changes in accordance with the priorities of different monarchs and especially new ideas concerning religion. The success of the Tudor revival of royal therapeutics meant that by 1603 the ceremony was a central feature of English life, by contrast to its precarious position in 1485. This helps to explain why James VI and I persuaded himself to practise the royal touch despite his initial misgivings.

94 *CSPV* ix. 505, 238.
95 *CSPV* vi. 437.
96 For the exalted nature of the Tudor monarchy see David Starkey on the bedchamber: 'Representation through intimacy: a study in the symbolism of monarchy and court office in early modern England', in I. Lewis (ed.), *Symbols and sentiments: cross-cultural studies in symbolism*, London 1977, 187–224; for progresses, pageantry and art see R. Strong, *The cult of Elizabeth*, London 1977, and S. Foister, *Holbein in England*, London 2006. For a discussion of all aspects of representations of the Tudor monarchy see Sharpe, *Selling the Tudor monarchy*.

3

The Royal Touch and the Stuart Monarchy, 1603–1688

The Stuarts touched greater numbers of people and with greater regularity than had any of their predecessors, meaning that, although the royal touch originated in the Middle Ages, in terms of its vitality it was primarily a seventeenth-century phenomenon. The ceremony was at its most popular during the Restoration, with Charles II touching an average of 4,000 people each year until the 1680s, when both he and James II administered some 6,000 a year. These huge figures are even more astonishing when it is recalled that between 1530 and 1532 Henry VIII is recorded as having touched just sixty-five scrofulous people. Did this mean that scrofula became more prevalent during the Stuart age, or that the Stuarts had greater pretensions to sacral monarchy than any of their forebears, or that the appeal of the royal touch greatly increased during the seventeenth century? Although scrofula was widespread in pre-modern Europe, whether its prevalence increased during the seventeenth century is not known; but even if it did, it is unlikely to have done so in proportion to the numbers that sought the royal touch. Whilst it is obviously the case that healing the sick in imitation of Christ could bolster royal authority, none of the political tracts that advocated absolutism discussed royal therapeutics.[1] Furthermore, enthusiasm for the royal touch reached such levels that all the Stuart monarchs struggled to control the demand for it. The Stuarts put more effort into holding back and regulating the crowds of ill people than in promoting themselves as thaumaturgic sovereigns.

In order to understand the great upsurge in popularity of royal therapeutics its increased appeal to sick people must be privileged. The first seventeenth-century reforms of the ceremony that improved its credentials by making it more Protestant date from James VI and I's reign. Initially James had spoken against the practice but eventually he decided to touch for scrofula. The second set of reforms was Charles I's bureaucratic measures which sought to bring greater order to the royal touch, especially the healing calendar. Their effectiveness varied, so great was the demand for the touch. Order broke down during the Civil War, with the king sometimes touching without liturgy or gold; yet the appeal of his therapeutic touch did not diminish, for

[1] M. Goldie, 'Restoration political thought' in L. K. J. Glassey (ed.), *The reigns of Charles II and James VII and II*, London 1997, 12–35 at p. 16.

reasons that can be connected to the cult of Charles the Martyr. The royal touch ceased to be practised in England during the Interregnum, although the future Charles II did perform the rite on the continent throughout his exile. Once the Stuarts were restored there was a big reaction in favour of thaumaturgic monarchy, which will be placed in its political and religious contexts. In 1666 the Irish JP Valentine Greatrakes became renowned in England as a 'stroker' who healed by touch: often described as a threat to Charles II, this was an exaggeration. The succession of the Roman Catholic James II in 1685 did nothing to diminish the appeal of royal therapeutics, despite widespread, virulent anti-Catholicism.

Every Stuart monarch, from James I to James II, was committed to providing their subjects with the royal touch, even if some guarded their prerogative more jealously than others. This means that the Stuarts were competent performers of public ceremony and were not as overshadowed in this area by their Tudor predecessors as is sometimes thought. Indeed, it seems that the key public role of the Stuart monarchs was that of healer, meaning that their religious and medical duties were of paramount importance. Although it has been suggested that the execution of Charles I in 1649 'desacralised' the monarchy, which in turn had a terminal effect on the idea of the body politic,[2] this chapter argues that the opposite was true. The architects of the regicide were a radical minority with no popular mandate, which helps to explain the unprecedented enthusiasm for royal therapeutics during the Restoration. Connected to this, an idea that originated during the Civil Wars came into its own during the Restoration, namely that by healing individual suffering the king could heal the body politic. This chapter asserts that the relationship between politics and medicine was at its most intense during the Restoration, hence the great numbers of people touched. These totals peaked at times of political crisis, which further reinforces the idea that the king's touch was thought to be able to heal the sick nation.

James VI and I: scepticism as the impetus for reform

When James VI and I succeeded to the English throne in March 1603 he was initially sceptical of the royal touch and refused to practise it, claiming that it was 'superstitious'; but within six months he had changed his mind and began performing the ceremony, having found an intellectual solution to his misgivings. He then touched for scrofula throughout his reign, and he reformed the practice, making it more Protestant, emphasising the importance of prayer and providence. This was very popular, which helps to explain why the numbers who sought the royal touch increased during his reign.

---

[2] K. Sharpe, *Politics and ideas in early Stuart England*, London 1989, 28–31; Zaller, 'Breaking the vessels', 757–78.

This in turn explains why James faced a new problem that would preoccupy the crown until royal therapeutics ceased in 1714, namely controlling the crowds of ill people who came to the royal court to be healed.

As soon as he became king of England James was expected to touch for scrofula, which indicates that by the end of Elizabeth's reign the ceremony was well established. But during his initial months as king of England James stated twice in public that he would not practise royal therapeutics. His public articulation of scepticism towards the ceremony, as far as is known the first of its kind ever spoken by an English monarch, was an extraordinary break with tradition.

Travelling south from Scotland to London in the spring of 1603, James was expected to touch people with scrofula *en route*, but declined. The Venetian ambassador Giovanni Carlo Scaramelli reported that on arriving in England James announced that he did not wish 'to arrogate vainly to himself such virtue and divinity, as to be able to cure diseases by touch alone'.[3] So although James's journey south was largely a joyous occasion – he knighted a significant number of subjects and participated in numerous celebrations – in terms of his medical role the progress was a disappointment. But the pressure must have been kept up, with people assuming that the new king would touch for scrofula once he was crowned, because in June, during the preparations for the coronation, Scaramelli noted that James stated he would not practise royal thaumaturgy 'as the age of miracles is past, and God alone can work them'.[4] James's scepticism might seem surprising given that he was an eloquent proponent of divine right monarchy,[5] but he had been brought up a Calvinist and so was cautious about miracles, and he had already ruled Scotland for nineteen years, a country that had no tradition of thaumaturgic monarchy.

By the autumn James had changed his mind and began to touch for scrofula. The prevailing interpretation is that although James did not believe in his ability to heal by touch, he recognised the political value of the ceremony to the monarchy once it was explained to him by his English advisors.[6] This included the English crown's claim of suzerainty over France, some early modern commentators maintaining that English sovereigns practised

---

[3] Rome Archives, ser. 1, general series from Vatican and other sources, TNA, PRO 31/9/88.

[4] CSPV x. 44.

[5] James VI, *The trew law of free monarchies*, Edinburgh 1598, and *Basilicon doron*, Edinburgh 1599.

[6] A. Wilson, *The history of Great Britain, being the life and reign of King James the First*, London 1653, 289; *The autobiography and diary of Mr James Melville, with a continuation of the diary*, ed. R. Pitcairn, Edinburgh 1842, 657–8; H. N. Paul, *The royal play of Macbeth*, New York 1950, 372–3; Crawfurd, *The King's evil*, 82; Bloch, *The royal touch*, 191 (336–7); Thomas, *Religion and the decline of magic*, 193.

the royal touch due to this prerogative.[7] This political reading of James's motives is pertinent – although whether the canny Scot really needed the ceremony's political importance explaining to him by English ministers is questionable. However, the key to understanding James's change of heart is the way in which his intellectual misgivings concerning miracles were overcome by emphasising the role of prayer and providence in the ceremony, in much the same way that Protestants reframed exorcism.[8]

James's emphasis on prayer and providence is evident from an examination of the circumstances in which he first touched for scrofula, at Woodstock Palace in September 1603. The timing and location are significant because the royal touch was not usually practised in London during the summer due to the hot weather and its association with plague;[9] but it could be practised in the provinces if the monarch was on progress, provided the locality was free from infection. In fact, plague had broken out in the capital during the summer of 1603, meaning that it was sensible for James to touch first in the autumn, outside London.

Scaramelli reported that by the autumn James had taken an interest in the 'ancient custom' of the royal touch and so it was arranged for a number of people with scrofula to be presented to him in his ante-chamber at Woodstock.[10] The ceremony began with prayers that were said by a Calvinist minister, after which James departed from the usual custom and made a speech explaining his actions in light of his earlier sceptical comments.[11] He began by acknowledging the longevity of English royal healings and said that, although he did not want to withhold any 'comfort' from his subjects, he was anxious to avoid the two extremes of 'superstition' and contempt for his people. The king then built up a case against the royal touch by arguing that it was not miraculous but 'superstitious', a term that in a Protestant country was associated with Roman Catholicism. 'Superstition' has always been a pejorative rather than analytical word, but the fear of committing a 'superstitious' act provoked great anxiety because what was at stake was one's

---

7   CSPV ii. 465; Diary of Mr James Melville, 357–8; W. Brenchley Rye, England as seen by foreigners in the days of Elizabeth and James the first, London 1865, 151–2.

8   See pp. 19–20 above.

9   'A proclamation concerning the kings evill', Whitehall, 25 Mar. 1616, in SRP i. 358–9.

10   Rome Archives, ser. i, general series from Vatican and other sources, TNA, PRO 31/9/87, fos 362–3; CSPV x. 92; CSPD, 1603–10, 38; J. Nichols, The progresses, processions and magnificent festivities of King James the First, his royal consort, family and court, London 1828, i. 257–8; Illustrations of British history, biography and manners in the reigns of Henry VIII, Edward VI, Mary, Elizabeth and James I, ed. Edmund Lodge, London 1838, i. 21; Crawfurd, The king's evil, 83.

11   Previous commentators have overlooked this speech. See TNA, PRO 31/9/87, fos 362–3; James I's 'extempore speech at the first touching of a diseased child of the king's evil', BL, MS Add. 22587, fo 4. See also S. Brogan, 'The royal touch', History Today lxi/2 (Feb. 2011), 46–52.

immortal soul. It was generally thought that those who worshipped God incorrectly had committed a heinous sin, part of the devil's plan to reduce mankind to damnation.[12] James said that belief in miraculous healings was problematic for three reasons. First, he argued against the idea of an interventionist, miracle-working God and instead advocated belief in providence:

> I doe not think that because I am a King therefore I can cure diseases or because I am a King of England I can cure this disease [scrofula] for that were to attribute more to myself than belongeth unto any man for miracles are ceased and god doth work by ordinary meanes.[13]

James was sceptical because he subscribed to the Protestant doctrine of the cessation of miracles. According to this, miraculous healings were not possible because, although miracles had been performed by Old Testament prophets and by Christ and his disciples, they had ceased soon after the Apostolic Age or at the latest by about AD 600. This was because by that time the Christian Church had become established and so God did not need miracles to be worked to convince people of the truth of Christianity. Protestant polemic insisted that all medieval and contemporary Roman Catholic miracles were either shams or diabolical illusions, and so not surprisingly the doctrine of the cessation of miracles generated much debate.[14]

James then stated that there was no biblical mandate for the royal touch, but that he favoured the doctrine and practices of the Early Church;[15] this comment reveals that the assertions of apologists such as William Tooker arguing for the biblical mandate had not convinced everyone.[16] After this, James turned to the liturgy. He thought that this had no operative value, refuting the idea of sacred language, which he described as putting 'confidence in sillables'. In his view belief in this was evidence of either 'popery' or witchcraft.[17] The reference to popery reflected the Protestant belief that the deference shown by Roman Catholics to the spoken word of prayer, for

---

[12] A. Walsham, 'Recording superstition in early modern Britain: the origins of folklore', in S. A. Smith and A. Knight (eds), *The religion of fools? Superstition past and present*, Oxford 2008, 178–206 at p. 182; H. Parish and W. G. Naphy (eds), *Religion and superstition in Reformation Europe*, Manchester 2002, 1–21.

[13] BL, MS Add. 22587, fo. 4r.

[14] D. P. Walker, 'The cessation of miracles', in I. Merkeland and A. G. Debus (eds), *Hermeticism and the Renaissance: intellectual history and the occult in early modern Europe*, Cranberry, NJ 1988, 111–24; A. Walsham, 'Miracles in post–Reformation England', in K. Cooper and J. Gregory (eds) *Signs, wonders, miracles: representations of divine power in the life of the Church* (Studies in Church History xli, 2005), 273–306.

[15] W. B. Patterson, *King James VI and I and the reunion of Christendom*, Cambridge 1997, 41.

[16] See p. 61 above.

[17] BL, MS Add. 22587, fo. 4r.

example during the mass, was analogous to a magical utterance or spell.[18] The reference to witchcraft invokes a topic in which James had been inter-ested at least since the North Berwick case of 1590 to 1591, when a group of witches had apparently sought his death, after which he wrote his treatise *Daemonologie* (1597). After this James paid less attention to witchcraft, and he later began to become sceptical of it, not least because of his involve-ment in the exposure of a number of fraudulent cases.[19] But the royal touch speech reveals that in 1603 James still thought of both witches and Roman Catholics as his enemies. This reflects the invocation of models of binary opposites which characterised much early modern thought, meaning that as God's chosen king James had a special role in opposition to witches and Catholics who served the devil and AntiChrist.[20]

James's speech then changed direction and he addressed his desire to avoid showing contempt for his people, many of whom expected their king to touch for scrofula. James knew that it was important for kings to uphold traditions which were associated with ruling justly.[21] As king, James had to uphold the mystique of monarchy and respect the custom of the royal touch, but he was also answerable to God for his subjects' salvation, and so had to avoid leading them into 'superstitious' practices. He overcame this problem by explaining that although 'miracles doe yet cease … in some cases prayer … is [the] best fair remedy'. He said that as God listened to even the 'meanest' sort of person when they prayed, the prayers of the king were given special attention by God and so James would not withhold them from his people

James concluded his speech by saying that

> As I find this my duty and your duty to pray for any afflicted creature I doe desire you all to pray with mee for this diseased child [and] if it please god to hear us he shall in wholle glory: [grant] the child the benefitt of our faithfull requests. And soe endeavouring to yield this accord from all the superstition hereof I will not refuse to satisfy my peoples desires.[22]

After James had made his speech he 'turned his eyes towards the Scotch

---

[18] Thomas, *Religion and the decline of magic*, 33, 42, 182, 194; cf. Scot, *Discoverie of witchcraft*, 303–4.

[19] Christine Larner, 'James VI and I and witchcraft', in A. G. R. Smith (ed.), *The reign of James VI and I*, London 1973, 74–90, 89; S. Clark, 'King James' *Daemonologie*: witchcraft and kingship', in S. Anglo (ed.), *The damned art: essays in the literature of witchcraft*, London 1977, 156–81 at pp. 161–2; L. Normand and G. Roberts, *Witchcraft in early modern Scotland: James VI's Demonology and the North Berwick witches*, Exeter 2000.

[20] Clark, 'King James' *Daemonologie*', 173–6; 'Inversion, misrule and the meaning of witchcraft', *P&P* lxxxvii (May 1980), 98–127 at p. 117; and *Thinking with demons*, 31–79.

[21] *The trew law of free monarchies*, in King James VI and I, *Political writings*, ed. J. P. Somerville, Cambridge 1994, 64.

[22] BL, MS Add. 22587, fo. 4v.

ministers around him, as though he expected their approval of what he was saying, having first conferred with them'.[23] This is a salient reminder that James had to negotiate with his Scottish subjects as well as his English ones.

Once James had found an intellectual solution to his scepticism he was prepared to touch for scrofula so long as he was not expected to condone miracles. He was willing to perform a ceremony that upheld monarchical authority and reverence to God, and might heal the sick, but was not prepared to tolerate miracles, which explains his emphasis on prayer and providence. Moreover, he did actually touch for scrofula rather than just pray for people's recovery, as he had decided that it was his duty to do so. Thus James found a middle way to keep himself and his ill subjects happy. Just as he knew the difference between the theory of divine right monarchy and the everyday cut and thrust of politics, so he balanced reformed theology with the need to uphold certain traditions. This was in keeping with his role as *Rex pacificus* and his preference for moderation and the *via media* whenever possible.[24]

His rationale was the same as that of Elizabeth I. The monarch acted as a conduit for God during a ceremony that was structured around prayers and there was no suggestion that the sovereign had an intrinsic ability to heal in the way that Christ had. But James's speech is important because he expressed himself in greater detail than his predecessor and no other English monarch explained their understanding of the royal touch in such lucid terms. The speech also helps to explain the changes to the ceremony that were instigated by James.

James introduced two changes to the imagery of his Angel coins (*see* Plate 6), which were first minted in October 1604. Since Mary Tudor's reign the reverse of the coins had borne the legend 'A Domino Factum Est Istud Et Est Mirabile In Oculis Nostris' ('This is the Lord's Doing and it is Marvellous in Our Eyes': Psalm cxviii.23), accompanied by a depiction of the ship of state in full sail, the central mast of which had a cross beam referencing Christ's cross. James abbreviated the inscription to 'A. Dno. Factum Est. Istud.'('This is the Lord's Doing'), thus removing the word 'Mirabile' ('marvellous' or 'miraculous'), in keeping with his view that the age of miracles had passed.[25] The cross beam from the mast was also removed: although this might initially seem surprising as the image of the cross was acceptable to Protestants, it was probably removed because the Angel was worn around the neck and Protestants saw the wearing of crosses as 'popish'.

James's other modification concerned the ritual itself. His predecessors, whether Roman Catholic or not, had made the sign of the cross over the

[23] TNA, PRO 31/9/87, fos 362–3.

[24] J. Wormald, 'James VI and I: two kings or one?', *History* lxviii/223 (1983), 187–209 at pp. 197–8; Patterson, *James VI and I*, 35–43, 50–74.

[25] Farquhar, 'Royal charities, I', 106–7; Bloch, *The royal touch*, 192 (338–9).

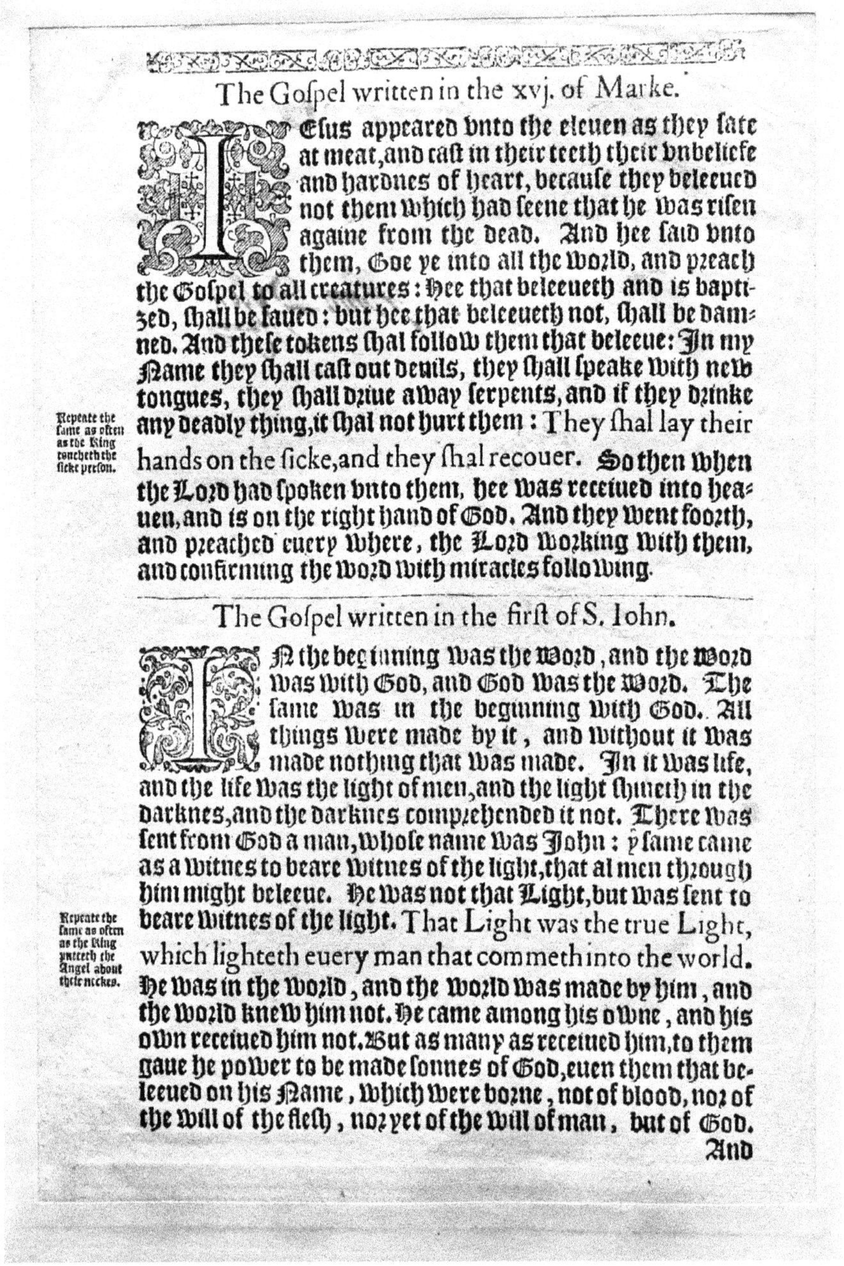

The Gospel written in the xvj. of Marke.

Esus appeared vnto the eleuen as they sate at meat, and cast in their teeth their vnbeliefe and hardnes of heart, because they beleeued not them which had seene that he was risen againe from the dead. And hee said vnto them, Goe ye into all the world, and preach the Gospel to all creatures: Hee that beleeueth and is bapti-zed, shall be saued: but hee that beleeueth not, shall be dam-ned. And these tokens shal follow them that beleeue: In my Name they shall cast out deuils, they shall speake with new tongues, they shall driue away serpents, and if they drinke

Repeate the same as often as the King toucheth the sicke prefon. any deadly thing, it shal not hurt them: They shal lay their hands on the sicke, and they shal recouer. So then when the Lord had spoken vnto them, hee was receiued into hea-uen, and is on the right hand of God. And they went foorth, and preached euery where, the Lord working with them, and confirming the word with miracles following.

The Gospel written in the first of S. Iohn.

IN the beginning was the Word, and the Word was with God, and God was the Word. The same was in the beginning with God. All things were made by it, and without it was made nothing that was made. In it was life, and the life was the light of men, and the light shineth in the darknes, and the darknes comprehended it not. There was sent from God a man, whose name was Iohn: y same came as a witnes to beare witnes of the light, that al men through him might beleeue. He was not that Light, but was sent to

Repeate the same as often as the King vntieth the Angel about their neckes. beare witnes of the light. That Light was the true Light, which lighteth euery man that commeth into the world. He was in the world, and the world was made by him, and the world knew him not. He came among his owne, and his own receiued him not. But as many as receiued him, to them gaue he power to be made sonnes of God, euen them that be-leeued on his Name, which were borne, not of blood, nor of the will of the flesh, nor yet of the will of man, but of God. And

Figure 4. James VI and I's liturgy, *The offices or prayers to be used at the ceremony of touching for the king's evil* (1618?), Lemon Collection, Society of Antiquaries, London, broadside 161.

And the same word became flesh, and dwelt among vs, and wee saw the glory of it, as the glory of the onely begotten Sonne of the Father, full of grace and trueth.

LOrd haue mercie vpon vs.
Chrift haue mercie vpon vs.
Lord haue mercie vpon vs.
Our Father which art in heauen, halowed be thy Name, Thy Kingdome come, Thy will be done in earth, as it is in heauen, Giue vs this day our dayly bread, And forgiue vs our trespasses, as we forgiue them that trepasse againft vs, And lead vs not into temptation:

Anfwere.

But deliuer vs from euill. Amen.

Minifter.

O Lord faue thy feruants.

Anfwere.

Which put their truft in thee.

Minifter.

Send vnto them helpe from aboue.

Anfwere.

And euermore mightily defend them.

Minifter.

Helpe vs O God our Sauiour.

Anfwere.

And for the glory of thy Names fake deliuer vs, be mercifull vnto vs finners for thy Names fake.

Minifter.

O Lord heare our prayers.

Anfwere.

And let our crie come vnto thee.

ALmighty God the eternal health of all fuch as put their truft in thee, heare vs wee befeech thee on the behalfe of thefe thy feruants for whom we call for thy mercifull help, that they receiuing health, may giue thankes to thee in thy holy Church, through Jefus Chrift our Lord, Amen.

THe peace of God which paffeth all vnderftanding, keepe your hearts and minds in the knowledge, and loue of God, and of his Sonne Jefus Chrift our Lord: and the bleffing of God Almighty, the Father, the Sonne, & the holy Ghoft, be amongft you, & remaine with you alwayes, Amen.

75

scrofulous sores of the person whom they touched, but James removed this gesture from the ceremony. This is known from two sources, the first being a broadside in the collection of the Society of Antiquaries in London, on which is printed the royal touch liturgy, dated 1618 (*see* Figure 4).[26] This is the earliest extant liturgy in English, and is notable because, unlike the Tudor ones, it makes no mention of the sign of the cross. The other source is retrospective. In 1659 the theologian and historian Hamon L'Estrange published one of the earliest studies of the Church of England's liturgy, in which he noted that James had ordered the sign of the cross to be removed from the royal touch ceremony because many people objected that it was a 'mysterious operation', which presumably meant that it was thought to be implicitly Roman Catholic. L'Estrange argued that the sign of the cross had no operative quality because the royal touch had not become less efficacious after its removal from the ritual.[27]

Also interesting in this connection is an occasion when James touched the son of the Turkish Ambassador in November 1618 in the first Banqueting House. There are contradictory accounts by English courtiers who witnessed this event; one says that the king made the sign of the cross over the sores whereas the other does not.[28] This incident is especially noteworthy because on this occasion it was a Muslim who had recourse to a Christian healer, indicating that the royal touch was not necessarily limited to Christians. If James did make the sign of the cross over the youth's sores it might have been in order to emphasise the Christian nature of the ceremony, given the young man's religion and because there was no chaplain present to read the liturgy, suggesting that the proceedings were impromptu. That James was willing to continue without prayers is remarkable given his earlier emphasis, but it is possible that any reservations that he had were in part overcome by his taste for attractive young men: when the king saw the youth approaching he laughed heartily. It was later reported that the young man was initially

---

[26] *The offices or prayers to be used at the ceremony of touching for the king's evil* (1618?), broadside 161, Lemon Collection, Society of Antiquaries, London. This is transcribed in Crawfurd, *The king's evil*, 85–7. See *A catalogue of printed broadsides in the possession of the Society of Antiquaries of London*, comp. R. Lemon, London 1866, 49.

[27] L'Estrange *The alliance of divine offices*, 250. For three other brief references to James's reforms see T. Fuller, *The church history of Britain*, London 1655, 146; P. Heylyn, *Examen historicum*, London 1659, 47–8; and Wiseman, *Several chirurgical treatises*, 240.

[28] John Finet says that James made the sign of the cross over the sores: *Finetti philoxenis: some choice observations of Sir John Finet Knight*, ed. J. Howell, London 1656, 58. Justinian Povy, auditor of the exchequer and accountant general to Anne of Denmark, wrote to Dudley Carlton (1574–1632), diplomat and ambassador to The Hague, and made no mention of the gesture: Nichols, *Progresses, processions and magnificent festivities*, iii. 494; cf. HMC, *Report on the manuscripts of the most honourable the marquess of Downshire, preserved at Easthampstead Park, Berkshire*, London 1924–95, vi.573, which does not mention the gesture.

sceptical of the efficacy of the royal touch, but, when cured by it, it was rumoured that he had converted to Christianity.[29]

How did people respond to James's reform of the royal touch? In November 1604 Nicolo Molin, the Venetian ambassador in London, was ambivalent, reporting that 'yesterday, after the sermon … his majesty touched a number of sufferers for scrofula; it remains to be seen with what result'. By Easter 1606, however, these doubts had passed: another Venetian ambassador noted that James had 'touched many for Scrofula, they say with hope of good effects, remembering the earlier cases of healing conferred by his hand'.[30]

There is no doubt that James's reforms were popular as he touched far larger numbers of people than had the Tudors. Thus in 1617 he travelled to Scotland, staying at Lincoln and York: on the way, at Lincoln, he touched fifty people in the cathedral and another fifty-three in St Catherine's Priory, and at York he touched seventy people in the minster.[31] It has been estimated that James spent an average of £435 *per annum* on Angels, which by his reign had a value of 10s. each, meaning that on average the crown minted 870 Angels each year.[32] It cannot be assumed that this total equals the exact number of people who were touched, but it provides a useful approximation.

The popularity of Jacobean thaumaturgy is attested by the problems the government had in controlling the demand for it. A proclamation issued in March 1616 stated that the seasonal healing calendar had broken down and that people were coming to court to be touched 'indifferently at all times'. Proclamations were used by the crown to speed up the execution of the law, being read out from the pulpit and then displayed in market squares and other prominent places.[33] James's notice sought to reintroduce the schedule whereby people did not come to court to be touched between Easter and Michaelmas due to the heat and the fear of plague.[34] This is the first proclamation of its kind, and it reinforces the view that James's court could at times be relatively relaxed; more important, it reminds us that James was an accessible monarch.[35] This was an ideal quality for a royal healer.

Another problem was that sometimes the king had an insufficient number of Angels to hand. In 1624, when James was again on progress, people complained to him that there were not enough Angels to distribute at Copthall, Middlesex. Sir Randolph Cranfield, the master of the mint, was

[29] HMC, *Downshire manuscripts*, vi. 581.

[30] CSPV x. 193, 344.

[31] Nicols, *Progresses, processions and magnificent festivities*, iii. 264–5, 273.

[32] H. Symonds, 'Mint marks and denominations of the coinage of James I as disclosed by the trials of the pyx', *BNJ* n.s. ix (1912), 207–27 at p. 223.

[33] K. Sharpe, *The personal rule of Charles I*, London 1992, 412.

[34] 'A proclamation concerning the kings evill', Whitehall, 25 Mar. 1616, in *SRP* i. 358–9.

[35] For James's accessibility see M. Lee, Jr, *Great Britain's Solomon: James VI and I in his three kingdoms*, Urbana 1990, 129–64.

blamed for this serious oversight and his brother advised him to find out 'who was at fault, so that he may make just excuse'.[36]

The enthusiasm for James's reformed practice of the royal touch partly explains why Shakespeare mentioned it in *Macbeth*, thought to have been written in 1606. In act four, scene three, Malcolm and Macduff are in England at the palace of Edward the Confessor, where they meet a doctor and ask him about the king's whereabouts. The doctor replies:

> there are a crew of wretched souls
> That stay his cure: their malady convinces
> The great assay of art; but at his touch —
> Such sanctity hath heaven given his hand –
> They presently amend.

Macduff then asks what the disease is and Malcolm replies:

> 'Tis call'd the evil:
> A most miraculous work in this good king;
> Which often, since my here-remain in England,
> I have seen him do. How he solicits heaven,
> Himself best knows: but strangely-visited people,
> All swoln and ulcerous, pitiful to the eye,
> The mere despair of surgery, he cures,
> Hanging a golden stamp about their necks,
> Put on with holy prayers: and 'tis spoken,
> To the succeeding royalty he leaves
> The healing benediction.[37]

It is a telling description, accurate in its account of prayers while omitting any mention of the sign of the cross, although it is obviously anachronistic concerning the Confessor. The implication that the royal touch was the last resort for patients for whom surgery had proved ineffective supports the comments to the same effect noted in the previous chapter.[38] However, the scene is irrelevant to the drama and is usually omitted from performances of the play; it was probably inserted for topical reasons.[39] Shakespeare no doubt wanted to flatter James, who would have been pleased with this section of the play because he sought ways to represent himself as the lineal descendant of English kings.[40]

---

[36] Draft of a letter by the earl of Middlesex to his brother Sir Randall Cranfield, Copthall, 1 Apr. 1624, in HMC, *Fourth report: the manuscripts of the of the Right Hon. the earl de la Warr at Knole Park, Co. Kent*, calendared by Alfred John Horwood, London 1874, 313.

[37] W. Shakespeare, *The tragedy of Macbeth*, ed. N. Brooke, Oxford 1994, 188–9.

[38] See p. 60 above.

[39] Paul, *Royal play*, 367.

[40] A lesser known paean is the poem published in 1612 by the theologian James Maxwell (b.1581), an ardent supporter of James, which states that, just as the king cured scrofula,

Lastly, what of James's attitude towards the royal touch? Earlier writers have concentrated upon the king's initial scepticism, implicitly taking the view that James remained unconvinced of the efficacy of the royal touch throughout his reign.[41] This view was shared by at least one of James's contemporaries, the courtier and historian Arthur Wilson (1595–1652). He wrote that James knew that the royal touch had aggrandised the English monarchy 'when miracles were in fashion', though the king himself thought that the cures were due to the power of suggestion.[42] Wilson was secretary to the earls of Essex and Warwick and so had first-hand experience of James's court.[43] His account of James's views on the royal touch is retrospective, written during the Civil War, and as an ardent Protestant Wilson might have thought that the age of miracles had passed, and projected this onto his account of James. It is interesting that the power of the imagination was suggested as an explanation for the cures: this is not as antithetical to belief in the royal touch as might be thought, because it was usual to think that faith was needed for medicine to work.

More pragmatically, it is known that James was squeamish about touching inflamed glands. In June 1611 Otto, Prince of Hesse, witnessed James perform the royal touch at Greenwich Palace and wrote that the king only 'laid two fingers upon them', while another observer on another occasion said that the ritual was distasteful to James to the point that he would have liked to abolish it. James's distaste for physical contact with his sick and poor subjects is further evident in his Maundy Thursday practices: he broke with tradition and did not wash the feet of the poor, instead having the archbishop of Canterbury do it in his name.[44]

The problem with the view that James was sceptical of the royal touch throughout his reign is that after 1603 he kept his thoughts on the ceremony private, while such an interpretation fails to do justice to his reform of the rationale and practice of the ritual. James was committed to his therapeutic duties. In his speech of October 1603 he implied that he would follow the established custom of the royal touch but his reforms and the numbers that he touched each year indicate that he did far more than that. Reports of the efficacy of his touch, such as those made by the Venetian ambassador, would have appealed to James's ideas of kingship and his intellectual vanity. James might have found touching scrofulous sores distasteful, but his emphasis on prayer and providence 'Protestantised' the ceremony and rendered it more

---

so he brought peace to England and Scotland and harmony to the Church: *A poem shewing the excellencie of our soveraigne King James his hand*, in *The laudable life and deplorable death of … Prince Henry*, London 1612, B3–E.

[41] Crawfurd, *The king's evil*, 82–90; Bloch, *The royal touch*, 191–2 (336–9); Paul, *Royal play*, 383; Shakespeare, *Macbeth*, 72.

[42] Wilson, *History of Great Britain*, 289.

[43] G. Parry, 'Wilson, Arthur (*bap.* 1595, *d.* 1652)', ODNB.

[44] Rye, *England*, 132, 144, 151–2; Paul, *Royal play*, 383.

acceptable to him and his subjects. James's successful handling of the royal touch fits with his historiographical rehabilitation more generally. The Whig interpretation of James as an incompetent ruler who put England on a high road to civil war has been revised: the king is now viewed as being a far more politically astute and capable ruler than his successor.[45]

Charles I: further reform and the quest for order

Charles I succeeded to the throne in March 1625; in May and June of that year he issued two proclamations addressing the royal touch, both of which reveal the disordered condition into which the ceremony had fallen by the end of his predecessor's reign. The main issue was that demand outstripped supply, which produced three major problems. The first was the healing calendar: oddly, Easter and Whit Sunday had become the key times of year at which James I had touched, and not Easter and Michaelmas as stated in the proclamation of 1616. Charles announced his return to the usual calendar of Easter and Michaelmas, thus avoiding the summer and equalising the time between ceremonies. His proclamations stressed that he would not touch outside this schedule. Secondly, not everyone who came to be touched had scrofula, and thirdly, some people were touched more than once. To address these issues Charles introduced the requirement that people needed to provide a certificate, written and signed by their minister or churchwarden, confirming that they had scrofula and had not been touched before. Thus regular medicine (confirmation that someone had scrofula) buttressed a miraculous healing ceremony. The certificate could also act as a travel permit, necessary because of the fear of plague-carriers. Charles would go on to issue a total of twenty-two proclamations, the last in 1639, all of which reinforced the schedule and criteria for royal therapeutics, while some also cancelled ceremonies, usually due to the plague.[46]

These notices, and other evidence, make it abundantly clear that because people were sick and hoped for a cure they did not always adhere to the rules. That Charles had to repeat his directives so often indicates that it was one thing to issue orders, but quite another to enforce them. Indeed, these three issues preoccupied the Stuarts until the royal touch ceased to be practised in 1714. This last problem, people being touched more than once,

---

45 Wormald, 'Two kings or one?', 187–209.

46 These are summarised in Brogan, 'Royal touch' (dissertation), appendix 1. They are sourced from SRP, and Crawfurd, The king's evil. For the timetable see proclamations dated 17 May, 18 June 1625; 18 June 1626; 28 June 1629; 6 Apr. 1630; 25 Mar. 1631; 20 June 1632; 28 July 1635; 1 July 1638; for cancellations see 17 June 1628; 13 Oct., 8 Nov. 1631; 22 Apr., 23 Sept., 14 Dec. 1634; 5 Mar., 7 Apr., 6 Sept. 1636; 5 Mar., 3 Sept. 1637; 2 Sept. 1638; 24 Sept. 1639; for certificates see 17 May, 18 June 1625; 18 June 1626; 28 June 1629; 6 Apr. 1630; 25 Mar., 13 Oct. 1631; 28 July 1635; 1 July 1638.

was particularly difficult for the crown. It meant that the crowd was larger than it need be and hence more difficult to manage, and it was costly in terms of providing Angels to people who had already received them. Those who sought a second touch have been described as seeking another Angel for profit, yet during the Restoration there were occasions when the surgeons themselves recommended that supplicants obtain a second touch if the first had not worked.[47]

A further innovation introduced by Charles in order to tighten up the entry process to the ceremony was the admission token. These were made for the royal surgeons to give to supplicants who met the required conditions. Along with these practical reforms, in 1625 Charles changed the inscription on the Angel from James I's 'A. Dno. Factum Est. Istud.' ('This is the Lord's doing') to 'Amor Populi Praesidium Regis' ('The Love of the People is the King's Protection'), alluding to his role as a *pater familias*.[48] It might have been necessary to remind people of this role given that Charles's bureaucratic reforms limited the times of the year when his touch was available.

Judith Richards has suggested that Charles used his many proclamations to withhold the royal touch from the populace, and that this was part of his wider policy of detachment from the public between 1625 and 1640, which contributed to the onset of the Civil War. She maintains that Charles was not interested in royal therapeutics until after 1640, at which time he began to touch larger numbers of people than previously as a way of canvassing support.[49] Whatever the reasons for the outbreak of civil war, Richards is wrong because a close reading of the evidence shows that Charles was committed to the royal touch, administering on an even larger scale than had James I. This lessens the need to concentrate on whether or not 1640 was a watershed in the practice. In any case there are no germane administrative records for the war period, making an accurate comparison impossible. It is also worth noting that during the Restoration the crown issued at least thirty-six announcements that sought to bring order to the royal touch, yet as we will see, there is no suggestion that either Charles II or James II sought to avoid their therapeutic role.

In order fully to understand the royal touch during Charles I's reign three key issues will be addressed: the desire for order from which his reforms stemmed; the regularity with which he touched and the problems that his rigid schedule caused; and the size of his ceremonies. Charles's obsession

[47] See p. 166 below.

[48] Farquhar, 'Royal charities, I', 120. I am grateful to Barrie Cook, curator of medieval and early modern coinage at the British Museum, for clarifying that this happened in 1625.

[49] J. Richards, '"His nowe majestie" and the English monarchy: the kingship of Charles I before 1640', *P&P* cxiii (Nov. 1986), 70–96 at p. 93. For convincing counter-arguments to Richards see Sharpe, *Personal rule*, 630, and *Image wars*, 239–42, and M. Kishlansky, 'Charles I: a case of mistaken identity', *P&P*, clxxxix/4 (Nov. 2005), 41–80.

with order and decorum was part of his wish to return to the harmony of an idealised past, while bureaucratic efficiency was thought to be a feature of a Godly commonwealth.[50] Christian thought maintained that since the Fall man had lived in a state of sin and Charles's reformist measures sought to regenerate the body politic and allow him to rule as a good Christian.[51] As well as reforming the royal touch, Charles brought more propriety to the royal court: the 'bawds, mimics and catamites' of James I's reign fell from favour, for better or worse, while the Venetian ambassador noted that 'the nobles do not enter his apartments in confusion as heretofore, but each rank has its appointed place and he has declared that he desires the rules and maxims of the late Queen Elizabeth [to be observed]'.[52] Charles's respect for tradition is evident in that he did not touch for scrofula until he had been crowned and anointed;[53] during the coronation he was invested with the regalia of Edward the Confessor, as custom demanded, thus making clear his reverence for the saint thought to be England's first thaumaturgic king.[54]

Given Charles's respect for the past and his taste for exalted sovereignty, he was unlikely to have withheld the key manifestation of mystical kingship – the royal touch – from his subjects. This is borne out by the regularity and size of his healing ceremonies. The former is apparent from Charles' proclamations. If it is assumed that between 1625 and 1639 the royal touch was practised at Easter and Michaelmas unless it was cancelled or post-poned by a proclamation then these two periods of seasonal therapeutics occurred on twenty-two out of a possible twenty-nine occasions. Six out of the seven cancellations were a result of the usual problems of plague, smallpox or hot weather; only once, in September 1639, did the king cancel due to unnamed 'speciall causes', a reference to the First Bishops' War.[55] At Easter and Michaelmas, ceremonies were held daily for fourteen days, which allowed ample time for large numbers to be touched.[56]

The weakness in Charles's more regulated system was that, if ceremonies were cancelled at Easter or Michaelmas, it could mean that people had to wait six or twelve months before they could be touched. Yet it was difficult to enforce this system, as the crown itself acknowledged.[57] Sick people could

---

[50] Sharpe, *Personal rule*, 32–3, 195–6.

[51] W. H. Greenleaf, *Order, empiricism and politics: two traditions of English political thought, 1500–1700*, Oxford 1964, 14–57.

[52] L. Hutchinson, *Memoirs of the life of Colonel Hutchinson*, ed. C. H. Firth, London 1885, i. 119–20; CSPV xix. 21.

[53] *SRP* ii. 35.

[54] C. Carlton, *Charles I: the personal monarch*, London 1983, 78; Strong, *Coronation*, 232–74.

[55] Brogan, 'Royal touch' (dissertation), appendix 1.

[56] *SRP* ii. 621, 693.

[57] See proclamation dated 1 July 1638, *SRP* ii. 621–2.

arrive at court regardless of the season, because most of them were desperate for a cure (while some might have wanted an Angel), and, unsurprisingly, the therapeutic schedule was not always popular. In a revealing example of the pressure that could be put on the king to touch the sick 'out of season', at Greenwich in June 1629 a petition was left for Sir Sidney Montagu, Charles' Master of Requests, to deliver to the monarch 'for 120 poor people to be cured of the Evil'.[58] The date of this is significant because it indicates that the people did not want to wait until the autumn to be touched; unfortunately the outcome is not recorded. However, at times the king did give in to pressure and abandon his own schedule: sometimes he touched at Christmas and Whitsun as well as Easter and Michaelmas.[59]

Aside from popular pressure, the ministers responsible for drafting and publishing proclamations could remind the king of the unfairness of cancelling ceremonies at short notice. When the Attorney-General Sir John Bankes wrote to the Secretary of State Sir John Coke on 7 April 1636 to explain that the royal touch was cancelled that Easter, he was anxious because the draft proclamation did not say that the rite would resume at Michaelmas:

> It is an act of piety and charity worthy of your Honour to put his Majesty in mind that there be divers of these diseased persons already come up to London from remote places ... to know his royal pleasure concerning them.[60]

This oversight was corrected that very day because the proclamation dated 7 April was amended to say that there would be no ceremonies until the autumn 'unless His Majestie shall hereafter declare any shorter time for that purpose'.[61]

The restrictions of Charles's schedule may partly explain a further problem that emerged in the 1630s, the appearance of three rival healers of scrofula, all of whom claimed to be seventh sons.[62] The idea that seventh sons, or seventh sons of seventh sons, or sometimes seventh daughters, could heal a variety of ailments by touch was found in many parts of Europe from the sixteenth century onwards and reflected the belief that seven was a mystically significant number.[63]

---

[58] HMC, *Fourth report*, 369.

[59] *SRP* ii. 349. For December healings see the proclamations dated 13 Oct. 1631 and 23 Sept. 1634; for Whitsun see 18 June 1625, 18 June 1626, 28 July 1635.

[60] HMC, *Twelfth report: the manuscripts of his grace the duke of Rutland K.G., preserved at Belvoir Castle*, London 1889, iii. 112–13.

[61] *SRP* ii. 2, 505.

[62] Thomas, *Religion and the decline of magic*, 200–1; Brogan, 'Royal touch' (dissertation), 98–105.

[63] J. Primrose, *Popular errours*, London 1651, 434–42; T. A., XEIPEΞOKH: *The excellency or handy work of the royal hand*, London 1665, 2–3; Bloch, *The royal touch*, 168–76 (293–308); Thomas, *Religion and the decline of magic*, 200–2; M. Hunter, *The occult laboratory:*

In January 1632 the Privy Council became aware of one James Philip Gaudre, a French knight living in London, who was imprisoned for debt in the Marshalsea where he had touched 200 people since 'midsummer last'. Subsequently, in October 1637, the Privy Council learned that one James Leverett, a Chelsea gardener aged about sixty, was healing scrofula, dropsy, fevers, agues and sores by touch. Leverett was said to minister to between thirty and forty people a day, including some whom the king had touched without success. The gardener was investigated by the Royal College of Physicians through a procedure that included providing people for him to cure as a way of testing his powers. Leverett was unable to cure these people, although he was said to have made disparaging remarks about the royal touch and even suggested that he take over the role of royal healer in order to save Charles I from the task. The third healer was an unnamed blacksmith in Wiltshire who also claimed to heal scrofula by touch, attracting supplicants with connections at the royal court.[64]

The Privy Council found that Gaudre and Leverett were frauds. Gaudre's fate is unknown but Leverett was whipped and sent to Bridewell prison for six weeks.[65] Leveret's chief crime was *lèse majesté*: he slighted royal therapeutics by declaring that anyone might have the gift to cure by touch; he cured someone whom the king had been unable to; and he had offered to take over the job of performing the royal touch. The fate of the third healer, the blacksmith, is unknown.

Charles I may have been partly responsible for the emergence of these healers, as becomes evident if the timing is considered. Gaudre came to the notice of the authorities in January 1632: during the previous autumn Charles had cancelled healings due to the plague and in November announced that he would not touch until Lent 1632.[66] When Leverett was interviewed in October 1637, Charles had not healed at Easter or Michaelmas of that year due to the plague, and in September he announced by proclamation that he would not heal until the following spring.[67] With regard to the blacksmith, his case dates from 1638, when the king announced that he would no longer touch when on progress, a move which may have provided an impetus for

---

magic, science and second sight in late seventeenth-century Scotland, Woodbridge 2001, 17, 87, 100, 105.

[64] For Gaudre see CSPD, 1631–33, 252, 347–8; for Leverett see C. Goodall, *The Royal College of Physicians of London founded and established by law; as appears by letters patents, acts of parliament, adjudged cases, &c. And an historical account of the college's proceedings against empiricks and unlicensed practisers in every princes reign from their first incorporation to the murther of the royal martr, King Charles the First*, London 1684, 446–63; for the blacksmith see CSPD, 1637, 506, and CSPD, 1638–9, 63, 68.

[65] *Privy Council registers preserved in the Public Record Office*, London 1967–8, ii. 437, 515.

[66] Crawfurd, *The king's evil*, 169–71, 173–4.

[67] *SRP* ii. 552–3, 574–5.

this provincial healer.[68] On the other hand, the punitive measures enforced by the crown against Leverett reveal that Charles guarded his prerogative jealously. During the Tudor and Jacobean age provincial healers had touched for scrofula without being prosecuted by the government, probably because they also healed other diseases, and because the royal touch was more accessible.[69]

Moving on to the increased demand for Charles's touch, this can be explained in two ways. First, it rested on the popularity of his predecessor's reforms that 'Protestantised' the ceremony. Secondly, Charles' numerous proclamations must have had an effect that was unforeseen and unappreciated by the government: they inadvertently advertised the royal touch.[70] On average Charles touched three times the number of people annually that James I had done, between 1625 and 1642 spending between £1,000 and £1,500 each year on Angels.[71] At a value of 10s. each, the inference is that Charles touched approximately 2–3,000 people *per annum*, whereas James's probable annual total was around 870.[72] This is borne out by a manuscript now in the National Library of Medicine, Washington, which contains information concerning the cost of providing Angels between 1628 and 1635.[73] (*see* Table 4) Also suggestive of the large numbers touched by Charles I are the orders for admission tokens for the ceremony: between 1635 and 1636 the crown ordered 5,500 of these, and between 1638 and 1639 it ordered 1,557 tokens.[74]

There are small pieces of evidence concerning the scale of the royal touch ceremonies that were performed when Charles was on progress. These were part of the panoply of early modern monarchical splendour: when the king and his court visited the provinces he stayed at the homes of important members of local elites, often knighting various prominent men and attending public church services.[75] In June 1633, after Charles's coronation

---

[68] *SRP* ii. 621–2.

[69] However, the earlier healers were harried by the church courts: Thomas, *Religion and the decline of magic*, 200–2.

[70] Richards, '"His nowe majestie"', 90.

[71] Farquhar, 'Royal charities, I', 132.

[72] See p. 77 above.

[73] 'King's evil: a collection of items pertaining to the royal touch for the healing of scrofula 1628–1712', National Library of Medicine, Washington, DC, MS f115, unfoliated. This manuscript has been transcribed in F. H. Garrison, 'A relic of the king's evil in the Surgeon General's Library (Washington DC)', *Proceedings of the Royal Society of Medicine* vii (1914), 227–34.

[74] H. Symons, 'Charles I: the trials of the pyx, the mint marks and the mint accounts', *Numismatic Chronicle* 4th ser. x (1910), 380–98 at p. 395.

[75] *The Fairfax correspondence: memoirs of the reign of Charles I*, ed. G. W. Johnson London 1848, i. 281–2; Sharpe, *Personal rule*, 217, 219, 230, 630–1, 702.

Table 4 Charles I's expenditure on Angels, 1628–35

	Expenditure	Number of angels (at 10s each)
Michaelmas 1628	£600.00	1,200
Easter 1629	£110.00	220
Michaelmas 1629	£200.00	400
Easter 1633	£550.00	1,100
Easter 1634	£350.00	700
Easter 1635	£600.00	1,200

in Edinburgh, he touched 100 people in the chapel at Holyrood House.[76] In York, in 1639, he touched 200 people at one ceremony in the minster and then held two more rituals there, at each of which he touched 100 people.[77] A few days later he arrived at Durham where he touched 'divers for the Evil' at the castle.[78] Also suggestive of the popularity of Charles's thaumaturgic practice is an engraving of him touching the sick that was bound into a copy of the *Book of Common Prayer*, which is noted in an inventory of St George's Chapel, Windsor, dated 21 September 1641. Unfortunately the book appears to have been lost during the first years of the Civil War when the Parliamentarians occupied Windsor Castle, and no other copies of the image have been found.[79]

Despite all of Charles' measures, the evidence suggests that the management of the royal touch did not improve but rather got worse, reaching a nadir in 1635 when it seems that admission tokens were being forged and used by people who wanted an Angel. The scale and consequence of the problem is evident in a note written by Charles to the warden of the mint dated 1 April 1635:

> a great abuse has been committed by the people who, to gain the gold, have counterfeited the Serjeant Surgeon's tokens, which were cast in a mould made by a Freemason, whereby his Majesty has not only been deceived of so

[76] Sir James Balfour's notes connected to Charles I's state visit to Edinburgh, 1633, National Library of Scotland, Edinburgh, Advocates MSS 15.2.17, fo. 23.

[77] F. Drake, *Eboracum: or, The history and antiquities of the city of York, from its original to the present time; together with the history of the cathedral church and the lives of the archbishops*, London 1736, 137; Nichols, *Progresses, processions and magnificent festivities*, iii. 273.

[78] *Fairfax correspondence*, i. 282.

[79] I am grateful to Eleanor Cracknell, Assistant Archivist at St George's Chapel Archives and Chapter Library for this information. See *The inventories of St George's Chapel, Windsor Castle, 1384–1667*, ed. M. F. Bond, London 1947, 242, and E. Ashmole, *The institution, laws and ceremonies of the Most Noble Order of the Garter*, London 1672, 496.

many angels, but the number has been many times increased to be more than was appointed for the day, and many that were appointed wanted their angels, and the royal presence was disturbed by their outcry.[80]

One can only imagine Charles's indignation at the lack of decorum resulting from people forging admission tokens to gain entry to the ceremony, and there not being enough Angels for everyone. By way of response, the crown sought to make it harder for people to use forged tokens by instructing the Mint to make a specific number of different types of tokens, of 'brass, copper and other such metal', some the same size as an Angels, others square. Specific tokens were then to be used on specific days, after which they were to be collected and given back to the Mint to ensure that their number equalled the number of Angels which had been distributed.[81]

Two of Charles's tokens have survived, both of which are the same size as Angels. Their designs emphasise that the healing power originated with God. One is brass and bears the legend 'he touched them' on the obverse, with an image of a hand descending from a cloud onto a man's head; the reverse is inscribed 'and they were healed', alongside an image of a crown, a rose and a thistle, signifying Charles's two kingdoms of England and Scotland, Ireland being omitted (*see* Plate 7).[82] The other token is copper and has on its obverse an engraving of Henry VIII seated – which is a little strange – with the legend 'Hoc Opus Dei', 'This is God's work'; the reverse is inscribed 'Annunciatio Beatae Virginia 1640'. This refers to Lady Day, 25 March 1640, the celebration of the Annunciation of the Virgin, and so this token must have been made specifically for a ceremony to be held on that day.[83]

If 1635 was a watershed in the crown's efforts to regulate the public ceremonies, it seems that people with connections at court could still access the small, private ones that were held for the elite with relative ease. At Easter 1636 Nathan Walworth, steward to the third earl of Pembroke, noted that although he had journeyed to Whitehall forty times, he could not obtain a touch for his friend at a public healing as 'the sicknesse begins in London and the King will suffer no diseased person to come neere him, yet there were some healed, but it was such as had some noble mans letter, and it was done privatelye in the garden'.[84]

---

[80] *CSPD*, 1635, 1.

[81] Ibid.; Lord Chamberlain's department: miscellaneous records: warrant books: 'Declaration concerning the healing of the evill sett up at court gate', 1635, TNA, LC5/133, 1.

[82] Farquhar, 'Royal charities, I', 120–7. For earlier identifications of the token as a brass Angel see Pettigrew, *On superstitions*, frontispiece, figs 7, 8, and Symonds, 'Charles I', 395.

[83] D. Allen, 'An admission ticket to the ceremony of touching?', *Numismatic Chronicle*, 5th ser. xviii (1938), 292–4.

[84] *The correspondence of Nathan Walworth and Peter Seddon of Oxford, and other documents chiefly relating to the building of Ringley Chapel*, ed. J. S. Fletcher, Manchester 1880, 41–2.

The Civil War and disorder

In 1642 Charles I abandoned London and moved his court to Oxford due to the political crisis which would result in the Civil Wars. The social and political strife of the 1640s meant that Charles's attempts at reforming the royal touch gave way to even more disorder. The initial problem was that of access: as the king was in Oxford, Londoners complained that they could not get to their thaumaturgic sovereign. Once the conflict began, the apparatus of the ceremony became precarious: Charles was unable to distribute Angels and sometimes had no clergyman to read the liturgy, while the healing schedule was eventually abandoned, as was the vetting process. Once Charles was captive, the same problems continued. Yet none of this reduced the popularity of the royal therapeutics. During the last two years of Charles's life large crowds flocked to him seeking his touch, and despite the mixed views of his opponents on the subject, they allowed them access to the king right up until he was detained at Windsor in December 1648 prior to his trial.

Beginning with the king's move to Oxford, an anonymous pamphlet published in London in February 1643 entitled *The humble petition* complained that 'divers hundreds' of the king's scrofulous subjects no longer had access to him.[85] The author was motivated in part by his keen feeling for the king's absence as Easter approached, usually one of the busiest periods for royal therapeutics. The pamphlet ended with a plea that the king return to London to tend to his sick subjects, and a pragmatic reminder that some of the sick were 'young men and women in the prime of youth who may hereafter doe your Majesty good service'. The author hoped that the king's return would bring about the 'cure of our infirmitie', as well as 'the recovery of the State, which hath languished of a tedious sicknesse since your Highnesses depar-ture … and can no more be cured of its infirmitie then wee, till your gracious return'.[86] Although the date of the petition coincided with a truce of twenty days which had just been brokered between the king and parliament, there is no evidence that the king visited London, or that the petitioners travelled to Oxford.[87] In fact, it is likely that the king's preoccupation with war meant that he did not want to touch scrofulous people at that time: on 26 March 1643 *Mercurius Aulicus* reported that the king had notices posted up at the 'Court gates' forbidding anyone to come to be touched until Michaelmas.[88] The king did not return to London until December 1648, when his trial prevented him from touching the sick.

---

[85] *The humble petition of divers hundreds of the kings poore subjects, afflicted with that grievous infirmitie, called the kings evill*, London 1643.

[86] Ibid. 7–8.

[87] *Mercurius Aulicus*, 26 Mar. 1643.

[88] These notices have not survived: Farquhar, 'Royal charities I', 128.

How should *The humble petition* be interpreted? Marc Bloch stated that it cannot be taken at face value because it was royalist propaganda.[89] It certainly could function as propaganda for the crown, and, as it was published in London, it is hardly surprising that the author chose to remain anonymous. But as the Greenwich petition of 1629 showed, this was not the first time that people with scrofula had appealed to Charles to make the royal touch available. Bloch was evidently unaware of the earlier petition, and the problem with his interpretation of the second one is two-fold. It overlooks the possibility that some Londoners might really have scrofula and wanted the king to cure them, while assuming that belief in royal therapeutics was limited to royalists: Bloch stated that supporters of the Long Parliament rejected belief in the royal touch.[90] Certainly, as opinion hardened later in the 1640s some Parliamentarians did reject belief in the royal touch, but early on in the conflict the evidence suggests that this was not the case. One key source is a permit to travel that was authorised on 15 February 1643 for a child of Sir Charles Berkeley (1599–1668), the royalist MP and landowner, to be conveyed in a horse litter from Bruton, Somerset, to Oxford in order to be touched.[91] The date of this permit coincides with that of *The humble petition*, revealing that Londoners were not the only people seeking contact with their less-accessible king. The problem of travelling to the king was greater during the Civil War, particularly if the sick person lived in or needed to pass through an area controlled by Parliament. Berkeley's permit is noteworthy because it demonstrates that, at least in the early years of the war, Parliament was willing to authorise travel to the royal healer; as such it provides evidence of belief in the royal touch even amongst some of those who were fighting against him. In sum, although *The humble petition* has a mildly subversive flavour because it was published in Parliament-controlled London, it needs to be viewed within a context of widespread belief in the royal touch. As a petition it speaks to the disorder of the 1640s.

During the Civil Wars the royal touch ceremony underwent various modifications due to the contingencies of the conflict and Charles's difficult circumstances during his captivity. Knowledge of this period is greatly reliant on retrospective accounts written after the Restoration; although they contain an obvious royalist bias, they are consistent on fundamental problems.[92]

Not surprisingly, the most immediate change to the ceremony was that Angels ceased to be distributed. Parliament took control of the Mint in

---

[89] Bloch, *The royal touch*, 209 (372–3).

[90] Bloch notes that some parliamentarians thought that relics of the dead Charles I had healing properties: ibid. 402 n. 180 (372, 375).

[91] House of Lords Records Office, journal office, main papers, 1509–1700, HL/PO/JO/10/1/143.

[92] T. A., *Excellency*, 8–10; Wiseman, 'A treatise of the king's evil', 241; Browne, *Adenochoiradelogia*, 133–49.

1642, and although the king set up a new one in Oxford his penurious position meant that the production of gold Angels ceased in 1643.[93] From then on the king distributed silver Angels until he was imprisoned and he could not obtain them, at which point he gave out silver two pence coins.[94] These were worth far less than the Angels and yet there are no reports of people complaining that they received a less valuable coin. Sometimes Charles could not even provide silver two pence coins, so people brought their own coins for him to use, as well as ribbons to hang them on.[95] Sometimes he even touched people and no coins were given out at all.[96] Turning to the liturgy, it seems that this was read by clergymen if they were present, but otherwise the king made do without it. One memorialist specifically stated that the king touched without the liturgy;[97] however, another source reports that when Charles was captive on the Isle of Wight, two bishops officiated at the ceremony.[98] In terms of the healing schedule, the last administrative reference to this is the notice dated 26 March 1643, while anecdotal evidence reveals that the timetable was abandoned during the king's captivity, if not before. The requirement that sick people produce certificates was also dropped, and so not surprisingly we hear of people with a range of illnesses seeking access to the king.

It might be thought that the touch of a defeated, captive king whose ceremonies included no Angels and perhaps no liturgy would have little appeal to the populace. This was not so. After his defeat by parliament Charles experienced an upsurge in popularity: at this stage a political settlement was unthinkable without him; his defeat and suffering meant that he was no longer a threat and was viewed sympathetically; the experience of war, including dearth, high taxation and predatory soldiers, meant that many argued that rule by Charles was the lesser of two evils. Some even thought that the king took on a Christ-like role in captivity, even though he was duplicitously trying to play off his enemies against each other, hoping to divide and rule.[99]

This perceived Messiah-like quality was aided by the popularity of Charles's royal touch. From the king's point of view, this last vestige of sacral monarchy was a way of canvassing support and doing good, whilst it afforded those who were sympathetic to him the opportunity to pay their respects and possibly be healed. It also points to the central position of the royal touch

93 Woolf, 'The sovereign remedy', 103.

94 T. A., Excellency, 8; Browne, Adenochoiradelogia, 141, 144; Wiseman, 'Treatise', 241.

95 Browne, Adenochoiradelogia, 147–8; C. M. Clifford Fielding, Royalist father and roundhead son, being the memoirs of the first and second earls of Denbigh, 1600–1675, London 1915, 249.

96 Browne, Adenochoiradelogia, 134, 143, 146; Wiseman, 'Treatise', 241.

97 Fielding, Royalist father, 249.

98 Browne, Adenochoiradelogia, 145.

99 J. Miller, A brief history of the English Civil Wars, London 2009, 142–3.

within English culture at this time and thus raises two further issues. First, contemporaries on either side of the political divide commented that the body politic was sick. By touching ill people, Charles could claim not only to be healing individual suffering but also the political wounds caused by the recent strife. That the king was willing to touch without the usual ceremony – which is remarkable given Charles' personality – and that people were willing to participate too, is indicative of the charisma of office. It appears that as Charles's political powers diminished, his thaumaturgic ones were thought to increase, hence the enthusiasm for an abbreviated ceremony. The strongest examples of this date from the end of Charles's captivity, when his guards finally proscribed the royal touch. At this juncture, people in need of royal thaumaturgy instead sought Charles's blessing as he travelled past them, and so in extreme circumstances his benediction replaced the full ceremony.[100] The explanation for the apparent increase in Charles's charisma despite his dire circumstances must be in part due to the view that, regardless of Charles's personal situation, he was still king and England was a very hierarchical country. It is also worth noting that the fact that crowds flocked to Charles even when he had no Angels to distribute also gives the lie to those who suggest that the gold was the primary motivation of those who sought the royal touch.

Anecdotal evidence concerning Charles and the royal touch between 1646 and 1648 is revealing in terms of the popularity of the rite. At the beginning of February 1647, travelling south from Newcastle to Holmby House in Northamptonshire, the captive king found that his road was lined with cheering crowds: en route he touched large numbers of people.[101] Indeed, so many ill people flocked to him that on 9 February the commissioners in charge of him drew up a declaration which sought to keep the throng away. The crowds understandably posed a security risk, but the declaration focuses on the king's need to avoid catching a disease.[102] The implication is that the vetting process had ceased, presumably as Charles was not attended by sufficient medical staff, so the fear of contagion may well have been genuine. The declaration had little or no effect. On 20 April, during Easter week, the commissioners wrote to the House of Commons because they could not control the huge numbers who came to Holmby House to be touched at this popular time. The Commons set up a committee to draft 'a Declaration to be set forth to the People, concerning the Superstition of being Touched for the

100 Browen, *Adenochoiradelogia*, 134, 143. For the charisma of office see also R. Herrick, 'To the king to cure the evil', in *Hesperides, or, The works both humane and divine of Robert Herrick Esq.*, London 1648, 66.

101 A *joyful message for al loyall subjects: sent from the kings majesties royall court at Causam*, London 1647, sig. A3; *Journal of the House of Commons*, V: 1646–1648, London 1830, 151–2; Browne, *Adenochoiradelogia*, 148–9.

102 *Journal of the House of Lords*, IX: 1646, London 1802, 5.

Healing of the King's Evil'.[103] This use of the word 'superstition' is revealing as some Puritans did indeed view the royal touch this way. The proclamation has not survived, but clearly Parliament had the same problem managing the huge demand for the royal touch as had the king prior to 1642.

Despite the best efforts of those parliamentarians who did not want the king to touch the sick, Charles continued to do so. In the summer of 1647 the press reported that while Charles was at Lord Craven's house he 'touched abundance for the Kings Evill, and healed many'.[104] Charles touched while a prisoner at Hampton Court and Windsor, at various places on the Isle of Wight, and at intervals during journeys to and from different prisons.[105] Although on one occasion the king's guards on the Isle of Wight treated a man who sought the royal touch harshly, the impression is that Charles's guards had to accept that their political prisoner was also a healer and to allow controlled access to him.[106] In fact, Charles touched so many people during his captivity that his guards gave him the nickname 'the Stroker'.[107] This helps to explain why the poet and waterman John Taylor stated that he gained easy access to the king – although Taylor only wanted to kiss the royal hand – and mentioned six women and one man whom the king had recently touched and healed.[108]

Who were these people who sought Charles' touch? No doubt many were royalists or at least sympathetic to the king, so it is no surprise that a monarchist like Taylor the water poet believed in the king's touch; but it seems that people from across the political and ideological spectrum came to be touched. Retrospective accounts of Charles's captivity mention him touching a Quaker woman and a Puritan woman, as well as a woman who brought her daughter to be touched despite having 'no great Opinion' of the ceremony.[109] An unnamed senior parliamentarian brought his only child, who had scrofula, to be touched by Charles when he was a prisoner at Hatfield House at the end of June 1647 – apparently the child was cured the next day.[110] These accounts suggest that the pragmatic desire for a cure could sometimes over-ride religious and political divisions; the results could potentially stimulate reconciliation and reinforce the view that the king's touch could heal the nation's ills. Thus the cases of religious minorities, doubters

---

[103] *Journal of the House of Commons*, v. 151–2; cf. Browne, *Adenochoiradelogia*, 148–9.

[104] *Kingdome's Weekly Intelligencer*, 6–13 July 1647.

[105] Browne, *Adenochoiradelogia*, 141, 142, 144 (for Hampton Court), 134, 145 (Isle of Wight), 143–3 (Windsor), 143 (journeys).

[106] Browne, *Adenochoiradelogia*, 134–5.

[107] *Mercurius Elenctius*, 7 Feb. 1649.

[108] J. Tailor, *Tailors travels from London to the Isle of Wight, with his returne, and occasion of his journey*, London 1648, 10–12.

[109] Browne, *Adenochoiradelogia*, 141 (for the Quaker), 144 (the Puritan), 148 (sceptical woman).

[110] T. A., *Excellency*, 8.

and parliamentarians all seeking the royal touch had a propaganda value for monarchists, proclaiming that the benevolent king could alleviate even his enemies' suffering. This view was put forward in publications during the Restoration and so it seems possible that during the 1640s it was discussed orally.

In December 1648 Charles was moved to Windsor in preparation for his trial. He touched many people *en route*, but once he was within the castle the royal touch was finally supressed. This was announced in the press: 'The *King* touched some of the *Evill* as he came [to Windsor], (as before) but now others are not admitted to come to him with the *Evill*....'[111] As Charles approached his denouement Parliament had to quash his therapeutic activities once and for all, no doubt for both ideological and security purposes. Despite this, on the day that Charles was moved from Windsor to London to stand trial, a woman in the crowd at Windsor called Helena Payne pressed forward and held the king's coat 'humbly supplicating His Majesties Sacred Touch'. This action was surely an allusion to the Gospel account of the woman who had suffered haemorrhages for many years, who was healed by touching the hem of Christ's cloak (Matt. ix.20). Although Charles explained that he had no gold, Helena Payne was not concerned about this and insisted that he touch her, and, remarkably, he did.[112] This was the last recorded incident of Charles touching for scrofula, and it can be dated to 19 January 1649, just eleven days before he was executed as a war criminal.

Interregnum radicalism

The regicide, and the abolition of the House of Lords and the Church of England were traumatic events pushed through by a radical minority with no popular mandate. It seems that the bulk of the nation wanted peace and a return to the old ways.[113] This helps to explain the cult of Charles the Martyr, and the huge popularity of *Eikon basilike*, the book published immediately after Charles's execution that presented him as a moderate man as

---

[111] *Perfect Occurrences*, 27 Dec 1648.

[112] Browne, *Adenochoiradelogia*, 142–3.

[113] C. Hill, *The world turned upside down*, London 1972; F. McGregor and B. Reay (eds), *Radical religion in the English Revolution*, Oxford 1984; F. D. Dow, *Radicalism in the English Revolution*, Oxford 1985; G. E. Aylmer, *Rebellion or revolution? England, 1640–1660*, Oxford 1986; J. Walter, 'The impact on society: a word turned upside down?', in J. Morrill (ed.), *The impact of the English Civil War*, London 1991, 359–91; J. Morrill and J. Walter, 'Order and disorder in the English Revolution', in J. Morrill (ed.),*The nature of the English Revolution*, London 1993, 359–91; P. Baker, 'Rhetoric, reality and the varieties of Civil War radicalism', in J. Adamson (ed.), *The English Civil War: conflict and contexts, 1640–1649*, Basingstoke 2009.

well as a saint, which went through thirty-five editions in 1649 alone.[114] This presentation of Charles was contentious though, as it can be argued that he was largely responsible for his own downfall. At the end of the first Civil War regicide was unthinkable but within a mere two years Charles's duplicity had hardened a small determined group of his opponents, transforming them into king-killers. Yet at the same time, within the broader population, sympathy for Charles increased, and the cult of Charles the Martyr began in 1646. Immediately after Charles's execution the handkerchiefs and other objects that had been dipped in Charles's blood were said to heal scrofula miraculously.[115]

The most publicised of these cases was that of the 'Mayd at Detford', aged about thirteen, who had had scrofula since she was a year and a half, and had been blind for a year as a result of the disease. Her story was told in three pamphlets published in 1649, all of which have very similar narratives and references to biblical healings.[116] Mistress Bayly, her mother, had not thought to get her daughter touched while the king was alive for reasons not divulged, but after his execution she obtained a handkerchief soaked in Charles's blood from a draper. The maid's eyes were then rubbed with the 'bloody side' of the relic; her scrofula soon disappeared and her sight was restored.[117]

The authors of the pamphlets went to great lengths to assert the authenticity of their accounts. The title page of the first pamphlet, A miracle of miracles, states 'the truth hereof many thousands can testifie', and the copy in the British Library, which is in the Thomason Tracts, has 'this is very true July 5th' written by hand (probably by Thomason) underneath. The second pamphlet, A letter sent into France, contains more elaborate attempts to assert authenticity, the subtitle stating that 500 people could attest to the certainty of this miracle. In the text the author explained that he had written down Mistress Bayly's and her daughter's account verbatim, or 'as near I could', and that the event had been witnessed by 'Mr Thomas Bret' a gentleman of 'knowne truth and integrity'. The account was then read aloud to all three so that they could vouch for its accuracy, after which they signed it.[118]

This strong desire for authenticity suggests that the healing was contro-

---

114 Eikon basilike, London 1649; Sharpe, Image wars, 391–403; A. Lacey, The cult of King Charles the martyr, Woodbridge 2003.

115 Browne, Adenochoiradelogia, 109, 150–5; T. A., Excellency, 9–10.

116 A miracle of miracles: wrought by the blood of King Charles the First, of happy memory, upon a mayd at Detford foure miles from London, who by the violence of the disease called the kings evill was blinde one whole yeere, London 1649; Letter sent into France to the lord duke of Buckingham His Grace: of a great miracle wrought by a piece of a handkerchefe, dipped in his majesties bloud, n.a., London 1649; A second letter to the lord duke of Buckingham his grace at the court of France, London 1649; cf. Brown, Adenochoiradelogia, 151.

117 Miracle of miracles, 5; cf. Letter sent into France, A3r.

118 Letter sent into France, A2v.

versial, and in October 1649 *A second letter* was published which explained the reasons for its author's anonymity: the publication of the first pamphlet resulted in a warrant for his apprehension, which he only avoided by escaping to the country, where he still lived. The purpose of *A second letter* was to inform its readers of a further twenty-two scrofula cures effected by the blood of Charles I, twenty-one of which were brought about by a handkerchief owned by one 'Mrs Hunsdon' of St Martin in the Fields. The last case was described in more detail. One Elizabeth Man had scrofula and was blind too, like the Maid of Deptford; so she went to the maid's home and stayed there while Mistress Bayly wiped her eyes with the relic. After a few days her scrofula disappeared and her eyesight returned, though the young woman was cautious about saying that she had experienced a miraculous cure because Mistress Bayly had initially wiped her eyes with some medicinal water before applying the relic; this caution was probably intended to portray the young woman as reliable. The young woman also said that while she resided in Deptford she saw several other scrofulous people come to be treated by the relic, who were all cured.[119]

Why were these cures so contentious? First, there are Protestant attitudes towards relics. They occupied an ambiguous position. Some Protestants did collect and treasure relics, for instance those associated with the Marian martyrs. The instinct to acquire any physical remnants of those who had suffered heroically for their beliefs transcended the divisions of the Reformation. But Protestant doctrine maintained that relics had a semiotic rather than sacramental value; the objects had a spiritual and emotional importance, but were not meant to possess thaumaturgic properties. In other words, relics could not work miracles but they could provide comfort and inspiration. Yet in reality there was potential for slippage as comfort and inspiration could aid faith, which could bring about subtle idolatry or even miracles.[120] The handkerchiefs soaked in Charles I's blood were a rare example of a Protestant relic thought to have thaumaturgic properties, even if the authors of the pamphlets maintained that the miraculous cures were brought about by providence. Second, these cases marked a radical new development because there was no precedent for royal body fluids producing miraculous cures. The handkerchiefs were accepted as genuine relics, unlike Roman Catholic ones, even if their properties were debated. Thirdly, the cases had a strong political message: Charles's posthumous miracles were meant to open the eyes of the king's opponents, just as they restored sight to the blind.

Charles I's relics appear to have set a precedent as there is evidence of belief in the ability of blood relics of the future Charles II to effect cures of scrofula. After the battle of Worcester in 1651, when he was in hiding at

---

[119] *Second letter*, A2–3.

[120] A. Walsham, 'Skeletons in the cupboard: relics after the English Reformation', in A. Walsham (ed.), *Relics and remains* (*P&P* supplement v, 2010), 121–43, esp. pp. 131–8.

Moseley, he had a nose bleed and exchanged his bloody handkerchief for a clean one from the Catholic priest Father Huddleston Samuel.[121] According to Pepys, to whom the king later dictated an account of his escape, the handkerchief was given by the priest to a kinswoman who 'kept it with great veneration and used it as a remedy for the King's Evil'.[122] It is also interesting that, while in hiding in Trent, Dorset, Charles spent time boring holes into gold coins which he gave to those who helped him escape.[123] Presumably the mementoes reminded people of Angels.

Oliver Cromwell did not practise the royal touch as Lord Protector because he was not a hereditary monarch, nor had he been anointed on the hands; the ceremony was also heavily associated with the Stuarts. However, the future Charles II did touch for scrofula during his exile throughout the 1650s. In doing so, he privileged hereditary thaumaturgy over consecration, and thus asserted his right to rule. In some respects though, his therapeutic practices suffered from a continuation of the disorder of the 1640s because Charles was politically disempowered and penurious; he had no Angels to dispense and so often bestowed silver coins or relied upon people bringing their own.[124] On the other hand, the vetting process for supplicants was robust.[125] All of this meant that during the 1650s people who wished to obtain the royal touch had a number of options: they could go to Charles II in exile, or alternatively they could go to Louis XIV, or find a blood relic of Charles I. Yet this situation could be problematic. In May 1650 one Mrs Sherard, aunt of Sir Ralph Verney, wanted to take her daughter to France as she had scrofula, and it was thought that the touch of Louis XIV would be more efficacious than that of the un-anointed 'wanderer and exile', Charles Stuart. This implies that consecration was privileged over heredity. Unfortunately, when Sherard arrived in Paris she found that Louis had not yet been crowned and so her daughter was not touched. Interestingly, her daughter was eventually touched in the autumn of 1653 even though Louis was not crowned until June 1654, suggesting that pragmatism won the day over ideology.[126]

The Interregnum government's attitude towards Stuart thaumaturgy was not as hostile as might be thought. The administration took measures against

---

[121] T. Blount, *Boscobel, or, The history of his sacred majesties most miraculous preservation after the battle of Worcester, 3 Sept. 1651*, London 1660, 35; *A summary of occurrences relating to the miraculous preservation of our late sovereign lord, King Charles II*, London 1688, 19–20.

[122] *An account of the preservation of King Charles II after the Battle of Worcester drawn up by himself*, London 1766, 31.

[123] R. Ollard, *The escape of Charles II*, London 1986, 78.

[124] Browne, *Adenochoiradelogia*, 157; Lower, *Relation*, 76.

[125] Browne, *Adenochoiradelogia*, 156–60.

[126] *Memoirs of the Verney family during the seventeenth century*, ed. F. Verney and M. M. Verney, London 1907, i. 497, 499, 509.

those who advocated Charles I's blood relics in print, but it did not try to stop people travelling to the continent to access the royal touch. Presumably this is because controlling travel was difficult, while people who were touched by Charles in Europe appear not have made a loud noise about it. In the 1680s John Browne, the king's surgeon who wrote an important book on the royal touch, stated that an enterprising Scottish merchant even organised boat trips so that people from Scotland and Newcastle could access Charles on the continent.[127]

A further issue that illustrates the Interregnum government's ambivalence towards healing by touch is the proliferation of sectarian healers during the 1640s and 1650s. During the Civil Wars the breakdown of Church and State and the expression of radical opinion became mutually reinforcing and a large number of radical Protestant sects were founded in England and Wales, such as the Quakers and Baptists.[128] The Reformation had emphasised the individual's direct relationship to God; some sectarians took this to extremes, claiming to have such a strong contact with the Almighty that they could heal by touch in the same way as the monarch. Other healers maintained that their powers were due to their being seventh sons. What is interesting is that both royalists and radical sectarians could believe in healing by touch – the common thread being that religion underpinned health and medicine – though both were hostile to the other's claims.[129] For the royalists and those sympathetic to the crown, the sectarian healers represented a dramatic break with the past, the destabilisation of the Church of England and the social order, a rejection of the distinction between the laity and clergy, and a threat to the sacred touch of the king. Yet for others, the sectarians were another option for those who could not travel to Europe to obtain the royal touch.

During the first years of the Restoration one of the royal touch apologists looked back on this problematic state of affairs, condemning the sectarian healers and suggesting that their rise represented the sinfulness of the nation. The main thrust of his denunciation was that the sectarian healers who claimed to cure scrofula by touch had only appeared because England had been without a thaumaturgic monarch for a decade.[130] The new healers filled this gap, just as the healers of the 1630s had done. The sectarians were castigated as 'seducing jugglers', 'seventh sons, [and] stroakers'. It was claimed that they courted fortune in the hope of success and that, unlike the king, they had no 'warrant from God' to heal. The apologist said that the purpose of his treatise was to expose these healers as fraudsters, not least because they had deceived the masses. This was probably an oversimplification because

127 Browne, *Adenochoiradelogia*, 156–60.

128 Dow, *Radicalism in the English Revolution*, 59, 65.

129 The religious underpinnings of medicine are discussed at pp. 11, 19, 21–2 above.

130 T. A., *Excellency*, 1; cf. *Mercurius Publicus*, 28 June–5 July, for 27 June 1660; Primrose, *Popular errours*, 434–42.

in the 1630s people of all ranks showed an interest in artisan healers when they were unable to access the royal touch.[131]

The apologist went on to further denigrate the sectarian healers in some remarkably frank passages that denied that they wrought miraculous healings. Some of this condemnation could in theory have undermined the royal touch, though of course the apologist stressed again and again that royal therapeutics were genuine. The first comment made was that although the sectarian healers supposedly cured scrofula, this was not itself miraculous as it was a disease which could be cured by medicine. Secondly, the powers of seventh sons were denied as 'according to … Philosophy, a number hath no operative vertue'. Thirdly, with regard to the physical act of touching a sick person in order to heal them, the apologist said that 'the [sectarian] Touch, as Touch, hath only the power of Touch', contrasting their 'Manual Touch' with the sacred touch of the king. This meant that the touch of the healers was purely physical, whereas the king's acted as a conduit for God's healing powers. If the 'manual touch' of the healers seemed to bring about a cure, the apologist insisted that this was because they had touched 'simple wounds' which in time would have healed anyway, and so their 'forged miracles' were nothing more than coincidence. The attack on these healers concluded with a condescending remark on their social position: the apologist said that it was not 'lawful for ordinary persons to assume so great a power, their skill in healing is not the Gift of God, as appeareth by the quality of the persons, who are generally ignorant, and prophane'.[132]

Evidently the sectarian healers were considered a threat by the royal touch apologists, even in the early years of the Restoration. In one respect this is surprising, given the extreme popularity of the royal touch throughout the Restoration; but it is a reminder of the extent to which the social order had been destabilised, and the extreme anxiety that this provoked in many contemporaries. It is also a reminder that English culture had changed, not least because during the second half of the seventeenth century England and Wales experienced large number of miraculous healings, often wrought by people from the lower ranks of society.[133] Partly for these reasons, apologists for the royal touch may have overestimated the threat of sectarian healers of scrofula when they looked back on the English Republic from the safety of the Restoration.

---

[131] T. A., *Excellency*, 1, 2, 5, 11.
[132] Ibid. 1–5; cf. Primrose, *Errours*, 441–2.
[133] Shaw, *Miracles*, 3–50, 52–64.

The Restoration reaction

Once the Restoration of the Stuarts was secured, Charles II touched more than 300 people for scrofula at The Hague and Breda before embarking for England. Prior to this, Charles had publicly forgiven the English parliamentary commissioners who visited him to request pardon.[134] Both of these gestures – healing the sick and forgiving his enemies – were an imitation of Christ that signified that, once restored, Charles intended to use his authority wisely and to be merciful. In fact, he was aided by the English Parliament which had just sent him a chest of Angels and 10s. pieces, meaning that the English royal touch ceremony was performed by Charles with its full ritual splendour for the first time in almost twenty years.[135]

Once the king reached England at the end of May 1660, the numbers touched rose dramatically. At least 2,000 sick people had congregated in the capital, seeking the king's touch. Despite Charles's demanding schedule, in his first month as king he touched 900 people – a figure equivalent to an annual total for James I. The press reported that thousands more were arriving in London, and in an attempt at crowd control the government announced in June that healings would only take place on Fridays and that the numbers would be limited to 200, but they would continue until everyone had been touched.[136] This turned out to be too stringent, as shortly afterwards it was announced that healings would occur on both Wednesdays and Fridays.[137] Within six months the new king had touched some 6,000 people, an unprecedentedly large number.

When assessing the numbers touched by Charles II, it is extremely fortunate that the staff of the Chapel Royal, who were responsible for providing the correct number of Angels for each ceremony, kept a register of the numbers touched from May 1660 to September 1664, and from May 1667 to April 1683; the gap in the data can be attributed to the Great Plague and the Fire of London. John Browne, the king's surgeon, published the registers in 1684 as a way of evidencing the great appeal of royal therapeutics. The total for Charles's reign is 96,796 (*see* Figure 5 and Table 5).[138]

---

134 van Wicquefort, *Relation*, 78; Sharpe, *Rebranding rule*, 151.
135 Farquhar, 'Royal charities, II', 100–1.
136 *Mercurius Publicus*, 28 June–5 July, for 27 June 1660; see chapter 1 above.
137 *Parliamentary Intelligencer*, 16–23 July 1660; *Mercurius Publicus*, 19–26 July 1660.
138 The registers are in Browne, *Adenochoiradelogia*, 197–9, although the pagination stops at p. 197. It should be noted that the total for 1683 is only for the months from January to April, while the total for 1684 is at p. 79. There are also problems with some of Browne's arithmetic because sometimes the twelve monthly totals for a year do not add up to the annual total provided. I have rectified the totals and modernised the calendar.

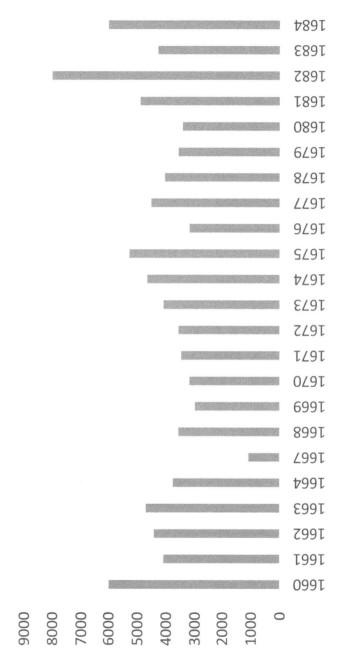

Figure 5. The number of people touched for scrofula by Charles II, 1660–84.

Table 5 The number of people touched for scrofula by Charles II, 1660–84

Year	Modernised calendar total
1660	6,005
1661	4,075
1662	4,443
1663	4,706
1664	3,753
1667	1,086
1668	3,563
1669	3,004
1670	3,171
1671	3,457
1672	3,577
1673	4,092
1674	4,665
1675	5,307
1676	3,178
1677	4,512
1678	4,021
1679	3,582
1680	3,409
1681	4,908
1682	7,993
1683	4,289
1684	6,000
Total	96,796

Three manuscripts survive which provide similar data from Charles's reign, all of which verify the overall reliability of Browne's figures.[139] This data is remarkable, similar in detail to the records from Edward I's reign.[140] The low point in 1667 represents the aftermath of plague and fire, though the total of

---

[139] BL, MS Egerton 806, fos 59r–60r gives a total of 1,640 for April–November 1668, compared to Browne who gives 1,709. The Folger Shakespeare Library, Washington, DC, holds MS Folger 266450 which records that Charles touched 4,566 people between January and July 1683 on thirty-one occasions, providing exactly the same monthly totals as Browne for the period January to April 1683 (and I am grateful to Michael Hunter for drawing my attention to this source). TNA, E407/85/1 records the numbers touched between April 1669 and December 1685, though the data is not complete for every year.

[140] See p. 36 above.

1,086 is still very high compared to earlier reigns. There is some correlation between high annual totals and political crises. During the Second Anglo Dutch War of 1672–4 the numbers increase, peaking at 4,665, while during the Popish Plot of 1678 there is another high total of 4,021. The following year's lower total of 3,582 is surprising given that the Exclusion Crisis raged, but Charles II was seriously ill during the summer and so was unlikely to have touched. The numbers then peak during the Tory reaction. The annual total in 1682 is the greatest of all, an astonishing 7,993, the context for which is the earl of Shaftesbury fleeing to Holland, and the duke of Monmouth touring England on a quasi-royal progress. It is tempting to speculate that during times of political emergency either the crown decided to touch more people or people voted with their feet and sought the royal touch in larger numbers, or both. The ceremony allowed people to show their loyalty to the king who, it was hoped, would cure scrofula and alleviate the nation's ills.

The enormous annual totals raise the question of the unprecedented enthusiasm for the royal touch. Obviously the Restoration government was keen to revive the royal touch in order to assert the prestige of the monarchy, and the populace evidently responded positively to this as there had been no royal healer in England for more than a decade.[141] But the numbers are so great that a closer examination is required.

The initial passion for royal therapeutics during the first few years of the Restoration was part of the groundswell of popular royalism that overtook a significant proportion of the population. Bonfires, public toasts and the singing of ballads were just some of the ways in which that people cele-brated the return of the Stuarts.[142] Notwithstanding the merriments, the Restoration was widely understood in providential terms, while the different expectations that various religious groups had of the new administration reveal a very complex situation. Presbyterians wanted a comprehensive church settlement with a limited episcopacy but no toleration of radical sects. Roman Catholics and sectarians put their trust in the promise that Charles made in his Declaration of Breda, just prior to the Restoration, that he would provide 'liberty to tender consciences'. In theory Anglicans were hostile to all of this, expecting much of the political and religious innova-tions of the last twenty years to be dismantled.[143] It is clear that, despite Charles's personal desire for comprehension and toleration, he was to be thwarted by parliament, which passed a number of punitive laws and codes against religious minorities, the first of which was the Act of Uniformity of May 1662. But in the first two years of the Restoration Charles touched all

---

[141] Bloch, *The royal touch*, 211–12 (378–9).

[142] Tim Harris provides an excellent discussion of this: *London crowds in the reign of Charles II*, Cambridge 1987, chs ii–iii (for dissent see pp. 36–7, 50–51).

[143] Ibid. 61.

who came to him regardless of their religious or political affiliations,[144] which indicated his benevolence and his preference for toleration; in the same way those who sought his touch could show their allegiance despite differences of belief. This continued after the punitive legislation had been passed, and was a continuation of the approach to royal therapeutics taken by Elizabeth I and Charles I that included religious minorities and political opponents.

In 1661, when hopes for a comprehensive religious settlement were still high, the first of three books devoted to the royal touch during the Restoration period was published. They all shine much light on the enthusiasm for the rite. In 1661 appeared *Ostenta Carolina, or The late calamaties of England with the authors of them*, written by John Bird (c. 1604–65). After the failure of the religious settlement came the publication of *XEIPEΞOKH: the excellency or handy work of the royal hand* (1665), written by 'T.A.'.[145] And then, much later, in 1684 John Browne published *Adenochoiradelogia*, which will be dealt with separately.[146]

Bird was an Oxford graduate and lay Presbyterian who welcomed the Restoration of the Stuarts for the reasons outlined above.[147] His book was printed by Francis Sowle who was responsible for printing most of the Quaker literature in London, which itself hints at the broad appeal of the royal touch in the early 1660s.[148] Bird's interest in the royal touch also stemmed from his royalism during the Civil Wars, as well as his interest in medicine and healthcare. Between 1629 and 1632 he was examined by the Royal College of Physicians on a number of occasions for practising medicine without a licence; and he died of the plague in 1665, having first tended those with the disease.[149]

The second book, *The excellency or handy work of the royal hand*, poses a problem of authorship. The only clue is the dedication to the duke of York that is signed 'T.A. M.D.'. In the early eighteenth century, the surgeon William Becket said in his book on the royal touch that the author was Thomas Allen (d.1684), the physician of Bethlem Hospital and Fellow of the Royal Society.[150] However, the two copies of *The excellency* in the British

---

[144] See pp. 155–6 below.

[145] J. Bird, *Ostenta Carolina, or The late calamities of England with the authors of them*, London 1661; T. A., *Excellency*.

[146] See pp. 157–60 below.

[147] R. A. Hunter and I. Macalpine, 'John Bird on "Reckets" (London, 1661)', *Journal of the History of Medicine* xiii/3 (1958), 397–403 at p. 402.

[148] H. R. Plomer, *A dictionary of the booksellers and printers who were at work in England, Scotland and Ireland from 1641 to 1667*, London 1907, 168.

[149] Hunter and Macalpine, 'John Bird', 402–3; Bird, *Ostenta Carolina*,'The epistle to the reader'; *The obituary of Richard Smyth, secondary of the Poultry Compter London*, ed. H. Ellis (Camden Society, 1849), 68.

[150] Becket, *Free and impartial enquiry*, 58. See also S. Halket and J. Laing, *Dictionary of anonymous and pseudonymous English literature*, Edinburgh 1926–62, i. 324. For anonymous

Library both bear handwritten inscriptions that the author is Thomas Harris (sometimes spelt Arris), a physician, and the MP for St Albans.[151] Both Allen and Harris were M.D.s (Harris, Oxford, 1651; Allen, Cambridge, 1659) and there is no internal evidence within the book that assists with solving the problem of attribution, so it seems best to refer to the author as 'T.A.'.

Both books saw the rationale for the royal touch of the restored Stuarts as resting on the biblical healing mandate that had been explained by William Tooker at the end of Elizabeth I's reign.[152] But the specific circumstances of the Restoration gave rise to further theories that concentrated on the diseased body politic and sin, as well as on the redemption offered by the return of the king.

The body politic and sin

Bird and T.A. both heralded Charles II as a divine-right monarch and healer, and their books discussed the state of the English nation in the 1660s. The extreme trauma of the Civil War, regicide and the failure of the Interregnum government after Cromwell's death was usually understood in providential terms, which brought about collective anxieties concerning the sinful nature of the nation, against the background of a profoundly millenarian mood. This brought the idea of the body politic into sharp relief.

In pre-modern Europe it was widely thought that, just as God was sovereign in the universe or macrocosm, so a similar sovereignty existed in the microcosms of both the human body and the body politic (human society). This 'argument by correspondence' meant that the body politic and the physical human body lent themselves to analogies, as between the head and the monarch, bodily health and social well-being, the circulation of blood and money, or the rule of the rational soul and political sovereignty. The theory maintained that the better the health and well-being of each person, the better the health and well-being of the nation. As the social order was thought to be structured by God, the theory maintained that monarchy was

---

early modern publications see Marcy North, 'Ignoto in the age of print: the manipulation of anonymity in early modern England', *Studies in Philology* xci/4 (1994), 390–416. For Allen see W. Munk, *The roll of the Royal College of Physicians of London*, London 1878, i. 361; T. Birch, *The history of the Royal Society of London for Improving Natural Knowledge*, London 1756–7, ii. 246; and M. Hunter, *The Royal Society and its Fellows, 1660–1700: the morphology of an early scientific institution*, 2nd edn, Oxford 1994, 182.

[151] See the books in the BL catalogued as 1187.i.1.3 and 1187.i.1.3. Note that Wing's Short title catalogue says that the attribution to Allen is uncertain, and the author could be Harris. I am grateful to Peter Elmer for discussing both Allen and Harris with me, and the problem of attribution; he has also informed me that two other possible candidates are Thomas Allen's son, also called Thomas, and the physician Thomas Ady (although Ady rejected belief in witchcraft, so may have had doubts about royal therapeutics).

[152] See p. 61 above.

the best form of government: the king ruled his people and upheld laws and customs, just as the head ruled the human body through reason.[153]

This meant that physical or psychological disorder within individuals was thought directly to influence the state, and *vice-versa*, and so a direct parallel was drawn between the conditions of the body politic and that of the king's subjects. Disease and 'passions' had to be cured and controlled by medicine and reason if individual and collective order was to be maintained. One way of creating concord was for monarchs to interact harmoniously with their subjects, for example during thaumaturgic ceremonies. The body politic was no mere metaphor.

Many commentators in England in 1660 maintained that the body politic was diseased and corrupted. The execution of Charles I had severed the head from the body politic, leading to disorder and the rule of 'fanatics'. The failure of the Rump Parliament lent itself to witty analogies with a disordered body, especially excremental.[154] The prevalence of scrofula was one way of ascertaining the poor health of the body politic, as was the idea that the nation was bewitched.[155] Corporeal readings of the sick body politic abounded in 1660.[156] Bird spoke for many when he asserted that the illness was due to recent 'state physicians', that is, the republican administrations, which had brought about an era of iniquity. This was a direct consequence of the regicide and the abolition of the monarchy, which led Bird to describe viscerally the body politic as having 'wounds' and 'putrefying sores', the symptoms of scrofula.[157] T. A. went further, saying that rebellion against the monarch was analogous to gangrene, which 'menaceth to eat out the Life and Soul of the Monarchy and Religion'.[158]

Bird, T. A. and many other commentators identified the root cause of the diseased body politic as sin, the ascendancy of the will in fallen man. John Spurr has convincingly argued that Restoration England was consumed with fears concerning its sinful nature. Sin was usually discussed pragmatically rather than in abstract form, and so the everyday sins of individuals were thought to be responsible for the social problems of the country – a sick body politic – which in turn caused the wrath of God. This is a pertinent reminder that belief in an active and providential God was the essential core to reli-

---

[153] E. Forsett, *A comparative discourse of the bodies natural and politique*, London 1606, 89–103; Greenleaf, *Order, empiricism and politics*, 21–2.

[154] M. Jenner, 'The roasting of the rump: scatology and the body politic in Restoration England: reply', *P&P* cxcvi (Aug. 2007), 273–86.

[155] P. Elmer, *The miraculous conformist: Valentine Greatrakes, the body politic, and the politics of healing in Restoration Britain*, Oxford 2013, 120.

[156] Ibid. 111–24.

[157] Bird, *Ostenta Carolina*, 51.

[158] T. A., *Excellency*, 36.

gious orthodoxy at this time, as was a causal relationship between human sin and its divine consequences.[159]

As well as believing that sin was a disease, it was widely believed that disease and misfortune were punishments from God as a result of wrong-doing. God was thought to punish whole communities or nations for the sins of a few people, which were their collective responsibility. This helps to explain the view of the relationship between scrofula and sin. During the Restoration, people with scrofula were thought to bear the collective weight of the nation's sins; fortunately they were not demonised as particularly sinful individuals themselves. None of the commentators blamed people with scrofula for their condition; Bird pointed out that almost everyone in England had suffered because of the action of a small number of people who ruled during the Interregnum, thus aligning medical, economic and social problems.[160]

In light of this preoccupation with sin, it is not surprising that the Great Plague in 1665 and the Fire of London of 1666 were seen as warnings that God wished England to have a moral regeneration; the numerology of 1666, a year which included the number of the AntiChrist, added to the millenarian fever.[161] The clergyman Richard Perrinchief was typical of many preachers when in November 1666 he lamented that the miseries which used to come singly now fell upon the nation 'with as much speed as hasty messengers'.[162] The theology behind this was that God punished the wicked, while the righteous, if punished, would be rewarded for bearing their suffering.[163] Thus the Christian doctrine of salvation through suffering was asserted.

Godliness, the nation's remedy

The sinful and diseased body politic required medicine. Moral regenera-tion was identified as the remedy and could only be achieved by individual godliness, as preached by ministers of the Church of England, with athe-ists, papists, dissenters and apathetic Anglicans in their sights.[164] Of course, collective moral rejuvenation was not a new concept – Tudor homilies had stated that the populace should acknowledge themselves before God as

[159] J. Spurr, *The Restoration Church of England, 1646–89*, London 1991, 269–70; M. Hunter, *Science and Society in Restoration England*, Cambridge 1981, 163–4.

[160] Bird, *Ostenta Carolina*, 51.

[161] Spurr, *Restoration Church*, 53.

[162] R. Perrinchief, *A sermon preached before the honourable House of Commons at St Margaret's Westminster on 7 November*, London 1666; cf. Spurr, *Restoration Church*, 54.

[163] *The works of Henry Smith*, ed. Thomas Fuller, Edinburgh 1867, ii. 241.

[164] Spurr, *Restoration Church*, 277–8, ch. vi.

miserable sinners, repent and ask for mercy – but the trauma of the recent past gave it a new urgency.[165]

The Stuart Restoration was greeted by many as the first stage of national redemption, with the new king and his therapeutic practices being central to this process. Hence the cult of kingship flourished as never before, partly as a reaction against the strife of the 1640s and 1650s, the body politic being ruled by its proper head once again. The restoration of the monarchy resurrected the body politic, with its head intact. More specifically, three key models of kingship bolstered reverence to the crown, increasing its sacrality. These were thaumaturgic, martyrological and Davidic.[166] The thaumaturgic model was the most important: nearly 100,000 scrofulous people came to Charles II hoping that he would cure them by his touch, and by implication, revive the body politic. The Presbyterian Richard Edes was typical when he expressed confidence in Charles's ability to heal. 'His Majestie is now become a Physitian, and the Lord make him a healer of his People', he wrote, 'I may say to everyone that is sick of this Evil … the King touches you, the Lord Cure you.' Edes went on to say that the healer king would purge the body politic of its 'malignant humour' and so restore peace.[167] Also noteworthy in this connection is the sermon preached before the king in June 1660 by the archbishop of Canterbury, Gilbert Sheldon (1598–1677). He emphasised that it was important to help those who had suffered in the recent past, especially 'the *sick*, the *maimed*, the *lame*, the *desolute*, *Widows* and *Children*'. This is significant both in its own right and because these were the types of people who sought the royal touch, and this cannot have been lost on Sheldon's audience. He then elaborated on the need to forgive and urged the new king to see his people as prodigals, returning at last to their father, the king.[168]

The thaumaturgic model of kingship was bolstered by the martyrological and Davidic archetypes. The martyrological emphasised that Charles II was particularly suited to his role of healer as he was the son of a sacrificial victim: the cult of Charles I was widespread and during the Restoration he was given near-saintly status. The *Book of Common Prayer* commemorated his execution with fasts and special services held on 30 January each year, alongside those that honoured the discovery of the Gunpowder Plot on 5 November and Charles II's accession on 29 May. The frontispiece to the best-selling *Eikon Basilike* (1649) depicted Charles I grasping a crown of thorns as

---

[165] *Certain sermons or homilies* (1547); and *A homily against disobedience and wilful rebellion* (1570): a critical edition, ed. Ronald B. Bond, Toronto 1987, 73.

[166] Goldie, 'Restoration political thought', 15. Goldie also discusses three other models: Augustan, Platonic and feudal.

[167] R. Edes, *Great Britains resurrection, or, Englands complacencie in her soveraigne King Charles II*, London 1660, 33.

[168] *In God's name: examples of preaching in England from the Act of Supremacy to the Act of Uniformity, 1533–1622*, ed. J. Chandos, London 1971, 551–2.

his earthly crown lay fallen on the ground, in keeping with royalist images of kingship that dwelt on the patient sufferings of Christ.[169]

The Davidic model of kingship emphasised the special qualities bestowed on Charles II as a result of his exile. Prior to his banishment, Charles had been miraculously preserved by God after his defeat at Worcester in 1651 and during his remarkable escape to France; he had suffered a decade of exile and relative poverty and yet returned to England without bloodshed or vengeance.[170] Once restored, numerous sermons drew on 2 Samuel xix–xxii, comparing the Old Testament king David, who was exiled by Saul before he returned to assume power, with Charles II.[171]

Bird drew on all three models, concluding that so great were Charles II's powers due to his exceptional circumstances, that he would heal his sick subjects and the body politic once and for all. Unlike his predecessors, he would actually eradicate scrofula. Of course Bird's hyperbole created a hostage to fortune – as the years passed and the numbers touched increased it must have been obvious that scrofula was not being eradicated, and in any case Charles would not wish to eliminate scrofula as this would deprive the crown of its thaumaturgic role. But Bird's sentiment reflected the euphoria of the early Restoration. He described Charles II's powers:

> He healeth the *Bruises* and *Putrified* Sores of those whom he toucheth, [and] will take away the *Falseness* of Doctrine and *Blasphemy* of Religion, Injustice, Oppression in the *State*, and *wicked living* from all. Which may well be signi-fied by *corruption* and *putrid Ulcers* …because these things proceed from a Diseased Soul, are *loathsome* and odious to God and man, and *stink* in their nostrils.[172]

Crucially, Bird noted that when Christ healed the sick he forgave their sins, as 'healing of men is interpreted [as the] forgiving of sins'. In the same way Charles II would bring mercy to the sick, regardless of their religious or political affiliations. To make sure that his readers fully understood him, Bird even associated Charles II with Edward the Confessor, not the most obvious comparison it must be said. But Bird observed that both had martyred fathers and had suffered exile before returning to rule, while the Confessor was thought to be England's first thaumaturgic king, whereas Charles would be its last. In one of his more eccentric passages, Bird went on to predict that Charles would travel to France and cleanse the French nation of scrofula too (apparently the French royal touch was less efficacious than the English

---

169 Goldie, 'Restoration political thought', 15.

170 Bird, *Ostenta Carolina*, 80, 86–7; T. A., *Excellency*, 18; *In God's name*, 554.

171 Goldie, 'Restoration political thought', 15; cf. M. Douglas, *Purity and danger: an analysis of the concepts of pollution and taboo*, London 1996, 97, who stresses the importance of a period of exile to the men in some primitive cultures who then return as healers.

172 Bird, *Ostenta Carolina*, 71.

because France was a Catholic country) after which the grateful French would convert to Protestantism.[173]

Valentine Greatrakes

Apologists for the royal touch went to great lengths to extol its relevance and efficacy, and to identify the exceptional qualities of Charles II. However, despite the enormous popularity of royal therapeutics at this time, in 1666 the Irish JP, healer and demonologist Valentine Greatrakes (1629–83) began to heal by touch in England (*see* Figure 6). Greatrakes ministered to thousands of people during his six months in England, stimulating much intellectual curiosity that precipitated a pamphlet debate. He has often been described as the most serious of all the rival healers to the Stuarts; but in fact he was only mildly subversive.

In 1662 Greatrakes, who lived in Ireland, had an 'impulse ... of mind' that he could cure scrofula by the laying on of hands, accompanied by prayers. This he did for three years, until a second 'impulse' revealed to him that he could cure diseases in general in this way, resulting in him tending to those who were ill with aches, agues, asthma, eczema, leprosy, rheumatism, arthritis, dropsy, deafness, warts and tumours.[174] Hundreds of people visited him, although like the king he was not able to cure everyone. He was invited

---

[173] Ibid. 36, 72–5, 83–4.

[174] V. Greatrakes, *A brief account of Mr Valentine Greatrakes and divers of the strange cures by him lately performed*, London 1666, 22, 28. The most up-to-date treatment of Greatrakes is Peter Elmer's excellent *Miraculous conformist* (see n. 152 above). Greatrakes has been discussed in relation to the royal touch in Crawfurd, *The king's evil*, 120–1; Bloch, *Royal touch*, 216 (384); Thomas, *Religion and the decline of magic*, 202–4; Weber, 'The monarch's sacred body', 67–76; and Shaw, *Miracles*,74–98. Useful works on Greatrakes include M. McKeon, *Politics and poetry in Restoration England: the case of Dryden's annus mirabilis*, London 1975, 208–15; J. R. Jacob, *Robert Boyle and the English Revolution: a study in social and intellectual change*, New York 1977, 164–76; E. Duffy, 'Valentine Greatrakes, the Irish stroker: miracle, science and orthodoxy in Restoration England', in Keith Robbins (ed.), *Religion and humanism* (Studies in Church History xvii, 1981), 251–73; N. H. Steneck, 'Greatrakes the stroker: the interpretation of historians', and B. B. Kaplan, 'Greatrakes the stroker: the interpretation of his contemporaries', *Isis* lxxiii/2 (1982), 161–77, 178–85; D. P. Walker, 'Valentine Greatrakes, the Irish stroker and the question of miracles', *Mélanges sur la literature de la Renaissance á la mémoire de V. L. Saulnier*, Geneva 1984, 343–56; *The Conway letters: the correspondence of Anne, Viscountess Conway, Henry More, and their friends, 1642–84*, ed. M. Hope Nicolson and S. Hutton, Oxford 1992, 244–308; Simon Shaffer, 'Regeneration: the body of natural philosophers in Restoration England', in C. Lawrence and S. Shapin (eds), *Science incarnate: historical embodiments of natural knowledge*, London 1998, 83–120, esp. pp. 106–16; C. S. Breathnach, 'Robert Boyle's approach to the ministrations of Valentine Greatrakes', *History of Psychiatry* x (1999), 87–109; and A. Marshall, 'The Westminster magistrate and the Irish stroker: Sir Edmund Godfrey and Valentine Greatrakes, some unpublished correspondence', *HJ* xl (1997), 499–505.

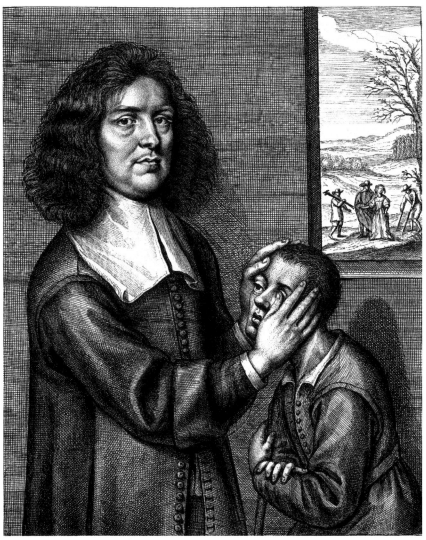

Figure 6. 'The true and lively pourtraicture of Valentine Greatrakes Esqr', frontispiece to A brief account of Mr Valentine Greatrakes.

to England by the philosopher Lady Anne Conway, in the hope that he would cure her of her migraines. Greatrakes arrived at her home at Ragley, Warwickshire, in January 1666, but was unable to cure her, although he tended to hundreds of other people; this resulted in the mayor of Worcester inviting him to that city, where he again stroked large numbers of people. As a result of this he was summoned to the royal court in London. Three patients were brought from St Bartholomew's Hospital for Greatrakes to cure in front of the king, as well as the monarch's friend, the poet Sir John Denham, who was temporarily insane; but Greatrakes was unable to cure any of them. Despite this, Greatrakes's healings remained popular although he returned to Ireland at the end of May 1666, apparently exhausted. However, he continued to heal by touch both there and on several subsequent visits to England until he died in 1683, although after 1666 he avoided the limelight.

The Greatrakes affair provoked a 'great discourse ... at the Coffee-houses, and everywhere', with views on the stroker ranging from conviction to disbelief: 'some take him to be a *Conjurer*, and some an *Impostor*, but others again *adore* him as an *Apostle*'.[175] The courtier George Walsh wrote to his cousin Henry Slingsby, a Fellow of the Royal Society and Deputy Master of the Mint, that 'some say they are better' for being stroked by Greatrakes, but that 'others are the worse'. More specifically, Walsh reported that Denham's condition had actually deteriorated after Greatrakes' ministrations, the poet being now 'stark mad'.[176]

Such conflicting views were reflected in the pamphlets that discussed Greatrakes, which are concerned with the origin of his powers: did he perform miracles or did he heal by natural means? This in turn raised the question of whether the age of miracles had indeed ceased and even whether biblical miracles, especially those of Christ, were natural or supernatural phenomena. Henry Stubbe, author, physician and political pamphleteer, published *The miraculous conformist*, an apology for the stroker in the form of an open letter to the preeminent natural philosopher Robert Boyle. In it, Stubbe maintained that Greatrakes's cures were miraculous in origin, but natural in implementation;[177] in other words, God granted Greatrakes a special power to heal, but nevertheless the Irishman had to physically massage his patients so as to restore their health. Boyle was very interested in Greatrakes and witnessed the stroker tending the sick. Although Boyle disagreed with Stubbe on a number of issues relating to Greatrakes's powers, he agreed with him that the stroker's cures were authentic, and he agreed with Stubbe's proposition. Thus both commentators allowed that Greatrakes had been given a special power by God, while their naturalistic interpretation

175 J. Glanvill, *A blow at modern Sadducism*, London 1668, 84–5.
176 HMC, *Sixth report of the Royal Commission*, London 1877, 339.
177 Stubbe, *Miraculous conformist*, 12–13.

of his cures left Christ's miracles inscrutable.[178] On the other hand, outright scepticism towards Greatrakes was expressed by David Lloyd, reader in the Charterhouse, in his *Wonders no miracles*.[179] Lloyd said that Greatrakes was a blasphemous imposter who charged gullible people for his services. This forced Greatrakes to publish his own account in which he refuted Lloyd and claimed that his powers came from God; he also provided witness statements to his cures from luminaries such as Boyle.[180]

Inevitably, the debate concerning Greatrakes' powers also touched on royal therapeutics. Both Stubbe and Lloyd discussed this, affirming their belief in the king's ability to heal by touch. Greatrakes did not mention it in his tract, presumably because he sought to avoid controversy. Stubbe's passage is brief, whereas Lloyd went into more detail: he denounced the nonconformists (whom he described as 'melancholy') who doubted the efficacy of the royal touch, claiming that when it worked it did so by the power of suggestion. Lloyd also castigated the other healers who tried to cure by touch 'as well as the King; levelling his Gift, as well as they would his Office'.[181] Thus, for Lloyd, the key issue was that the sectarian healers and the seventh sons who first appeared during the 1640s and 1650s, and now Greatrakes, were seditious because, now that the Stuarts were restored, only the king should cure scrofula by touch.

It is easy to assume from this that Greatrakes was a threat to the crown, which is the prevailing historiographical interpretation.[182] Peter Elmer argues more specifically that Greatrakes represented an implicit criticism of Charles II because the Irishman led a virtuous life, and attracted moderate 'Latitudinarians' and people who had done well during the Interregnum but now wished to be loyal to the Stuarts – and this was Greatrake's position too. By contrast, the king was dissolute, and parliament was dominated by cavaliers and had passed punitive legislation against nonconformity: Charles had not healed the nation's wounds despite touching thousands of sick people each year.[183]

---

[178] R.. Boyle to H. Stubbe, 9 Mar. 1666, in *The correspondence of Robert Boyle*, ed. M. Hunter, A. Clericuzio and L. M. Principe, London 2001, iii. 93–107.

[179] D. Lloyd, *Wonders no miracles, or, Mr. Valentine Greatrates gift of healing examined upon occasion of a sad effect of his stroaking, March the 7, 1665, at one Mr. Cressets house in Charter-house-yard*, London 1666.

[180] Greatrakes, *A brief account*.

[181] Stubbe, *Miraculous conformist*, 9; Lloyd, *Wonders no miracles*, 12–14, quotation at p. 14. This debate coincides with the publication of a short, inconclusive essay on the royal touch in the journal of the Royal Society: 'Some observations of the effects of touch and friction', *Philosophical Transactions* (1665–78), i. 206–9.

[182] Laver, 'Miracles', 35; Sturdy, 'Royal touch in England', 178; Thomas, *Religion and the decline of magic*, 203–4; Shaw, *Miracles*, 85, 97.

[183] Elmer, *Miraculous conformist*, chs iii–iv.

There is some truth in this, but it can be argued that Greatrakes was only a mild threat to Charles II. Certainly the king appears to have disliked the stroker: he was not invited to the royal court again after his failure to heal the four men there, while Walsh told Slingsby that Charles was 'far from having a good opinion of his person or his cures'.[184] The fact that Greatrakes initially touched for scrofula might have irked the king, and was probably tactless. But on reflection one can see the logic: Greatrakes tested his powers on scrofula presumably because it was the only disease in post-Reformation Britain that still had an official mandate to be cured miraculously by the laying on of hands.[185] Moreover, the king and the stroker were not the only two men in Britain in 1666 who cured scrofula by touch, despite this sometimes being implied in the secondary literature. Many of the healers of the 1640s and 1650s were still tending the sick during the Restoration. These were the people castigated by Lloyd, who even said that in Britain during the last fifty years, no less than fifty-seven Roman Catholic thaumaturgic healers were known.[186]

A comparison of the duration and scale of Greatrakes's ministry with the royal touch supports the view that the Irishman was not a serious threat to the crown. Greatrakes was only in England for the first six months of 1666, just after the ravages of the Great Plague and before the Great Fire. Not surprisingly, there is no evidence that Charles II touched for scrofula between 1665 and 1666.[187] This means that Greatrakes fulfilled the same role as the rival healers of the 1630s – he touched the sick at a time when the king was not available. As for the numbers treated by Greatrakes, although he was popular there is little hard evidence concerning the size of the crowds. He may have stroked 1,000 people during the month when he was at Ragley Hall, and thousands more when in London.[188] Yet this is insignificant compared to the king, who touched an average of 4,000 people every year for twenty-five years.

In relation to the curative practices of Greatrakes and the king, it is the differences rather than the similarities that are noteworthy. Although the Irishman began by touching for scrofula, he broadened out to a range of conditions and as such must have posed less of a challenge to the crown. If Greatrakes found that stroking was not sufficient to cure somebody, he would advise them to take medicine, or he would make incisions,[189] whereas the monarch did not.

---

184 HMC, 6th report, 39.
185 Walker, 'Greatrakes', 349.
186 Lloyd, Wonders no miracles, 6.
187 Browne, Adenochoiradelogia, 199.
188 Glanvill, A blow, 85; Elmer, Miraculous conformist, 81.
189 Stubbe, Miraculous conformist, 3.

A further reason that undermines the view of Greatrakes as a serious rival to the king is that the crown took no punitive action against the stroker. Unlike the healers of scrofula during the 1630s, Greatrakes was not, for a number of reasons, interrogated or persecuted by the government. Greatrakes differed from the healers of the 1630s in that he said nothing controversial about the royal touch; and he was an orthodox Anglican whose humility was evident in that he stated that his mission was to heal suffering bodies.[190] More broadly, many educated people were involved with a new culture of inquisitiveness, associated with the natural philosophers and the newly-formed Royal Society. This was an outlook shared by Charles II.[191] The curious, objective view of Greatrakes that was characteristic of the contemporary intellectual milieu can be glimpsed in a questionnaire compiled by Robert Boyle concerning the stroker's inspiration, methods and results.

Boyle asked if the Irishman used ceremony and prayers when stroking the sick:

> Whether before he applys himself to do a cure, he uses any Ceremony, or other words, or prayer; & if a Prayer whether he uses arbitrary words or some set Forme? and if the later what it is; As also whether whilst he is stroaking he imploy's any peculiar Rites, or words, or doe, or doe not, use to give thanks when he has done. And whether he require that Patient to doe, or say any thing, before & after he has stroakd.[192]

This is revealing as it suggests that Boyle wanted to compare Greatrakes's practices with those of the king, and that Boyle had the royal touch liturgy in mind. On the other hand, Boyle might have had in mind the many cunning folk who cured by touch, as it was commonplace for them to pray as they did so.[193]

Since at least the Reformation, the thaumaturgic sovereigns had touched people of various faiths and political persuasions, something that surely prompted Boyle to question 'Whether Mr. Greatrakes be able to cure Men of differing Religions, as Roman Catholicks, Socinians, [or] Jews'. Boyle must also have been aware of the view held by some people that if the royal touch worked it did so by psychosomatic means, as he asked whether the stroker

---

[190] It might be tempting to contrast the social status of Greatrakes, a JP, with the healers of the 1630s who appear to have been of a lowlier status – but the Frenchman was a knight and so this contrast is not helpful.

[191] Elmer, *Miraculous conformist*, 80; Weber, 'The monarch's sacred body', 76–7.

[192] 'Inquiries concerning Valentine Greatrakes', *Robert Boyles's 'heads' and 'inquiries'*, ed. M. Hunter (Robert Boyle Project occasional papers, i, 2005), 31–2, < http://www.bbk.ac.uk/boyle/researchers/works/Occasional_Papers/BOYLE%20Heads%20Revise3.pdf>

[193] For the cunning folk see Thomas, *Religion and the decline of magic*, 200. For healers of the 1630s see pp. 83–5 above.

had cured 'Infants, Naturalls, or destracted Persons to whose recovery the faith of the Patient cannot concurre'.[194]

Boyle's matter-of-fact questions betray no anxiety that Greatrakes undermined the crown; there is also no evidence that Greatrakes himself sought to do this – he was a law-abiding Anglican magistrate. It is true that during the 1650s he had held a military post for the Interregnum government, but Greatrakes came from a royalist family and worked for Cromwell purely for pragmatic reasons.[195] The most that can be said of him is that for six months he was a high-profile healer in England, which probably displeased Charles II.

James II: the problem of a Roman Catholic healer

Charles II died on 6 February 1685, having last touched 145 people for scrofula on 28 January; James II first touched for scrofula on 4 March even though he was not crowned until 23 April.[196] In 1686 James published what was claimed to be the Catholic royal touch liturgy of Henry VII as well as the cramp ring service dating from that reign. The suggestion is that James sought to reintroduce the Catholic form of the royal touch ceremony and to revive the cramp ring rite. Between May and June of 1686 James replaced his Church of England chaplains with his Jesuit confessors, in part to officiate at the Catholicised healing service.[197] One would imagine that a Roman Catholic king practising a Roman Catholic rite would be unpopular given the widespread anti-Catholicism of the day, but the evidence is more complex. It seems that James only used the pre-Reformation liturgy on occasion as it could cause hostility, to which he was sensitive.

The context for James's reforms are his aims concerning religion. He knew that he could not coerce the bulk of his Protestant subjects into becoming Catholic, so instead he sought to provide the pre-conditions for conversion. He sought to repeal punitive anti-Catholic legislation, and to promote Catholic men and policies. James had converted to Catholicism in the 1670s and he naively believed that others would too, if only the conditions were right.[198] Thus he reintroduced the Catholic liturgy for the royal touch, surely

---

[194] For the power of imagination see pp. 167–9 below.

[195] Elmer, *Miraculous conformist*, 37.

[196] Record of the numbers touched for the evil on various occasions, 1669–85, TNA, E407/85/1; *London Gazette*, 4 Mar. 1685.

[197] *The Flemings in Oxford*, ed. J. R. McGrath, Oxford 1904, ii, pp. xiv, xv, 2, 159; N. Luttrell, *A brief historical relation of state affairs, from September 1678 to April 1714*, Farnborough 1969, i. 376; cf. Crawfurd, who said that James published the liturgy but did not use it: *The king's evil*, 136.

[198] For James's Catholic policies see J. Miller, *Popery and politics in England, 1660–88*, Cambridge 1973, 196–264, and *James II: a study in kingship*, London 1978, 1989, chs ix–

hoping to expose thousands of people every year to its benefits; but against his enthusiasm for Roman Catholicism we have to weigh his pragmatism, in that he did not use the liturgy consistently because sometimes it was too divisive.

In 1686, when on progress in Winchester, James asked John Churchill what the people thought of his Catholic liturgy and Churchill told him it was unpopular.[199] This hostility could result in people withdrawing from the ceremony when they realised the king was not using the Church of England rite: this certainly occurred at Bath, in August 1687, when 220 people came to be touched.[200] James had not informed the bishop of Bath Thomas Ken, that he would use the Roman rite, which took Ken by surprise. This suggests that James did not use the Catholic liturgy all the time, and that on this occasion he sought to use it by stealth, but also that he anticipated problems. Ken had to give an account of this incident to Archbishop William Sancroft, indicating its contentiousness. Ken soothed the situation by saying that the abbey was the only place big enough to accommodate the crowd and that afterwards he preached on the subject of charity in order to calm tensions.[201] The next day James touched 140 people in the abbey. The sources are silent concerning which liturgy was used and any responses of the crowd, although the numbers present were significantly lower than the day before, which again suggests the unpopularity of the Catholic rite.[202]

Yet against this evidence must be balanced enthusiasm for the Catholic king's ceremonies, both before his changes in the summer of 1686 and afterwards. Between March and December 1685 James held thirty-eight ceremonies at which he touched 4,416 people, an average of 112 per ceremony.[203] Between January and June 1686 he held thirty-two ceremonies at which he touched 4,893, an average of 153 per ceremony.[204] In April 1686 the press reported that James had 'healed several Thousands' since the previous Michaelmas. After the summer of 1686 the evidence suggests either that the Catholic liturgy was not used very often, or that people's desire to be touched overruled any hostility that they felt towards it: in 1687 the press reported

xiv, and S. Sowerby, *Making toleration: the repealers and the Glorious Revolution*, Cambridge, MA–London 2013.

[199] A. Maynwaring, *The lives of two illustrious generals, John, duke of Marlborough and Francis Eugene, prince of Savoy*, London 1713, 19.

[200] Poley newletters, Beinecke Library, New Haven, OSB, MSS 1, box 2, folder 64. I am grateful to Robin Eagles for drawing my attention to this reference.

[201] E. R. Campana di Cavelli, *Les Derniers Stuarts à Saint-Germain en Laye: documents inédits et authentiques puisés aux archives publique et privées*, Paris 1871, ii. 108; A. Strickland, *The lives of the seven bishops committed to the Tower in 1688*, London 1866, 265–7.

[202] Poley newsletters, OSB, MSS 1, box 2, folder 64.

[203] TNA, E407/85/1.

[204] Document recording the numbers touched by James II on each of thirty-two occasions, 8 Jan.–20 June 1686, Wellcome Library, London, MS 5251.

that James had touched 'about 5000 Persons' whilst on a summer progress.[205] In 1687, when in Portsmouth, he touched 400 people in the chapel there; when in Oxford he touched between 700 and 800 people at one ceremony in the cathedral; and at Chester he held two ceremonies in the choir of the cathedral at which he touched 350 and 450 people respectively.[206] At times these large crowds taxed the king. In 1688 a strange break with custom occurred at one ceremony, in that when James was weary he would simply touch a piece of string that was around each sufferer's neck rather than stroke their sores. It was reported on the same occasion that Jesuits gave each person their touch-piece while the king touched their sores: it is noteworthy that Protestants would accept a touch-piece from a Jesuit, given the acute hostility to members of the Society.[207]

There is no concrete evidence of James's views on royal therapeutics, which is unfortunate; but James was cautious about miracles. He had a conversation to this effect with Thomas Ken in 1685, which was recorded by John Evelyn. James said 'he was so extreamly difficult of Miracles, for fear of being impos'd on, that if he should chance to see one himselfe, without some other witnesse, he should apprehend it some delusion of his senses'.[208] They then discussed a fraudulent miracle cure, as well as a number said to be authentic, including the healing of a blind woman by the blood of Charles I, after which they turned to the use of relics to cure diseases more broadly, and second sight.

In one respect, James's attitude towards his healing prerogative had more in common with that of Charles I than of Charles II in that he guarded it closely. After the ill-fated rebellion of the duke of Monmouth in 1685 was crushed, a bill of attainder was drawn up by parliament against the duke. This stated that Monmouth had been proclaimed king in Taunton by the people, had assumed the title of king, and had received the acclamation 'God save the king'. Most importantly, he had 'touched children off the king's evil'.[209] The duke had also touched for scrofula during his progress of 1680, when he toured Wiltshire, Somerset and Devon canvassing support from the Whig gentry as the 'Protestant successor' to Charles II; and he touched again in 1682 when touring Cheshire. From one point of view, Monmouth and his supporters used the royal touch to bolster his claim to

---

205 *London Gazette*, 8, 14 Apr. 1686; 19 Sept. 1687.

206 Poley newsletters, OSB MSS 1, box 2, folder 64; *Life and times of Anthony Wood*, iii. 231; E. Bernard to T. Smith, 4 Sept. 1687, Bodl. Lib., MS Smith 47, 46–7; T. Cartwright, *The diary of Dr Thomas Cartwright, bishop of Chester: commencing at the time of his elevation to that see, August M.DC.LXXXVI,; and terminating with the visitation of St Mary Magdalene College, Oxford, October M.DC.LXXXVII*, London 1843, 74–5.

207 Henri de Valburg Misson, M. *Misson's memoirs and observations in his travels over England*, trans. Mr Ozell, London 1719, 166–8.

208 J. Evelyn, *The diary of John Evelyn*, ed. E. S. De Beer, Oxford 1955, ii. 468–9.

209 T. B. Howell, *A complete collection of state trials*, xi, London 1811, cols 1059–60.

the throne, the context of which was the unprecedented enthusiasm for the ceremony during the 1680s. Yet the reality was that Monmouth never held actual healing ceremonies whilst on progress, and almost certainly did not do so in 1685. On both progresses one person approached the duke regarding scofula: in the West Country it was a young woman with scrofula, while in Cheshire a young man asked that his child be touched. Monmouth obliged each time, quickly touching the person but without liturgy or gold, simply saying 'God bless you'.[210] Whether these incidents were spontaneous or stage-managed is impossible to say, and there are no details at all concerning what happened in 1685. But as far as James II was concerned Monmouth was guilty of treason and *lèse-majesté*. There was no precedent for the heir to the throne touching for scrofula, let alone a royal bastard. Indeed, while Monmouth's therapeutic actions were no more than a very quiet echo of the royal touch, they might have done his cause more harm than good, as is suggested in a pamphlet that ridiculed his pretensions.[211] If Monmouth could touch for scrofula, then why not his half-sister too, which is exactly what happens in the satirical publication. It also mocked the 'black box' that was rumoured to contain the marriage certificate of Charles II and Monmouth's mother, Lucy Walter; the receptacle was an urban myth, but the pamphlet declared sarcastically that by healing scrofula Monmouth proved that 'God Almighty himself declare[d] for *The Black Box*'.[212]

Monmouth was executed for treason, not for touching the sick, but nevertheless James guarded his healing prerogative zealously, presumably because the royal touch was the most popular aspect of his kingship. His pro-Catholic policies were greatly disliked, yet thousands approached him each year to be touched for scrofula. This reminds us how deeply ingrained royal thaumaturgy was in English culture by this time, which in turn helps to explain why a Catholic king performed a Protestant ceremony. Moreover, despite the unpopularity of James's Catholic liturgy, for some people deference to the king must have taken precedence over religious differences.

The royal touch flourished during the Stuart age as in no other and was a central feature of English life at this time. The Stuarts touched ill people regardless of their religion, their political beliefs, or their nationality, while people sought the healing touch of both Protestant and Roman Catholic

---

[210] *His grace the duke of Monmouth honoured in his progress in the west of England in an account of a most extraordinary cure of the kings evil*, London 1680; *The Protestant (Domestic) Intelligence*, no. 86, Friday 7 Jan 1680; *CSPD*, 1682, 423.

[211] *A true and wonderful account of a cure of the kings-evil, by Mrs Fanshaw, sister to … the duke of Monmouth* (London 1681), scoffs at Monmouth's claims to heal. *An answer to a scoffing and lying libel put forth and privately dispersed under the title of a wonderful account of the curing of the kings-evil by Madam Fanshaw the duke of Monmouth's sister* (London 1681) exonerates the duke and blames his supporters for not realising that there is no precedent for an heir to the throne practising the royal touch.

[212] *A true and wonderful account*, 1.

kings. While it is true that monarchical authority was bolstered by royal thaumaturgy, the demand for the royal touch was so great that at times the process was difficult to manage. Sick people petitioned the crown in order to access the royal touch 'out of season' or when the king was absent from London; sometimes there was an insufficient number of Angels for the king to distribute at ceremonies; on occasion people had to wait for long periods in the capital before being touched; at other times the government had to organise extra ceremonies to accommodate large crowds of unwell people. Issues such as these reinforce the need to investigate the royal touch from both 'top down' and 'bottom up' perspectives in order to reveal the lived reality of the process.

Sacral monarchy survived the regicide as did the idea of the body politic. For republicans and monarchomachs the executioner's axe decapitated the man Charles Stuart as well as the mystical office of king, and in doing so killed the notion of the body politic as it was thought to be governed by the sovereign. But the king never dies and so the exiled Charles II immediately began to touch for scrofula on the continent, while the regicide was too extreme a denouement for most contemporaries. Once the Restoration was secured, extraordinary numbers of sick people flocked to Charles II to be touched. These people really were ill and sought relief, while at the same time the ritual process reasserted the re-capitation of the immortal office of king and the body politic. Thus politics, medicine and religion came together in corporeal form in the royal body and in scrofulous bodies to an extent hitherto unknown in England.

4

The Ritual Process of the Royal Touch, 1660–1688

This chapter analyses the actual administration of the royal touch during its Restoration heyday. It provides the first detailed social history of the process, comprising a 'bottom up' parochial investigation that shines light on the demand for royal therapeutics as well as a 'top down' interpretation that concentrates on monarchical authority. As more people were touched for scrofula during the reigns of Charles II and James II than at any other time in English history the evidence is especially plentiful from this period. We will examine the announcements made by the crown prior to the ceremony, the healing schedule, and the certificates written out by the clergy for parishioners who wished to be touched, stating that they did have scrofula and had not been touched before; the journeys that people made to the royal court; the assessments made by the king's surgeons to ensure that the supplicants did have scrofula; the ceremony itself; and the retrospective assessments made of it by officials and other eyewitnesses. The significance of the touch-pieces that were given to each ill person at the service will also be scrutinised.

During the Restoration people were ill with scrofula as in previous times, but the appeal of the royal touch was enhanced between 1660 and 1688 as it was seen as an antidote to the trauma of the Civil Wars, regicide and Interregnum. This chapter argues that the demand for the royal touch was so great during the reigns of Charles II and James II that there were times when all aspects of the ritual process were difficult to manage. The government was responsible for advertising the healing schedule, the clergy for granting certificates to parishioners who had scrofula, while the royal surgeons had to check that supplicants really did have the disease and had not been touched before, prior to granting admission to the ceremonies. Despite this orderly division of labour there were times when the procedure became chaotic, the evidence suggesting that the government was more efficient in its role than were the clergy and surgeons in theirs.

Prior announcements: the healing calendar, certification and registration

When Charles II entered London on 29 May 1660 some 2,000 people who were ill with scrofula had already congregated there because they wished to be touched by the king.[1] This was problematic because of the logistics of organising enough ceremonies to accommodate all these people: after all it had been almost twenty years since officials had last organised these services in London for Charles I, and never on this scale. Another problem was the season: the summer was approaching, bringing with it warm weather and the fear of infectious diseases such as the plague. Thus the government began to regulate demand for the royal touch by placing prominent notices in newspapers that announced the forthcoming healing schedule.[2] It was made known that henceforth the king would touch 200 people every Friday, usually in the Banqueting House, until everyone had received their therapeutic touch.[3] This proved inadequate though, and shortly afterwards it was announced that healings would occur on Wednesdays and Fridays until everyone had been touched.[4] During his reign Charles II issued at least thirty of these notices, reiterating that the royal touch was available for two to three week periods at Easter, Michaelmas and Christmas, or cancelling ceremonies due to hot weather.[5] James II issued at least six.[6] In 1662 the notices were supplemented by a proclamation which, unlike the newspapers, was to be read from every pulpit in the nation. It stated that healings would happen from the feast of All Saints (1 November) until a week before Christmas, and in the month before Easter.[7] Both types of notices reiterated the healing schedule that James VI and I and Charles I had tried to enforce.[8] It is worth remembering that, as during Charles I's reign, all of the Restoration notices also advertised the royal touch and so might have unintentionally increased the demand for it.

Charles II's serjeant surgeon John Browne published two registers of the numbers of people who were touched by the king. It is apparent, on revisiting these, that, despite the numerous notices in the press and the proclamation, the demand for royal therapeutics was so great that large numbers

---

[1] *Mercurius Publicus*, 28 June–5 July 1660; *CSPV* xxx/2, 182.

[2] For Restoration newspapers see J. Sutherland, *The Restoration newspaper and its development*, Cambridge 1986, and J. Raymond (ed.), *News, newspapers and society in early modern England*, London 1999.

[3] *Mercurius Publicus*, 28 June–5 July 1660; *CSPV* xxx/2, 182.

[4] *Parliamentary Intelligencer*, 16–23 July 1660; *Mercurius Publicus*, 19–26 July 1660.

[5] *Mercurius Publicus*, 28 June–5 July 1660; *Parliamentary Intelligencer*, 16–23 July 1660; *Mercurius Publicus*, 19–26 July 1660; *Parliamentary Intelligencer*, 30 July–6 Aug. 1660; *Mercurius Publicus*, 14–21 Feb. 1661; *The Kingdomes Intelligencer*, 29 Apr. 1661; *Mercurius Publicus* 2 May 1661; 3–10 April 1662; *London Gazette*, 4, 8 Apr. 1667; 13, 20 Apr. 1668; 14 Apr. 1670; 11 Apr., 18 Nov., 1672; 7, 10 Apr. 1673; 14 Dec. 1674; 12 Apr. 1675; 1 May 1676; 28 Apr. 1679; 21 May, 25 Apr. 1682; 5, 9 Apr., 24 May, 7 June 1683; 24 Jan., 20, 23 Oct. 1684.

[6] *London Gazette*, 2 Mar. 1685; 8, 14, 19 Apr., 7 Oct. 1686; 19 Sept. 1687.

[7] 'A proclamation for the better ordering of those who repair to the court for their cure of the disease called the kings-evil', Hampton-Court, 4 July 1662.

[8] See pp. 77, 80 above.

of people were touched throughout the four summers from 1660 to 1663; it was not until 1664 that summer healings stopped. Thus in the first years of the Restoration Charles II had to deal with a 'backlog' of scrofulous people who had been unable to be touched during the Civil Wars and Interregnum. The healing calendar was then closely adhered to between 1668 and 1679.[9] The greatest recorded demand for the royal touch was between 1680 and 1685, coinciding with the Tory reaction. This explains why in 1684 a second proclamation reaffirmed the autumn timetable and gave notice of the spring timetable. It also stated that Charles would touch for scrofula when on progress, so as to lessen the need for people in the provinces to travel to London and to alleviate some of the pressure on those in the capital who organised the ceremony.[10] To reinforce this, the archbishop of Canterbury instructed his bishops to tell their clergy to read out the proclamation in church and to display it in a prominent place.[11]

Although the crown announced the periods when healing ceremonies would occur, it did not say on which specific days they would happen: presumably people made their way to court and then waited for information concerning the exact dates. However, the reality seems to have been that the schedule was not always adhered to: why else were so many notices needed? The Lord Chamberlain also noted that Charles II sometimes held ceremonies without consideration of the calendar, and that these decisions needed to be publicised, often at short notice.[12]

The crown required those who wished to be touched to provide a certificate from their minister which stated that they had scrofula but had not been touched before, a policy that had been first introduced by Charles I in 1625.[13] The problem with people being touched more than once was three-fold. It lessened the mystique of the ceremony; it meant that the crowd was larger than it need be; and it provided an opportunity for a small number of people to obtain more than one touch-piece and so 'cheat the King of his Gold'.[14] The requirement to obtain a certificate was communicated to the public in the proclamations of 1662 and 1684, as well as in many newspapers.[15] The

---

[9] Browne, *Adenochoiradelogia*, 197–9. For the combined summer months of May, June, July and August Charles touched 2,765 people in 1660, 889 in 1661, 599 in 1662, and 1,520 in 1663. In May and June of 1664 he touched 1,217 with no further healings until September.

[10] 'At the Court at Whitehall', Whitehall, 9 Jan. 1684.

[11] West Sussex Record Office, Chichester, PAR94/7/7, an injunction from the bishop of Chichester (Guy Carleton) about an order in council relating to touching for the kings evil, 12 Feb. 1683/4.

[12] TNA, LC5/141, 33. This is one of the Lord Chamberlain's warrants, evidence that will be discussed in the last section of this chapter.

[13] See p. 80 above.

[14] Browne, *Adenochoiradelogia*, 87.

[15] See, for example, *Mercurius Publicus*, 14–21 Feb.

1684 proclamation further required ministers and churchwardens to keep a register of the certificates that they issued, and this too was announced in the newspapers.[16] If the period for healings was drawing to a close, the government sometimes told ministers not to issue any more certificates until further notice.[17]

The ministers and churchwardens who were required to provide certificates sometimes wrote out a *pro-forma* certificate in their parish registers, and it was here too that they often kept lists of the names of those to whom certificates were issued.[18] As wide a search has been carried out as is practicable and so far nineteen copy certificates have been traced from thirteen counties, dating from 1682 to 1687;[19] related lists have emerged in forty-six registers from seventeen counties dating from 1672 to 1714.[20] No actual certificates that were given to people with scrofula have surfaced and no material has emerged from the earlier part of the century. Although this is the largest body of royal touch administrative data yet surveyed, considering that the clergy were requested to keep scrupulous records, it is surprising that more evidence has not come to light. The reiteration of the govern-

---

[16] 'At the Court at Whitehall', Whitehall, 9 Jan. 1684.

[17] *London Gazette*, 24 May 1683.

[18] For parish registers see C. J. Cox, *The parish registers of England*, London 1910; W. E. Tate, *The parish chest: a study of the parochial administration in England*, Cambridge 1951; D. J. Loschky, 'The usefulness of England's parish registers', *Review of Economics and Statistics* xlix/4 (1967), 471–79; A. Smyth, *Autobiography in early modern England*, Cambridge 2010, ch. iv. For brief discussions of certificates and lists see F. H. Arnold, 'Sussex certificates for the royal touch', *Sussex Archaeological Collections* xxv (1873), 402–12, and Woolf, 'Sovereign remedy', 103–4.

[19] All Saints, Maidstone, parish chest accounts, 1667–1727, Kent History and Library Centre, Maidstone P241/12/11 (x2); Amersham, register of burials in woollen, 1678–1717, Centre for Buckinghamshire Studies, Aylesbury, PR4/1/3; Bampton parish register, 1653–97, Oxfordshire History Centre, Oxford, 1653–97, PAR16/1/R1/2, fo. 3b; Faccombe, parish register, 1678–1795, Hampshire Record Office, Winchester, 91M79/PR2; Grasmere, parish register, 1570–1687, Kendal Archive Centre, Kendal, WPR/92/1/1; Great Hormead, parish register, 1538–1724, Hertfordshire Archives, Hertford, DP55/1/1; Horton Kirby, parish register, 1671–1810, Kent History and Library Centre, Maidstone, P193/1/1; Maulden, parish register, 1678–1702, Bedfordshire and Luton Archives and Records Service, Bedford, P31/1/3; Much Wenlock general register, 1642–98, Shropshire Archives, Shrewsbury, P198/A/1/2; St Botolph, Boston, rough register, 1683–1769, Lincolnshire Archives, Lincoln, Par/1/4A; St Mary's, Lichfield, parish register, 1677–1754, Lichfield Record Office, Lichfield, D20/1/2; St Mary the Virgin, Kelvedon, parish register, 1653–1773, Essex Record Office, Chelmsford, DP/134/1/2; South Stoneham, parish register, Hampshire Record Office, Winchester, SRO/PR9/1/1; Welwyn, vestry minute book, 1658–1731, Hertfordshire archives, Hertford, DP119/8/3; Winterbourne Stickland, burials register, 1678–1750, Dorset History Centre, Dorchester, PE/WSD/RG4/1; Witley, All Saints parish records, 1653–1771, Surrey History Centre, Woking, PSH/WIT/1/1; BL, MSS Sloane 206 B, fos 61, 62; 2723, fo. 57.

[20] Brogan, 'Royal touch' (dissertation), appendix 2, 245–6.

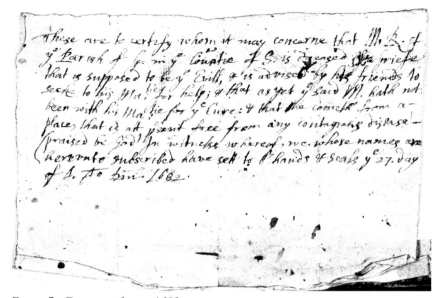

Figure 7. Copy certificate, 1682.

ment's administrative requests to the clergy indicates that it was aware that these tasks were not being properly carried out: people were arriving to be touched without providing certificates. This was a problem that was regularly addressed in the press.[21] The clergy were even accused publicly of committing a 'great neglect' of their duties.[22] However, there were no punitive consequences for them, so the extant records reflect the degree of conscientiousness of the local ministers.

A *pro-forma* certificate has survived at Witley, Surrey, dated 1682, which is suggestive of a real certificate (*see* Figure 7). It states that the bearer is 'advised by his friends to seeke his Majesty for help; and that as yet the said Mr hath not been with his majesty for the Cure; & that he cometh from a place that is att present free from any contagious disease (praised be God)'.[23]

In 1684 the government decided to standardise the certificates by publishing in the press the wording that it wanted ministers to use. This stipulates that the bearer has scrofula and had not been touched before:

We the Ministers and Church-Wardens of the parish of [——] in the City/County/Borough of [——] do hereby Certify that [gap] of this Parish [gap] aged about [gap] years, is afflicted as we are credibly informed with the Disease

---

[21] *Mercurius Publicus* 14–21 Feb. 1661; *London Gazette*, 18 Nov. 1672; 21 May, 25 Apr. 1682; 5, 9 Apr., 7 June 1683; 20, 23 Oct. 1684; 7 Oct. 1686; 19 Sept. 1687.

[22] *London Gazette*, 20, 23 Oct. 1684.

[23] All Saints, Witley, Surrey, PSH/WIT/1/1.

commonly called the Kings Evil; And (to the best of our knowledge) hath not heretofore been Touched by His Majesty for the said Disease. In Testimony whereof we have hereunto set our Hands and Seals this [——] day of [——] 168[——].[24]

This seems to have been a successful strategy: the wording is reflected in all the certificates that date from after this announcement.[25] Interestingly, there was no need for the named person to be able to read the certificate, and he or she was not required to sign it. The royal touch certificates are the earliest examples of certificates that relate to ill health, and the only examples of ones that relate to spiritual healing. As such they provide an incongruous combination of the bureaucratic and the mystical.

It is worth remembering that some people bypassed the whole certification procedure because the certificates were handwritten and so could be counterfeited.[26] In 1663 two women who lived in Westminster, Mary Lane and her daughter, were prosecuted for 'forging of false certificates pretending to have the disease called the Kings Evill, on purpose thereby to cheat his Majestie of his gold'.[27]

Once the certificate had been written out the crown expected a record to be kept including the recipient's name and the date that it was granted. These lists vary in scale from a memorandum recording that a single person had received a certificate, to an extensive list containing 200 or more names over a range of several years.[28] Certain lists are revealing in relation to the gender, age and status of those who sought the royal touch. Forty-six lists have been identified, containing a total of 623 entries, 68 per cent of which relate to women and 32 per cent to men.[29] This suggests either that the royal touch appealed more to women than to men, or that slightly more than twice as many women as men had scrofula. If the latter were the case, this might have been because one source of employment that was relatively open to women was dairy production and the bovine strand of the bacillus that caused scrofula was particularly robust. If more women than men had scrofula it could have been because they were more likely to have contact

---

[24] *London Gazette*, 20, 23 Oct. 1684.

[25] All Saints, Witley, Surrey, PSH/WIT/1/1; St Mary the Virgin, Kelvedon, Essex, DP/134/1/2; Welwyn, Hertfordshire, DP119.

[26] Browne, *Adenochoiradeogia*, 85.

[27] *Middlesex county records*, ed. J. C. Jeafferson, London 1886–92, iii. 334. I am grateful to Peter Elmer for this reference.

[28] For a single memorandum see Bagendon parish records, 1630–1742, Gloucestershire Archives, Gloucester, P33IN1/1, fo. 22; for the latter see St Nicholas, Deptford, composite register, 1638–1735, London Metropolitan Archive, P78/NIC/3/1–4.

[29] Brogan, 'Royal touch' (dissertation), appendix 2, 245–6.

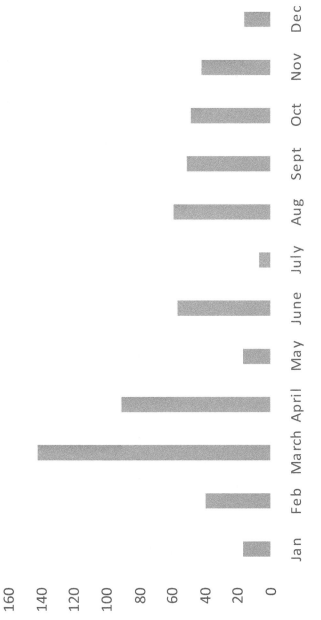

Figure 8. The healing calendar: the number of people touched for scrofula, 1673–1714.

with contaminated milk.[30] The lists also reveal that sometimes more than one person in a family had scrofula.[31]

In terms of age, the range within the sample is from a young child of 'about a year and a quarter' to a woman aged 'about 68 years'.[32] It is frustrating that people's occupations or roles are rarely recorded although some have come to light; we do hear of three husbandmen and a carpenter,[33] a labourer,[34] a glover,[35] a sergeant, a butcher, an inn keeper, a blacksmith and a cooper,[36] as well as two servants[37] and a butcher's daughter.[38] A small number of orphans were also given certificates.[39] Very occasionally a man was recorded as a 'gent' or 'Esquire',[40] while the parish register of Eton records the names of five scholars who were touched in 1686 by James II, including 'the Honourable Mr Charles Cecill', son of the earl of Salisbury.[41]

The extant lists indicate that there was greater registration during the three-year reign of James II than the twenty-five year reign of Charles II, which is indicative of the success of the government's drive to enforce the registration process that began with the proclamation of January 1684, and continued during the next reign.[42] The lists also reveal a general adherence to the seasonal healing calendar. A a total of 588 entries have been legibly dated for the period from 1673 to 1714[43] (See Figure 8).

It is striking that March has the largest total, followed by April, both of which relate to the regularity and popularity of the Easter ceremonies. July has the lowest total, in accordance with the crown's desire to avoid summer healings. It is worth noting that August's total would be barely higher than July's were it not for one healing ceremony undertaken by James II whilst

---

[30] See p. 17 above. For seventeenth-century attitudes to milk see J. C. Drummond, *The Englishman's diet*, London 1940, 148–9.

[31] Andover, Hampshire, register of burials, 60M67/PR4.

[32] Amersham, Buckinghamshire PR4/1/3; Whitchurch, Buckinghamshire, parish register, 1653–92, PR230/1/1.

[33] Stoke, Surrey, parish records PSH/STK/1/1.

[34] St Katherine's, Merstham, Surrey, parish records, 1538–1902, P23/1/1.

[35] Kempston, Bedfordshire, register book, 1680–1721, P60/1/9.

[36] All from Holy Trinity, Surrey, parish records, 1558–1812, PSH/GU/HT/1/1.

[37] Andover, Hampshire, register of burials, 60M67/PR4; Irnham, Lincolnshire, general register, PAR1/1, fo. 31.

[38] All from Maidstone, Kent, parish chest accounts, 1667–1727, P241/5/21.

[39] All Saints, Witley, Surrey, parish records, PSH/WIT/1/1.

[40] St Nicholas, Deptford, composite register, London Metropolitan, P78/NIC/3/1–4; Petworth, West Sussex, composite register, 1559–1794, WSRO Par 149/1/1/1, fo. 184.

[41] Eton, Buckinghamshire, parish register, 1653–1715, PR72/1/2.

[42] Brogan, 'Royal touch' (dissertation), 148.

[43] The monthly totals are 17 for January, 40 for February, 142 for March, 91 for April, 17 for May, 57 for June, 7 for July, 59 for August, 51 for September, 49 for October, 42 for November and 16 for December.

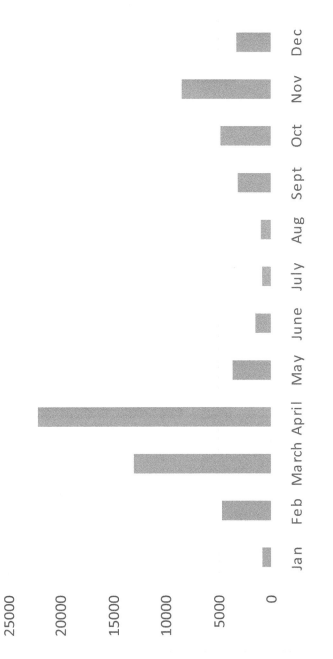

Figure 9. The healing calendar: the number of people touched for scrofula, May 1667–April 1682.

on progress in Lichfield in 1687, the demand for which produced thirty-five of the month's fifty-nine certificates, while another twelve were connected to his ceremony at Eton.[44] If these figures are correlated with Browne's data from *Adenochoiradelogia* and monthly totals from 1667 to 1682 calculated (the period 1660–4 has a number of months that have joint totals and so that data cannot be included), the popularity of the Easter ceremonies, and the small number of summer healings. is again notable (*see* Figure 9).[45] The conclusion is that the proclamations and newspapers continually reminding the population of the healing calendar during the Restoration period evidently worked, in that the king avoided touching large numbers of people during the summer, whether he was in London or the provinces.

The journey to the king

Once someone had acquired a certificate and been registered, they needed to journey to the royal court. The certificate could act as permit to travel or sometimes a separate permit was issued.[46] The lists draw attention to the geography of royal thaumaturgy. They indicate that the bulk of the people who sought the royal touch lived in the south of England and the midlands, and so had relatively easy journeys to London. On the other hand, Brown reported that people from England, Wales, Ireland, Scotland, France and Holland had all been touched by the king, and even from Russia and Virginia, America.[47] The French and the Dutch could have accessed Charles II's touch during his exile, but nevertheless some ill people made very long, arduous and expensive journeys to him. Monarchs spent a large proportion of their time in and around the capital and in April 1686 the press reported that in the last six months James II had 'Healed several Thousands, the greatest parts of which were habitants of *London*'.[48] On the other hand, during the summer the king was on progress, which gave people the opportunity to be touched without making an onerous journey to London.

A journey to the Stuart court could be costly, as could the provision of lodgings, and if this was beyond the means of a parishioner he or she could apply for financial help from parish funds. In 1663 the parish of Thornbury in Gloucestershire paid 5s. to 'Margrett Scott to goo to Bath to the King to have her Daughter Cured of the evill'.[49] No doubt this was less expen-

---

[44] St Mary, Lichfield, Buckinghamshire, parish register, D20/1/2; Eton, Buckinghamshire, parish register, 1653–1715, PR72/1/2.

[45] Browne, *Adenochoiradelogia*, 199–207.

[46] Pass for Anne Story and her daughter to travel from Carlisle to London to be touched by Charles II, 25 June 1681, BL, MS Sloane 2723, fo. 57.

[47] Browne, *Adenochoiradelogia*, 105, 139, 194–5.

[48] *London Gazette*, 8, 14 Apr. 1686.

[49] Thornbury, Gloucestershire, overseers' accounts, 1655–69, D688/1.

sive than sending her to London. In 1664 the parish of Cowden in Kent paid 15s. 10d. to two women 'John Stills Wife and Elizabeth Dimond', so that they could go 'to London to bee touched of the King's evill'; another payment of 6d. was made a few days later to Elizabeth Dimond so that her clothes could be mended – it was important to look as smart as possible in the presence of the king.[50] The parish might not pay the full amount required: in Tonbridge in 1671 it was specified that one Goodman Hayward received 10s. towards the cost of sending his apprentice to the court to be touched.[51] Part payments were also made at Kendal between 1661 and 1662 to John Shackley so that his wife could travel to London, and to Adam Sadler, both of whom received the sum of 30s. At the same time the same parish paid 25s. each to John Askew's wife and Elizabeth Rigge's daughter for the same journey, which may suggest that payments were means tested.[52] Aside from parish funds, a person who needed financial assistance could approach a friend, relative or other contact: in October 1669 a gentleman resident in Oxfordshire gave £10 'unto my Brother Roger towards his charges in goeing unto London to get the Kings Touch for the Evill'.[53]

The fact that parishioners received money from parish funds is indicative of the widespread belief in the possibility that the royal touch might cure scrofula. It seems improbable that money would have been given to assist someone to seek a remedy that was thought not to work. It also represents the desire of the parish and others to help those with scrofula return to good health in order that they could work and support themselves.

Accessing the royal touch

Once the travellers had arrived at their destination they had to make their way to the king's serjeant surgeons, who examined them to ensure that they had scrofula because so far this had only been affirmed by a minister. This is an early example of a public, government-regulated health process. The surgeons were appointed by the Lord Chamberlain. Originally three in number, the surgeons performed their royal touch duties on monthly rotation until their number was reduced to one in 1685.[54] Although the surgeons had

---

[50] Cowden, Kent, overseers accounts, 1599–1835, P99/12 /1; cf. Tong, Shropshire, Salop churchwardens' account book, 1630–80, P28/B/1/1/1.

[51] Tonbridge, Kent, parish chest accounts, 1670–1806, P371/12/1/6.

[52] Kendal, Cumberland, chamberlain's accounts, 1661–2, WSMB/K/1/5.

[53] *The Flemings in Oxford*, i. 453.

[54] J. C. Sainty and R. O. Bucholz, *Officials of the royal household 1660–1837*, I: *Department of the Lord Chamberlain and associated offices*, London 1997–8, 47–9, which includes a list of all the surgeons; Lord Chamberlain's department: miscellaneous records: warrant books: 'Orders for chyrurgeons at healings', TNA, LC5/140, 493–4.

to deal with large numbers of people their directives instructed them not to accept any payment from the public; however, one commentator did claim that money sometimes changed hands.[55] With the exception of travel and accommodation expenses, the royal touch was meant to be available free of charge.

During the Restoration the most renowned serjeant surgeon was Richard Wiseman (c.1620–76) whose *Several chirurgicall treatises* (1676) contained a study of scrofula and a brief discussion of the royal touch.[56] Wiseman held the view that the royal touch should be the last resort for particularly hard-to-treat cases of scrofula, to be used when all other methods had failed. When assessing people's scrofula sometimes he turned people away, recommending medicine rather than the king's touch.[57] A similar approach had occasionally been adopted by Elizabeth I's surgeons.[58]

From June 1660 onwards the medical examinations were scheduled to take place at the surgeon's house between one and three days before the ceremony, as was announced regularly in the press.[59] In the Tudor period the assessment had happened at court on the morning of the ceremony, and in the absence of any evidence from the first half of the seventeenth century it appears that this remained the case until 1660.[60] The new arrangements allowed the surgeons more time to assess large numbers of people and meant that those who were turned away were not at court when the ceremony occurred, which avoided the possibility of disturbances.[61]

In reality the situation was complex: there is evidence that because people were ill and wanted relief they were not always concerned about the niceties of diagnosis, or might prefer self-diagnosis. In 1682 although the daughter of the Lancashire gentlemanman Sir Thomas Preston had been diagnosed with chicken pox, his wife was certain that the swelling on her daughter's lip was scrofula: when Charles II was in Chester she was determined to take her daughter there so that she could be touched.[62] Browne mentioned people who self-diagnosed with scrofula and travelled great distances to the king, only to

---

[55] TNA, LC5/140, 493; T. A., *Excellency*, 30.

[56] Wiseman, *Several chirurgicall treatises*, pt IV, 248–306.

[57] Ibid. 250.

[58] See p. 67 above; *Charisma*, 93.

[59] *Mercurius Publicus*, 28 June–5 July 1660; *Parliamentary Intelligencer*, 16–23 July 1660; *Mercurius Publicus*, 19–26 July 1660; *Kingdomes Weekly Intelligencer*, 29 Apr. 1661; *Mercurius Publicus* 2 May 1661; *London Gazette*, 7 Oct. 1686.

[60] Tooker, *Charisma*, 94.

[61] *Mercurius Publicus*, 28 June–5 July 1660; *Parliamentary Intelligencer*, 16–23 July 1660; *Mercurius Publicus*, 19–26 July 1660; *The Kingdomes Intelligencer*, 29 Apr. 1661; *Mercurius Publicus* 2 May 1661; *London Gazette*, 7 Oct. 1686.

[62] T. Preston to R. Kenyon, Lancashire Archives, Preston, DDKE/HMC/434.

be turned away as they did not have the disease.[63] Presumably some of their symptoms were akin to scrofula, though on occasion the surgeons themselves were uncertain whether someone had the disease, and might err on the side of caution. The Norfolk physician Sir Thomas Browne (1605–82) wrote to his son in London concerning a neighbour who wished to be touched although the tumour on her throat was not 'the common Evil': Browne asked his son to direct her to the king's surgeons as 'the king toucheth many in the like case'.[64] Yet the medical assessment conducted by the royal surgeons was no mere formality: a rare surviving piece of evidence states that the surgeon must give 'tickets only to apparent cases [of scrofula]' and that if they were uncertain whether or not the person had scrofula they could be examined again at a later date.[65] In 1683 one Elizabeth Newman travelled from Hendon to London to be touched, but did not pass the medical assessment: a note in her parish register records that 'it did not appear to be the Evill and so she was not toucht'.[66]

If someone was assessed as having scrofula the surgeon then gave them an admission pass to the next ceremony. Originally these were metal tokens, some of which were similar to Angels; but a change occurred at some point whereby paper tickets were issued, which presumably had people's names written on them as well as details of the next ceremony, and so could not be used more than once. Dispensing these passes was not necessarily as straightforward as it sounds because Charles II did not always adhere to his own healing schedule, meaning that people could spend a long time in London waiting to be touched, which could be tedious and expensive.[67] Indeed, sometimes the surgeons themselves had to ascertain the date of the next ceremony by looking for announcements in the press.[68] The worst-case scenario was that someone had to wait so long that their finances were exhausted before they were touched. Thus William Denton, one of the king's physicians, lamented in November 1675 that it was impossible to know when the next ceremony would occur. He even had to lend 20s. to two people who had travelled 'above 100 miles' whose money had run out, so they could return home despite not being touched – and this was after he had spoken up for them at court.[69]

---

[63] Browne, *Adenochoiradelogia*, 86.

[64] Sir Thomas Browne to his son Edward in London, 29 Oct. 1679, in *The letters of Sir Thomas Browne*, ed. Geoffrey Keynes, London 1931, 154.

[65] *CSPD, 1661–2*, 428.

[66] St Mary's, Hendon, composite register, 1653–1744, London Metropolitan Archive DRO/029/001.

[67] Browne, *Adenochoiradelogia*, p. 88.

[68] HMC, *Seventh report: the manuscripts of Sir Harry Verney, Bart., at Claydon House, Co. Bucks*, calendared A. J. Horwood, London 1879, 493.

[69] Ibid.

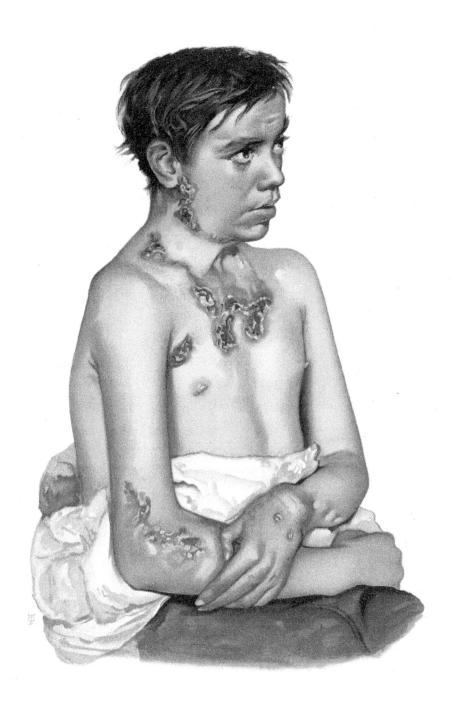

1. 'A young man with scrofula', from Bramwell, *Atlas of clinical medicine*, ii, plate 32.

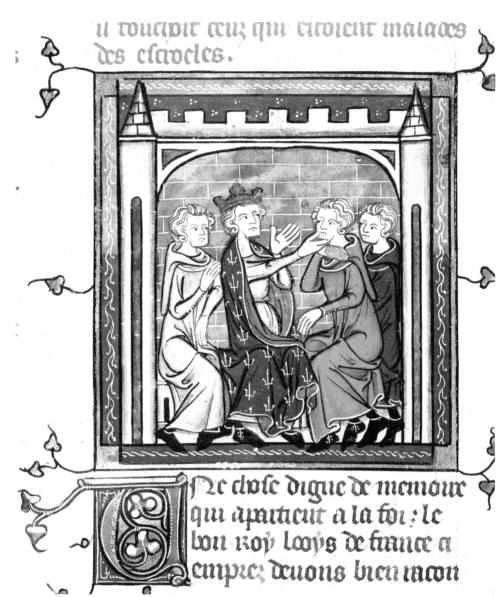

il touchoit ceuz qui eſtoient malades
des eſcroeles.

Ne choſe digne de memoire
qui apartient a la foi: le
bon roy loöys de france a
empres: deuons bien racon

2. 'Louis IX touches a scrofulous man', from *Les Grandes Chroniques de France*, BL MS Royal 16 G VI, fo. 424.

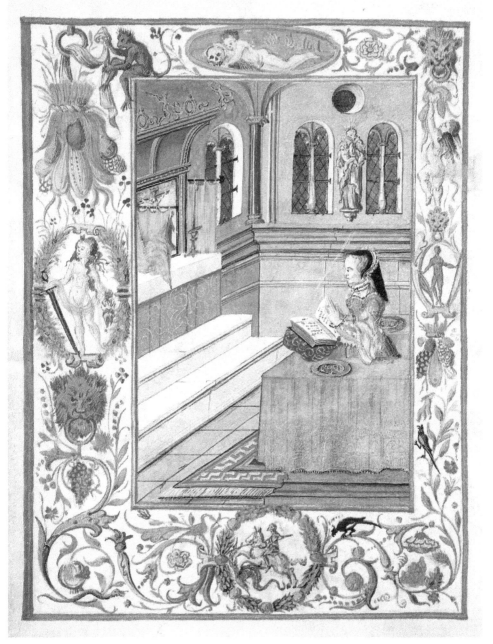

3. 'Mary Tudor praying in an oratory with a bowl of cramp rings to either side of her', Mary Tudor's missal, Westminster Cathedral Treasury, London, MS 7.

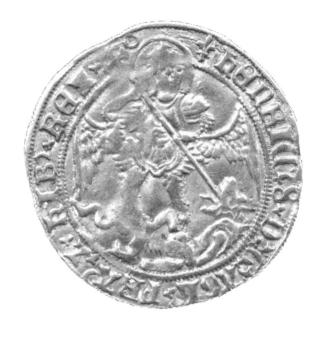

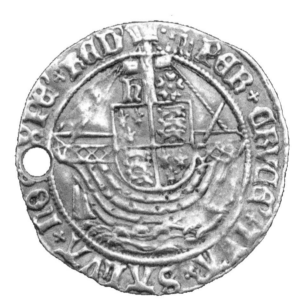

4. Henry VII Angel coin. 26mm. diameter.

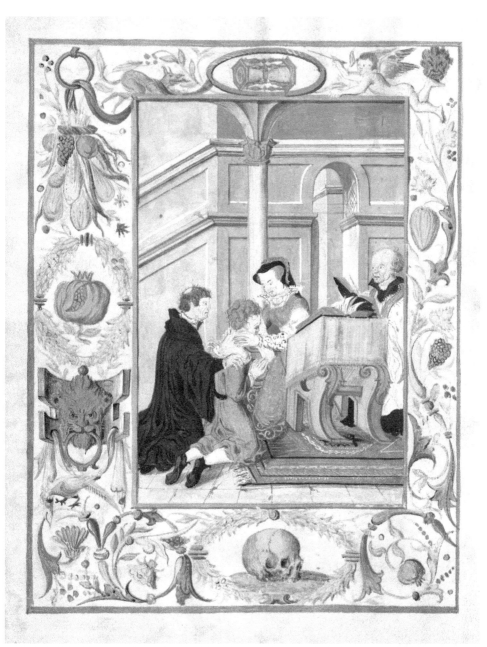

5. 'Mary Tudor touches a scrofulous boy', Mary Tudor's missal.

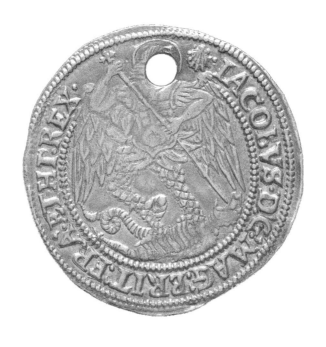

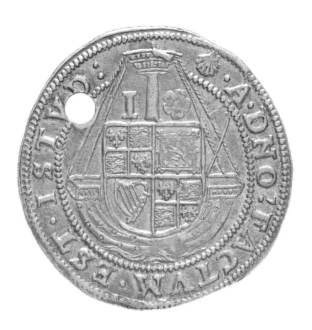

6. James VI and I Angel coin. 29mm. diameter.

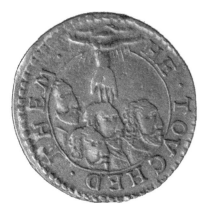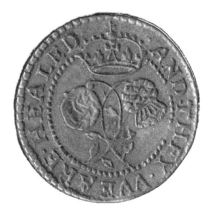

7. Charles I admission token to royal touch ceremony.

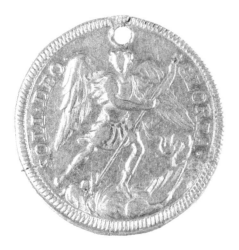

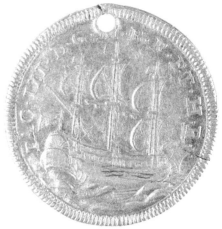

8. A rare gold touch-piece of James Stuart, the Old Pretender, styled James VIII and III. 20mm. diameter.

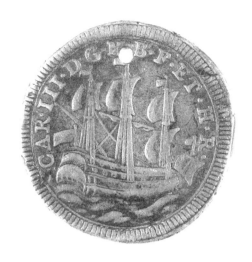

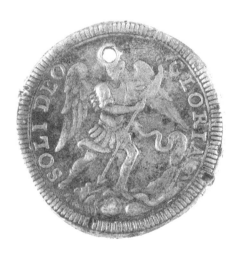

9. A touch-piece of Charles Edward Stuart, the Young Pretender, styled Charles III. 20mm. diameter.

The procedure for obtaining a pass was regularly described in newspapers in order to familiarise people with it. This extract from *Mercurius Publicus* is typical in telling those who wished to be touched

> first to repair to Mr. *Knight* his Majesties Chyrurgion, living at the Cross–Tavern, for their Tickets. That none might lose their labour, he thought fit to make it known, that he will be at his house every Wednesday and Thursday from two till six of the clock, to attend that service: And if any person of quality shall send to him, he will wait upon them at their lodgings, upon notice given to him.[70]

The 'quality' could thus arrange for the surgeon to visit them at home in order to avoid the long hours of waiting that were followed by frenzied activity once the procedure started. The consequences of this could be extreme. John Evelyn recorded an occasion in 1684, during the peak of demand for royal therapeutics, when the crush of people outside the surgeon's door was so great that several were killed.[71] Less dramatic was the comment made by Browne in the same year that 'it is harder to approach the Chirurgeon [to acquire a ticket for the ceremony], than obtain a Touch [at the ceremony itself]'.[72]

Not surprisingly, those with creative minds, money or contacts sought to circumvent the medical assessment and, if they were not well-connected enough to arrange for the surgeon to visit them, they still had a number of options. One way to speed up the process rather than bypass it was for a local physician to write to the king's surgeon informing him about someone coming from his parish with a certificate to be touched. The hope was to establish a relationship whereby the surgeon would trust the provincial certification process because it involved a minister and a doctor. This may be the manner in which Sir Thomas Browne in Norfolk operated: he wrote to his son that 'His Majesty cometh this day to newmarkett and I shall have occasion to write unto sirjeant Knight and send certificates for the evell for divers.'[73] If the sick person wished to avoid waiting at the surgeon's house then they could send someone to obtain a ticket on their behalf. This was problematic because it meant that the surgeon did not assess the sick person, and yet, as the surgeons received directives from the Lord Chamberlain instructing them not to operate in this manner, the suggestion is that it

---

[70] *Mercurius Publicus*, 28 June–5 July, for 27 June 1660. When the surgeon changed his address, a new announcement with the new address was made in the press: *Parliamentary Intelligencer*, 16–23 July 1660; *Mercurius Publicus*, 19–26 July 1660.

[71] *Diary of John Evelyn*, iv. 374.

[72] Browne, *Adenochoiradelogia*, 89.

[73] Sir Thomas Browne to his son Edward in London, 2 Oct. 1679, in *Letters of Sir Thomas Browne*, 151.

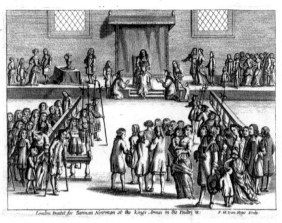

Figure 10. *The manner of his majesties curing the disease, called the kings-evil,* London 1679, BM 1849, 0315.31.

did sometimes occur.[74] Two other options involved using contacts at court, which could include circumventing the surgeons altogether. Some people appear to have found someone such as a courtier to intercede with one of the surgeons, or an official who was involved with the ceremony and had access to a small number of entrance tickets.[75] Samuel Pepys used his influence in May 1681 to obtain tickets for friends by writing directly to his friend James Pearce, a royal surgeon.[76]

The ceremony

There are a number of written sources that describe the ceremony, Browne's account in *Adenochoiradelogia* being the most detailed and trustworthy as he so often witnessed both public and private rites.[77] As well as textual sources it is fortunate that two printed images survive of Charles II touching for scrofula. The broadside entitled *The manner of his majesties curing the disease called the kings-evill* (1679), consists of an engraving of the ceremony by the Dutchman F. H. Van Hove, with the healing liturgy beneath it (*see* Figure 10).[78] In the year that it was produced Charles touched 3,582 people so the broadside could have been created as a memento for sale. The second image is Robert White's engraving 'The royal gift of healing', the frontispiece to *Adenochoiradelogia*, (*see* Figure 1), which is a more closely framed depiction than that on the broadside. This dates from 1684, a year in which Charles touched at least 6,000 people, one of the highest annual totals of his reign. White's frontispiece served to attract potential purchasers of Browne's book by illustrating the ceremony that was described in it. Both images were topical, the frontispiece depicting Charles at the height of the demand for his sacred touch.

Those who wished to be touched for scrofula had to make their way to the appointed building on the correct day at the right time. The ceremony might be held because it was the healing season, or on the whim of the king, or because 'ordinary' people had petitioned Charles to hold one, as when the

---

[74] Lord Chamberlain's department: miscellaneous records: warrant books: 'Orders for healings', TNA, LC5/144, p. 195.

[75] TNA, LC5/140, pp. 493–4; Browne, *Adenochoiradelogia*, 155–6, 171–2, 174.

[76] Samuel Pepys to James Pearce, 18 May 1681, Bodl. Lib., MS Rawlinson A194, fos 247v–248r.

[77] Browne, *Adenochoiradelogia*, 79, 83–103. See also van Wicquefort, *Relation*, 74–8; L. Magalotti, *Travels of Lorenzo the third, Grand Duke of Tuscany, through England, during the reign of King Charles II* (1669), London 1821, 214–16; *Diary of John Evelyn*, ii. 250–1; Misson, *Misson's memoirs*, 166–8; W. Shellinks, *The journal of William Schellinks' travels in England, 1661–1663*, ed. and trans. M. Exwood and H. L. Lehmann, London 1993, 72–3.

[78] *The manner of his majesties curing the disease called the kings-evill*. London 1679. At present three copies of this broadside are known: BM, 1849,0315.31; Ashmolean Museum, Oxford, Sutherland 114 (229); Bodl. Lib., MS Firth b.16 (1).

nobility solicited him to hold private ceremonies.[79] As in France the services were held in the morning,[80] while Browne informs us that by 1684 Charles's preferred day for them was Sunday (if he was not holding them more than once a week, as at Easter).[81]

The size of the crowd varied. During the first weeks of the Restoration Charles II touched between 200 and 600 people at any one ceremony,[82] though this was quickly limited to a maximum of 200 people.[83] Thereafter the numbers present ranged from 50 to 200 people, though occasionally it increased to as many as 335.[84] Wherever the ceremony was held it was necessary to have a room big enough to accommodate the crowd and the officials, and so the royal touch was usually held in the hall or chapel of a palace or in a cathedral. When in London, the Stuarts touched at the Banqueting House, where, according to Browne, Charles II 'doth most usually heal', and also in the great hall at Whitehall and the Chapel Royal at Windsor.[85] When on progress the Stuarts touched at the cathedrals in Lincoln and Lichfield, at Christ Church Oxford,[86] and at churches in Portsmouth and Holywell;[87] Charles II also touched in a non-palatial house in which he resided at Newmarket.[88]

The Lord Chamberlain was responsible for organising the ceremony but in practice he delegated the task to the surgeons, the clerk of the closet and the king's gentlemen ushers.[89] The gentlemen ushers prepared the room, and, given that Browne described the crowd as 'fetid to smell', one of their concerns was hygiene: sweet smelling parcels were regularly ordered to mask unpleasant odours.[90] The crowd that waited to be touched probably knew

[79] Browne, *Adenochoiradelogia*, 83–4.

[80] van Wiquefort, *Relation*, 75.

[81] Browne, *Adenochoiradelogia*, 95.

[82] *Mercurius Publicus*, 21–28 June 1660; *Parliamentary Intelligencer*, 18–25 June 1660.

[83] *Mercurius Publicus*, 28 June–5 July 1660; CSPV xxx/2, 182.

[84] Number of people touched Apr.–Nov. 1668, BL, MS Egerton 806, fos 59r–60r at fo. 59r; Wellcome Library, MS 5251. See also TNA, E407/85/1.

[85] *Mercurius Publicus*, 21–28 June, 28 June–5 July 1660; S., Pepys, *The diary of Samuel Pepys*, ed. R. Latham and W. Matthews, London 1970–83, i. 182; ii. 274; Browne, *Adenochoiradelogia*, 79, 176. I am grateful to David Baldwin, Serjeant of the Chapel Royal for information concerning the great hall at Whitehall, cf. *Adenochoiradelogia*, 90.

[86] *The life and times of Anthony Wood, antiquary, of Oxford, 1632–1695*, ed. A. Clark, Oxford 1891, i. 496, entry for 8 Sept. 1663; ii. 231, 234, entries for 4, 5 Sept. 1687.

[87] HMC, *Report of the manuscripts at Wells Cathedral*, London 1885, ii, pts III–iv, 376: September 1686, the manuscripts of Stanley Leighton Esq., MP.

[88] Browne, *Adenochoiradelogia*, 186; Magalotti, *Travels of Lorenzo the Third*, 214.

[89] TNA, LC5/140, pp. 493–4; LC5/141, p. 33; LC5/144, p. 195; Sainty and Bucholz, *Officials of the royal household*, 48–9, 56–7.

[90] Browne, *Adenochoiradelogia*, 102; Lord Chamberlain's department: miscellaneous

what the ceremony entailed as it was described in newspapers and depicted in printed images, and doubtless also discussed orally.[91] Sometimes the crowd needed patience though, as on one occasion Pepys wrote that Charles II did not arrive at the Banqueting House on time because 'it rayned so. And the poor people were forced to stand all the morning in the rain in the garden'.[92]

The king entered the room and sat hatless on his throne, which was usually on a dais and below a canopy which in the frontispiece to *Adenochoiradelogia* displays the royal coat of arms. He would have taken communion before-hand and heard a sermon, and he might have fasted prior to the ceremony.[93] These practices prepared the king for his thaumaturgic role and suggest that he needed to be purified in order to act as a conduit for God's grace.

Assembled next to the king were prominent courtiers and clergymen, sometimes including the archbishop of Canterbury.[94] In both images the courtiers are depicted in the background, discernible by their dress. Near to the king stood the royal chaplains who recited the healing liturgy and the clerk of the closet who held the touch-pieces, all of whom are visible in both images. The panoply of king, courtiers and chaplains projected the power of throne and altar, and not surprisingly people such as foreign dignitaries were invited to attend the ceremony, albeit discreetly so as not to draw attention away from proceedings.[95] The royal touch ranked alongside coro-nations, royal entries and other public regal events. Curious visitors would have wanted to observe the impressive sight of the king touching the sick, and possibly to compare it with the French ceremony. In 1669 Cosimo III of Tuscany watched the ceremony in the king's house at Newmarket, from an open side door.[96] In December 1673, just after the duke of York had married the duchess of Modena, the bride attended the royal touch with Prince Renaldo and 'Persons of Quality of their Train', all of them incognito.[97]

The crowd was escorted into the room by the yeomen of the guard, who can be seen in both images. Their job was to keep order and to guard the

records: order from Charles I to his apothecary, TNA, LC5/200, unfoliated (this dates from the 1630s).

[91] *Parliamentary Intelligencer*, 18–25 June 1660; *Mercurius Publicus*, 21–28 June 1660; *Mercurius Publicus*, 28 June–5 July 1660.

[92] Pepys, *Diary*, i. 182.

[93] Browne, *Adenochoiradelogia*, 96; van Wiquefort, *Relation*, 75. The seventeenth-century Stuarts might have fasted beforehand, though I have found no concrete evidence of this, but Anne did so and she often followed ceremonial precedents: see p. 197 below.

[94] Browne, *Adenochoiradelogia*, 96; van Wicquefort, *Relation*, 74; Shellinks, *Journal*, 91.

[95] Keay, *Magnificent monarch*, 117.

[96] Magalotti, *Travels of Lorenzo the Third*, 214–16.

[97] Lord Chamberlain's department: miscellaneous records: master of ceremonies: extracts from the notebooks of Sir John Cottrell, senior and junior, description of the duchess of Modena, Prince Renaldo etc viewing the royal touch ceremony incognito, TNA, LC5/2, p. 55.

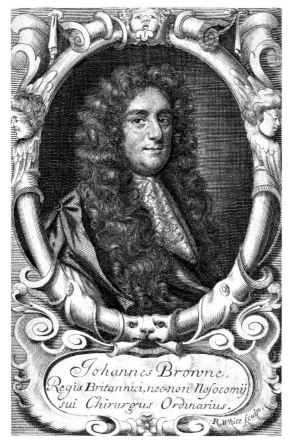

Figure 11. John Browne,
frontispiece to Browne,
Adenochoiradelogia.

king, who was in a potentially vulnerable position. Indeed, there is evidence
from James I's reign that people were searched on their way in to the ceremony, and although no similar evidence has emerged from later on, common
sense suggests that this precaution continued throughout the Stuart age.[98] As
for the crowd, Browne boasted that the royal touch was available to 'young
and old, rich and poor, beautiful and deformed'.[99] Many were frail. In June
1660 the press reported that 'a great company of poor afflicted Creatures
were met together, many brought in Chairs and Flaskets'.[100] In the broadside the people in the foreground waiting to be touched include a man on
crutches, three women with children and a man with a bandaged head. In
the frontispiece can be seen a man on crutches who is being assisted by

98   L. Andrewes, *Sermons*, ed. G. M. Story, Oxford 1967, 281.
99   Browne, *Adenochoiradelogia*, 84.
100 *Mercurius Publicus*, 21–28 June 1660.

138

another man with a stick who is himself stooping, and four children. As the bulk of the sick people in the images are facing the king rather than looking out towards the viewer, it is difficult at first to tell if they have scrofula. But on close inspection there are depictions of the symptoms. In the bottom left corner of the frontispiece the woman leaning down to attend to a young child appears to have a dark shadow on her right cheek. To her immediate left stands someone whose face also has dark patches on it. In the broadside, the man at the front with his arm in a sling has a dark patch on the side of his face, as does the man on crutches.

The formal proceedings began with the reading of the healing liturgy by the royal chaplains. The liturgy from the reign of Charles II was the same as that of James I and Charles I and it survives in three prayer books in the British Library, entitled 'At the healing'.[101] Presumably these were the actual prayer books that were used at the ceremony. The purpose of the liturgy was to provide structure for the service and to connect the royal touch directly with Christ's healing ministry. It attested to the importance of the spoken word of prayer as was to be expected of a Protestant rite.[102]

The ceremony began with the chaplain reading the passage from Mark xvi.14 that described Christ's appearance to his disciples after the Resurrection. One of the surgeons then led the first person to be touched up to the king along an approach to the throne that was guarded on either side by the yeoman warders. This is visible in both images, and in the broadside the approach is sectioned off by balustrades. The surgeons usually began with those who had travelled the furthest, though sometimes the guards arranged the order so that those who were most ill were presented first of all.[103] The surgeon made three low bows to the king after which he and the scrofulous person knelt in homage. The chaplain then read out Christ's words to his disciples: 'They shall lay their hands on the sick and they shall recover', at which the king used both hands to touch, stroke and press the scrofulous sores on the person's head and neck.[104] This was the key moment of the ceremony, which explains why both of the images depict the moment of physical contact between Charles II and the ill person before him. After this public intimacy, a second surgeon led the first person away to wait at one side – in the broadside he stands to the left of the dais, and in the frontispiece he stands to the right of the king. The surgeon in the frontispiece can be identified as John Browne, the author of *Adenochoiradelogia*, due to the resemblance between this figure

---

[101]   MacDonald Ross, 'Royal touch', 434 who cites BL, c.37.1.2 (1661), c.38.e.13 (1662) and 3406.f.9 (1680); cf. Sparrow Simpson, 'Forms of prayer', 209–301, and Crawfurd, *The king's evil*, 114–16. The liturgy is also found in the bottom half of the broadside.

[102]   For the parallel with exorcism see pp. 19–20 above.

[103]   *CSPD, 1661–62*, 428; Browne, *Adenochoiradelogia*, 96.

[104]   van Wicquefort, *Relation*, 76; Misson, *Memoirs*, 167; Magalotti, *Travels of Lorenzo the Third*, 215; Browne, *Adenochoiradelogia*, 96; *Diary of John Evelyn*, iii. 250; Shellinks, *Journal*, 73.

and Browne's portrait (*see* Figure 11). In the frontispiece, three people who have just been touched can be seen walking away to the right, behind the yeoman warders. The first person is bent over with his arm in a sling and walking with a stick; then a woman clasps her hands in prayer while looking upwards as though having a religious experience – she also has a patch of scrofula on her right cheek; and a third person stands in front, looking over his or her shoulder.

The first surgeon then presented to the king the second person to be touched in the same way, the chaplain recited the verse again, and this routine continued until everyone had been touched. Once this had happened, everyone who had been touched was presented to the king for a second time so as to receive their touch-piece which was threaded onto a strong white ribbon. These were handed to the king by the clerk of the closet, who between 1669 and 1685 was Nathaniel Crew (1633–1721), bishop of Durham, to whom Browne dedicated *Adenochoiradelogia*.[105] Crew was attended by Thomas Donkelley, the keeper of the royal closet, who kept records of how many touch-pieces were distributed.[106] Both images of the ceremony depict Crew holding touch-pieces, as can be ascertained by comparing these figures with the mezzotint portrait of Crew (*see* Figure 12).[107] The fact that the printed images of the ceremony included recognisable depictions of the people involved (the king, the surgeon, the clerk of the closet) adds to their verisimilitude and hints at their role in projecting a cult of personal monarchy. As people received their gold coins the chaplains recited passages from St John's Gospel which began 'That light was the true light which lighteth every man which cometh into the world' (John i.9).[108] Thus the two key moments of the ceremony, that of the royal touch and the gift of gold, were accompanied by readings from the New Testament.

All but one of the sources state that Charles II gave each person their touch-piece in the same way as had James I and Charles I, without making the sign of the cross over the sores in the manner of the Tudors. However, the broadside states that Charles did make this gesture. This is puzzling: surely commentators would have noted the reintroduction of this 'papist' action, so, strange as it seems, the suggestion is that the broadside description was wrong.

Once everyone had received their touch-piece the whole assembly knelt whilst the chaplains read further passages from St John's Gospel and said the Lord's Prayer, followed by other prayers.[109] This was followed by the

---

[105] Bucholz and Sainty, *Officials of the royal household*, i. 56; Browne, *Adenochoiradelogia*, Bb 2.

[106] Browne, *Adenochoiradelogia*, 94.

[107] BM, 1850, 0223.845, 338mm x 244mm, published by Pierce Tempest, 1675–1700.

[108] Browne, *Adenochoiradelogia*, 98.

[109] Ibid. 99–101.

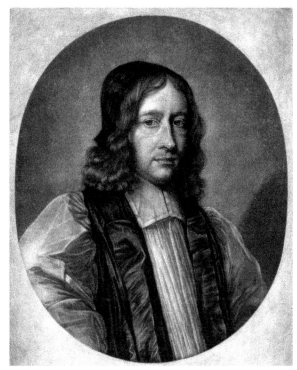

Figure 12. Nathaniel
Crew, artist unknown,
National Portrait
Gallery.

ritual cleansing of the king's hands. The gentlemen ushers presented the
Lord Chamberlain and two other prominent courtiers with a ewer of rose
water, a basin and a linen towel, and the three men bowed three times in
front of the king, knelt down and washed and dried his hands.[110] The Lord
Chamberlain can be seen in both images: in the broadside he stands to the
left of the dais, visible with his sash of office and a towel over his arm; in
the frontispiece he stands on the far left, to the left of the chaplain, behind
the ewer. The public cleansing of the king's hands was the important final
act of the ceremony: a lengthy healing rite required a formal ending that
signified that the king's thaumaturgic role had ended. This is borne out by
the prominent position of the ewer and basin in each of the healing images,
and by the fact the task was undertaken by noblemen rather than gentlemen
ushers. Once the king was ritually cleansed he retired, often to dine, and
everyone else was left to pray for him and to 'congratulate one another for
their recovery' before beginning their journeys home.[111]

---

[110]   Ibid. 101; van Wiquefort, *Relation*, 77–8; *Mercurius Publicus*, 21–28 June 1660.
[111]   van Wicquefort, *Relation*, 78; Magalotti, *Travels of Lorenzo the Third*, 216. For the
quotation see the last sentence of the broadside *The manner of his majestie*.

The significance of the gold touch-pieces

During the Restoration the crown distributed an average of 4,000 gold touch-pieces each year. Prior to the Restoration the crown distributed the prestigious Angels to people who were touched for scrofula, but this changed during Charles II's reign. In the early years of the Restoration no Angels were produced as the government was preoccupied with recalling the Interregnum coinage, which was no longer legal currency. This meant that between 1660 and 1665 the crown bought up Angels and also 10s-pieces from previous reigns and used them at the royal touch ceremony. In 1665 a new medal was issued to be distributed at the ceremony (*see* Figure 13). These differed from all earlier Angels in that they were not part of the regular currency; they were referred to in administrative records as 'healing medals' and are known today as touch-pieces.[112] However, the new medals were still referred to colloquially as Angels because, like the Angels from previous reigns, the new medals bore an image on their obverse of the Archangel Michael slaying the devil as well as the depiction of the ship of state in full sail on their reverse.

By 1665 the value of gold had increased and each touch-piece was worth 11s. 6d., a reminder of what a generous gift they were at a time when the average wage for a day labourer was one shilling.[113] Like the Angels, touch-pieces were made from twenty-two carat gold, thus containing more gold than any other English coin.[114] The value of the touch-piece changed in 1684 when they were commissioned with less gold in them, valued at 5s. 1d. each, a measure which reduced expenditure by just over 50 per cent.[115] The total expenditure for Charles's reign was £43,095.[116] Why did the crown spent such enormous sums on these touch pieces. What was the significance of giving a gold medal to each person who was touched?

The touch-pieces were not just souvenirs; they were an integral part of the ceremony. The Restoration medals broadcast the rationale for the healing in a manner that was more lucid and succinct than any Angel had done hitherto. The medal had a new legend on its obverse, 'Soli Deo Gloria' ('To God Alone the Glory'), which remained in place until the ritual ceased with the death of Queen Anne in 1714, after which it featured on the healing medals of the exiled Stuarts.[117] The new inscription reflected the government's wish to make clear the source of the healing power, in keeping with the rationale of the ceremony whereby the monarch acted as a conduit for God's healing powers. It must have

112 Farquhar, 'Royal charities, II', 95–183 at pp. 98–101, 118.
113 Ibid. 157; B. Coward, *The Stuart age*, London 1994, 56.
114 J. Craig, The *Mint: a history of the London Mint from A.D. 287 to 1948*, Cambridge 1948, 131.
115 Farquhar, 'Royal charities, II', 155.
116 Based on an annual total of £2,210.00 between 1665–84, and £1,110.00 for 1685.
117 Farquhar, 'Royal charities, IV', 159.

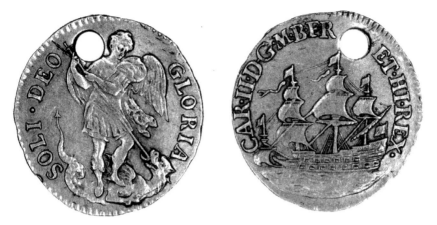

Figure 13. Charles II touch-piece. 22mm. diameter.

been especially necessary to broadcast this message given the huge numbers of people who were touched. English monarchs did not claim to be able to work miracles themselves in the way that Christ had; they maintained that they acted as a channel for God's grace only during the ceremony. This distinction was sometimes lost on 'ordinary' people as on the occasion of the incident with Elizabeth I at Gloucester, and as with the particular case of Arise Evans and Charles II.[118]

The images on the medal were equally important. The depiction of St Michael slaying the devil signified the triumph of good over evil, and of health over illness. It must have acquired extra significance given the widespread view that the Restoration marked the end of the turmoil and sin of the 1640s and 1650s. The ship of state had become a realistic depiction of the *Sovereign of the Seas*, the largest and most expensive vessel of its day, launched at Woolwich in 1637.[119] It is shown in full sail, emphasising the regenerated body politic that was a result of the Stuart restoration.

The gift of gold signified kingly munificence. The beauty, rarity and cost of gold meant that it was particularly associated with royalty and the gift of a touch-piece to scrofulous persons, some of whom were from the lower ranks of society, emphasised the benevolent and generous nature of the king. The gift was meant to forge a bond of allegiance between subject and monarch which would lessen the chances of political dissidence: the royal touch apologist T. A. said that the touch-pieces inclined 'the affections of the People to

[118] See pp. 62–3 for the Gloucester incident; p. 163 below for Arise Evans.
[119] Woolf, 'Sovereign remedy', 105–6.

their King'.[120] This must have been especially pertinent when people looked back on the traumatic 1640s and 1650s.

In occult sciences gold was connected to immortality because of its ability to resist decay, and it related to the sun and to the astrological sign of Leo, both of which associated it with kingship.[121] Gold symbolised perfection and purity, and so it was usual in the pre-modern world to think that if someone wore an object made from gold these qualities, as well as its beauty, would induce the wearer to be less sinful and lead a more virtuous life.[122] Because disease was associated with sin, this meant that they were more likely to recover from illness, which partly explains why, since Henry VII's reign, supplicants had been given a gold coin and expected to wear it constantly.[123] Some people thought of their touch-piece as an amulet that could cure scrofula on its own. Here it needs to be pointed out that the linking of disease and sin, and the idea that the king and his gold could alleviate both, is implicitly political; this helps to explain the contemporary belief that by curing scrofula the sovereign healed the ills of the body politic.

As well as influencing health via morality, gold was thought to be able to cure certain diseases and was sometimes even ingested as a panacea known as *Aurum potabile* (drinkable gold).[124] The virtuoso and antiquarian John Aubrey provided details of some specific medicinal uses of gold. He wrote that if 'pure gold' were bound to 'old ulcers or Fistulas' the treatment was successful because the gold drew out of the sufferer's body the mercury which was thought to cause these conditions.[125] He also said that if gold were worn on a tumour it cured the condition.[126] T. A. discussed the restorative properties of gold, giving a dramatic account of its use to heal the son of Henry Clinton (1568–1619), the second earl of Lincoln, who was ill with a 'malignant Fever' and unable to speak. The earl called for the renowned Dr William Butler (1535–1618). The doctor asked for some pieces of gold, and crammed as many of them into the boy's mouth as was possible; the earl was concerned in case his son choked, but after a while the doctor removed the gold from the boy's mouth and

120 T. A., *Excellency*, 20.
121 E. A. Wallis Budge, *Amulets and superstitions*, London 1930, 487; F. Gettings, *Dictionary of occult, hermetic and alchemical sigils*, London 1981, 126; C. H. V. Sutherland, *Gold: its beauty, power and allure*, London 1969, 18.
122 J. Evans, *Magical jewels of the Middle Ages and Renaissance, particularly in England*, Oxford 1922, 146–7.
123 See p. 150 above.
124 F. Anthony, *Medicinae chymicae et veri potabilis auri assertion*, London 1610; M. Gwinne, *Aurum non aurum*, London 1611; F. Anthony, *The apologie, or, Defence of a verity heretofore published concerning a medicine called aurum potabile*, London 1616; R. Boyle, *Of the reconcileableness of specifick medicines to the corpuscular philosophy*, London 1685.
125 J. Aubrey, *Remains of Gentilisme and Judaisme* (1686–7), in J. Buchanan-Brown (ed.), *Three prose works*, Fontwell 1972, 127–304 at p. 238.
126 Idem, *Observations*, ibid. 305–63 at p. 339.

it came out 'as black as Coal'. T. A. explained that 'the malignity thus spending it self, the Gentleman recovered'. Butler was known for using eccentric methods that aimed to shock his patients into recovery: on one occasion he cured a man of the ague by having him thrown from a balcony into the Thames, and the cramming of gold into someone's mouth might have been similarly unconventional.[127] Nevertheless, T. A. marvelled 'what wonders Gold will do', observing how its purity enabled it to cleanse the body of disease or impurity. There is a striking resemblance here between gold purifying a diseased human body and a sinful body politic. Thus T. A. said that 'Angel gold breathed life into fetid sores'.[128]

Retrospective assessments

Two types of retrospective assessment of the royal touch ceremony survive. First, there are the official appraisals of the Lord Chamberlain, taking the form of directives to the surgeons that sought to bring more order to the ceremony, and secondly, the records of observers who were mainly concerned with Charles II. The official assessments indicate that the ceremony did not always run as smoothly as has been described. This was partly because it was difficult to organise a service involving hundreds of sick people, many of whom were not used to the ways of the court, although there were problems even during private ceremonies. Two specific difficulties could lessen decorum, namely surgeons who were uncertain whether or not someone had scrofula when assessing them before the ceremony, and doubt concerning when the next ceremony would happen. These issues exasperated supplicants and officials and caused the former unnecessary expense.

Aside from these problems, it is surprising to find that during the ceremony itself surgeons sometimes argued with each other over diagnostic issues that should have been resolved beforehand, and that members of the public quarrelled concerning whether someone had been touched before. These public spats were incompatible with a service that re-enacted Christ's healing ministry and not surprisingly they incurred Charles II's displeasure. To make matters worse, they were reported in the press. In February 1661 *Mercurius Publicus* recounted that 'certain persons (too many one would think) who having the *Kings-Evill*, and have been *touched* by his Sacred MAJESTY, have yet the forehead [audacity] to come twice or thrice, alledging they were never there before, till divers witnesses proved the contrary'.[129] The article then goes on to stress the need for supplicants to provide certificates from

[127] Idem, *Brief lives*, ed. J. Buchanan-Brown, London 2000, 66; cf. Thompson Cooper, rev. S. Bakewell, 'Butler, William (1535–1618)', *ODNB*.
[128] T. A., *Excellency*, 26–7.
[129] *Mercurius Publicus*, 14–21 Feb. 1661.

their ministers stating that they have not been touched before, as a guard against such scenes.

The Lord Chamberlain issued three warrants that sought to address these and other problems, one in May and another in November 1674, when the numbers touched by the king were rising, and a third in February 1682, when they had increased dramatically.[130] These were directives for the surgeons, and suggest that the surgeons were the cause of many of the problems at the ceremony. The first warrant begins:

> many inconveniences & disorders have happened at publique and private Healings, by reasons of Differences & disagreements Between His Majesties Serjeant Chyrurgeon to the person & Chyrurgeon of the Household which many tymes have made a disturbance in His Majesties presence at the time of Healings.[131]

The overall effectiveness of the warrants is questionable, though, because in 1684 Browne devoted nine pages of his book to many of the same issues: that he thought it appropriate to do this publicly indicates the scale of the problems.[132]

The first directive of May 1674 addressed eleven problems. The first was the healing calendar, which was defined as being from Ash Wednesday until the end of May and from 1 September to 30 November.[133] It stipulated that whichever surgeon was on duty was responsible for informing people of last-minute cancellations of healings, or sudden decisions to hold one.[134] The other two warrants have nothing to say about the healing calendar, which suggests that things had improved by 1674 and remained fairly healthy in 1682, and that the crown's notices in the press were proving effective. But there must still have been problems at times because in 1684 Browne took a firm line on this issue, stating that the healing calendar and specific healing days should be advertised in advance so that those who came to be touched could obtain a 'quick dispatch' and not have to wait around in London until 'both their money and Credit is gone'.[135]

The problem of ensuring that only those with scrofula were touched was addressed in two of the warrants and by Browne, which indicates that this was an ongoing challenge for officials. The Lord Chamberlain and Brown both re-emphasised the need for certificates to be granted by ministers, and the warrants prohibited the surgeons from giving admission tickets to the

---

130 TNA, LC5/140, pp. 493–4; 'Chyrurgeons concerning healings' 1674, LC5/141, p. 33; 'Orders for healings', 1682, LC5/144, p. 195.
131 TNA, LC5/140, p. 493.
132 Browne, *Adenochoiradelogia*, 85–94.
133 TNA, LC5/140, 493.
134 TNA, LC5/140, 494, point 7.
135 Browne, *Adenochoiradelogia*, 88.

ceremony to any who did not bring certificates, suggesting that at times they did just that.[136] The certificates were meant to ensure that only people who appeared to have scrofula made their way to the royal court, meaning that in theory the surgeons' assessment was quicker and easier than that of the ministers. Browne went further than the directives, and recommended that, as certificates were easy to counterfeit, they should be printed rather than handwritten and blank ones sent to the bishops who could sign and seal them and then send them on to the clergy in their diocese. The clergy could then issue them and countersign them, and keep a register of those to whom they granted certificates.[137] Browne also suggested that those who wanted to be touched should take it upon themselves to be medically examined where they lived, rather than to wait until they got to London. Their certificates, he suggested, could then be countersigned by a doctor, and so ease the strain on the royal surgeons and prevent wasted journeys.[138]

Browne's suggestions were not taken up, though the government's require-ment that handwritten certificates should be sealed must have been an attempt to guard against counterfeited certificates. Some people forged these documents for mercenary reasons (they wanted to acquire a gold touch-piece), but presumably others were desperate to be cured of an ailment even if it was not scrofula, while some people might simply have wanted to see the king at close quarters. The problem of faked documentation seems to have worsened as Charles II's reign progressed because the 1684 proclamation required ministers and churchwardens to 'be very careful to examine into the truth before they give such Certificates'; at the same time Browne wrote that great care should be taken when writing and sealing certificates in order to help guarantee their authenticity.[139]

The lists kept by the ministers were also a way of ensuring that people were not touched more than once. However, sometimes this occurred with the surgeons' knowledge and approval, if a second touch was thought neces-sary to cure especially resistant scrofula. Both the Lord Chamberlain and Browne wanted the surgeons to keep a register too, which would allow for the close monitoring of names, necessary in part because if someone moved house they changed their parish.[140] No surgeons' register has come to light, so whether this idea was taken up cannot be known.

The warrants addressed other issues that reveal problems that occurred on occasion. The first stated that any differences of opinion that arose between the surgeons concerning diagnosis should be brought to the attention of the Lord Chamberlain; the surgeons were strictly forbidden from arguing in front

---

[136] TNA, LC5/140, 493; LC5/144, 195; Browne, *Adenochoiradelogia*, 84.

[137] Browne, *Adenochoiradelogia*, 85–6.

[138] Ibid. 86.

[139] 'At the Court at Whitehall', Whitehall, 9 Jan. 1684; Browne, *Adenochoiradeogia*, 85.

[140] TNA, LC5/140, 493, point 2; Browne, *Adenochoiradelogia*, 87–8.

of the king.[141] Surgeons were not to refuse entry to the ceremony to any of the officials who were meant to attend, and a procedure was drawn up to be followed should a surgeon be ill or absent when required to officiate; it was also important that they informed the king beforehand of the number of people that he was to touch, and gave plenty of notice of the next ceremony to the nobility so that they could attend.[142] Lastly, the surgeons were warned to follow their directives carefully on pain of being suspended from their duties.[143]

The directives reveal the problems that occurred at times. How effective were they in resolving them? The proclamation of 1684 and the periodic reiteration of its content in the press suggests that the main problems of certification and registration were not permanently overcome. Whether this means that these aspects of the royal touch were in a continual state of flux, or alternated between periods of satisfactory maintenance and relapse, is difficult to say. It is probable that measures were introduced after periods of especially noticeable disorder, but that they were not completely effective in the long term.

Turning to the second type of assessments, those of observers of Charles II. These all date from 1660 because of the topicality of the royal touch at that time, and because the new king was still relatively unknown. The commentaries were very favourable and reflected the euphoria of the Restoration.[144] A Venetian observer noted that the king showed 'exemplary patience' when touching large numbers of sick people and the press reported that:

> such was his princely patience and tenderness to the poor afflicted Creatures that though it took up a very long time, his Majesty being never weary of wel-doing, was pleased to make enquiry whether there were any more that had not yet been touch'd.[145]

The king would certainly need patience and stamina if he was to touch 200 sick people at one ceremony, let alone 600. If it took half a minute for each supplicant to be presented to the king and touched, and another half a minute for each to receive their touch-piece, then a ceremony involving 200 supplicants would have lasted at least three hours and twenty minutes. When we remember that many people were frail it is likely that ceremonies took longer than this.

Other assessments of the king emphasised his engagement with the ritual and his alertness to any misdemeanours. In July 1660 a newspaper noted his

---

141 TNA, LC5/140, 494.

142 TNA, LC5/140, 493–4; LC5/141, 33.

143 TNA, LC5/140, 494.

144 See pp. 2, 102–3 above.

145 *CSPV* xxx. II, 182; *Parliamentary Intelligencer*, 18–25 June 1660; *Mercurius Publicus*, 21–28 June 1660.

astuteness when someone who had not been touched joined the crowd of people queueing to receive their gold coin, reporting that 'his Majesty ... presently discovered him, saying, *This man hath not yet been touch'd*'.[146] The hot weather of July 1660 caused positive comment on the king's stamina because he continued to touch despite the heat and the associated fear of infection, and the same newspaper contrasted him with 'Physitions, Chirurgeons ... [and] Apothecaries' who did not attend their patients during the summer.[147]

The public role of healer was a key aspect of the Stuart monarchy. During the Restoration some 100,000 people passed through the ritual process of the royal touch. The ceremony directly linked the crown and the ill people to Christ's healing ministry and as such should have been performed with decorum. Yet the great number of supplicants, the problems of diagnosing scrofula, and people's desperation for a cure, a touch-piece, or just to see the king, made the process difficult to manage. This means that the official accounts of the ceremony are sometimes at odds with the assessments of it made by the Lord Chamberlain. The directives that he issued to surgeons, seeking to correct their disagreements and poor conduct, do not seem to have been completely effective. Indeed, the broadside image of the ceremony might have been disseminated so as to familiarise people with a well-organised service in the hope of improving behaviour at it. It probably would have been seen by more people than the frontispiece to Browne's book; it included the liturgy, which was almost correct, and an orderly image of the ceremony.

Although incidences of disorder were an issue for officials they obviously did not deter the supplicants. Indeed, the royal touch was connected to a cult of personal monarchy at this time. Sick people went to great lengths to access Charles II's therapeutic touch, which he was willing to provide. In some respects the ceremony was an excellent public relations exercise: it showed the king as compassionate and charitable and allowed thousands of people to pay him homage. Thus the two printed images of Charles touching the sick were probably produced to reflect and promote a cult of sacral monarchy. Further evidence for the role of visual culture in this veneration is provided by a third printed image of Charles II touching for scrofula produced by the print-maker Peter Stent, which unfortunately is not extant. It was advertised for sale in 1662, to coincide with the king's marriage to Catherine of Braganza, and again in 1673. A small image, it was sold to 'adorn Tobacco-boxes' and was 'much in use'.[148]

---

[146] *Mercurius Publicus*, 28 June–5 July 1660.

[147] Ibid. 12–19 July 1660.

[148] A. Globe, *Peter Stent, London printseller, circa 1642–1665: being a catalogue raisonné of his engraved prints and books with an historical and bibliographical introduction*, Vancouver 1985, 126, 184.

The complexities of lay belief are evident in that on the one hand people clamoured to attend a ceremony in which the king acted the part of Christ and attempted to heal them by his sacred touch. The religious aspects of the ceremony are self-evident. On the other hand some people were willing to forge certificates in order to attend, whether for mercenary or medical reasons. But despite the government's ongoing concerns it seems that the mercenary were only a small minority. After all, the Angel was first introduced by Henry VII yet throughout the Tudor age the numbers who sought the royal touch were far lower than during the seventeenth century. These different views on the royal touch – veneration and ambivalence – indicate that the ceremony was debated, and it is to that discourse that we now turn.

5

The Restoration Debate: The Rise of Ambivalence and Scepticism, 1660–1688

During the Restoration the Stuarts touched for scrofula on a vast scale, which partly explains why there is more evidence relating to the practice from this period than any other. This includes commentaries on the royal touch, which, although sometimes fragmentary, reveal a range of views – from belief to ambivalence to scepticism. It must be stressed that it was usual to believe in the efficacy of the royal touch, given the religious underpinnings of medicine, the sacral role of the sovereign, and the connection between people's individual health and that of the body politic. The increased scale and frequency of Stuart therapeutics only strengthens this view. Yet the royal touch was debated.

In fact, the royal touch must always have been discussed. The supplicants who turned to the crown wanted to be cured, meaning that the efficacy of the practice would surely have been assessed. Although the evidence of this debate prior to the seventeenth century is scarce, what survives is revealing. Three specific cases merit examination. In 1344 Thomas Bradwardine, chaplain to Edward III and future archbishop of Canterbury, wrote that the healings performed by the king were indeed scrutinised, being testified by 'the sick persons who had been cured, by those present when the cures took place, or who had seen the results of them, by the people of many nations, and by their universal renown'. Turning to those who doubted miracles, he went on: 'Christians, whoever thou art that dost discredit miracles still wrought in these very times … come into England to the present English king, bring with you any Christian who has the King's Evil no matter inveterate, how deep-seated and loathsome, and he will cure him in the name of Jesus Christ'.[1]

By the end of Elizabeth I's reign critics of the royal touch objected to it on three grounds: that prayer had no intrinsic efficacy; cures might be wrought by wearing the gold Angel rather than the royal touch, which was problematic for Protestants as it was suggestive of magic; or cures might be caused by the power of suggestion.[2] The Tudor debate was addressed briefly and frankly in 1584 by the MP Reginald Scot, in his sceptical book on witchcraft. In it he said that some people thought that the ability to heal resided in the

[1] Bloch, *The Royal touch*, 57, 310 n. 20 (99); Crawfurd, *The king's evil*, 39.
[2] See p. 63 above.

monarch's person; others that the powers were given by God; while some people said that the ceremony worked because of the prayers. The Protestant Scot emphasised the importance of prayer, no doubt because he thought the age of miracles had passed. He said that 'hir majestie onelie useth godlie and divine praier, with some almes, and referreth the cure to God and to the physician'.[3] This is reminiscent of Elizabeth's own words on the topic, spoken in Gloucestershire, which also emphasised prayer; the passage also fits with the views of James VI and I.

In 1610 Thomas Morton (1564–1659), the polemical anti-Catholic churchman and future bishop of Durham favoured by James VI and I, published *A catholike appeale for Protestants* in which he denounced Catholic miracles. Discussing the royal touch he maintained that 'it cannot be called a work properly miraculous', adding in a note:

> For these Kings in such healings do not absolutely intend a miraculous worke, the ordinary effect whereof is to cure perfectly and in an instant onely by power of speech and touching: but they do after prayer commend the diseased parties vnto the ordinary meanes of Gods ordinance, euen the cure of Physitions.[4]

Thus Morton echoes Scot, Elizabeth I and James VI and I, privileging providence and even medicine. The themes of these three cases are taken up in more detail by Restoration commentators. There was an intra-Protestant debate concerning the underpinnings and efficacy of the royal touch, as well as its status: just how miraculous was it? Those who believed that the practice could cure scrofula differed as to what the primary healing power was thought to be – was it the touch, the prayers or the gold? –- whilst doubt was expressed from a range of positions including religious, medical and intellectual. This was further complicated because whereas Christ's miracles had produced immediate cures, the ceremony was hardly ever described as doing so.

The fact that the royal touch was contested and its effectiveness scrutinised helps to explain why its apologists went to such lengths to extol its virtues: the idea that the monarch's sacred hands acted as a conduit for God's healing powers did not convince everyone. Indeed, if this had been the case then there would have been little need for such authors to write as much as they did. It seems that the debate intensified during the 1670s and 1680s as compared to earlier periods: more people were being touched than ever before, and more uncertainty was being expressed. This is why Browne's book attacks critics of the royal touch more forcefully than had Tooker eighty years earlier. The critical views can be contextualised in terms of the government's failure to find a religious settlement, the new intel-

3   Scot, *Discoverie*, bk 13, ch. 9, 303–4.
4   T. Morton, *A catholike appeale for Protestants*, London 1609, 428.

lectual culture that saw nature working by fixed laws, and the attacks on orthodoxy conducted by the wits.

Discussion of the debate will begin with an analysis of the doubts expressed during the first summer of the Restoration (which proved that not everyone was swept away by the fervour for the restored Stuarts), before going on to examine John Browne's *Adenochoiradelogia*, a key source for the full range of views on royal therapeutics, and then to the objections made by various groups and individuals. Some dissenters objected that the royal touch was 'superstitious' or Roman Catholic, and, alongside some doctors, they also argued that the ceremony worked by the power of suggestion as opposed to supernatural means. Other unidentified detractors maintained that so-called cures were really nothing more than the coincidence of scrofula going into remission of its own accord shortly after people were touched by the king. Further evidence of doubt was expressed in learned circles as recorded by the antiquarian John Aubrey, particularly in connection with occult beliefs and the new mechanical philosophy. Beyond this, the wits and scoffers who are sometimes said to typify the Restoration mocked the royal touch, although it is frustrating that their particular objections have not come down to us. Lastly, one cannot help wondering if, despite the huge numbers touched by Charles II, contemporaries speculated about his suitability for the role of sacral healer given his adventurous sex life.

The evidence used in this chapter indicates that even though some of the doubt concerning the royal touch was expressed in private correspondence, much of it was articulated orally. This means that it can only be accessed at one remove, through the attacks made on it in print by the apologists.[5] Issues were debated both publicly and privately and the written evidence that has survived provides only a partial history of what was discussed concerning royal therapeutics. Most free-thought was expressed orally as it was less perilous than committing ideas to print, but even oral heterodoxy could have dire consequences. The strangest case relating to the royal touch is that of the Presbyterian minister Thomas Rosewell. In 1684 he was found guilty of treason and sentenced to death for supposedly preaching against the king, and for having made comments that included one about people flocking to the monarch on the 'pretence of healing the king's evil, which he could not do'. But the evidence was weak and public opinion sided with Rosewell, so he was pardoned.[6] The case is interesting as it reveals the seriousness with which the establishment viewed public criticisms of royal thaumaturgy, while also hinting that public opinion was more tolerant of sceptical views about it.

---

[5]   Bird, *Ostenta Carolina*, 89–90; T. A., *Excellency*, 31, 36, 37; Browne, *Adenochoiradelogia*, 106–7, 113–26.

[6]   Howell, *State trials*, x. 147; J. Benedict, 'Rosewell Thomas (1630–92)', ODNB.

Apart from the pulpit, learned conversations and debates happened in the universities, parliament, Inns of Court, coffee houses and at dinner parties and other similar gatherings; ideas were discussed in inns and taverns, squares and streets, spinning bees, the workplace or around the fireside.[7] The elite, the learned and 'ordinary' people all discussed the royal touch, with belief, uncertainty and cynicism being expressed within each group.

Contemporaries attached great significance to oral heterodoxy as it was associated with the rise of irreligion and atheism. To deny the royal touch implied that God did not intervene in day-to-day events, a belief that would become one of the characteristics of deism; it also questioned a royal custom thought to be six hundred years old. Robert Boyle lamented men's 'licentious discourses' and the Boyle Lecturer Robert Bentley considered that atheism was much worse in his time because it was no longer 'buried in books' but found in taverns, coffee houses and other public places.[8] Orthodox responses to heterodoxy could be made formally from the pulpit and in the lecture hall, as well as less formally, and of course in print. The counter arguments of the royal touch apologists suggest that they had a good grasp of the ideas of their unnamed opponents, which is itself testament to the vitality of the oral culture of scepticism.

Refuting doubt in the first years of the Restoration

Restoration scepticism first comes to light in a ballad dating from 1660 which addresses mild criticism of the royal touch, and in a passage at the end of John Bird's *Ostenta Carolina* (1661) that refutes more serious denigrations. The ballad, *The loyal subjects hearty wishes to King Charles the second*, was one of about 120 ballads published in 1660 to celebrate the restoration of the Stuarts.[9] What is unusual about this one is that it discussed the royal touch,

[7] Michael Hunter, 'The witchcraft controversy and the nature of free thought in Restoration England: John Wagstaffe's *The question of witchcraft debated*' (1669), in Hunter, *Science and the shape of orthodoxy*, 286–307 at p. 287. See also B. Scribner, 'Oral culture and the diffusion of Reformation ideas', in his *Popular culture and popular movements in Reformation Germany*, London 1987, 49–70; A. Fox, *Oral and literate culture in England*, Oxford 2000; and A. Fox and D. Wolf (eds), *The spoken word: oral culture in England, 1500–1850*, Manchester 2002.

[8] R. Boyle, *The works of Robert Boyle*, ed. M. Hunter and E. B. Davis, London 1999–2000, iv. 151; Hunter, *Science and society*, 164.

[9] *The loyal subjects hearty wishes to King Charles the Second*, London, printed for John Andrews, n.d. The *Wing short title catalogue* suggests that the date of publication was 1660. For Restoration ballads see A. McShane,'"Rime and reason": the political world of the broadside ballad, 1640–1689', unpubl. PhD diss. Warwick 2004; 'Typography matters: branding ballads and gelding curates in Stuart England', in J. Hinks and C. Armstrong (eds), *Book trade connections from the seventeenth to the twentieth centuries*, London 2008, 19–44; and *Political broadside ballads of seventeenth-century England: a critical bibliography*, London 2011.

and during a time of unprecedented enthusiasm for the practice it registered anxiety about those who did not believe in it. It also questioned the sincerity of many of those who participated in the festivities that marked the Restoration. Like most ballads it is anonymous, but the preamble tells us that its author had fought for Charles I during the Civil War and for Charles II at the battle of Worcester. Like many popular ballads this one was to be sung to a military tune, such melodies being associated with loyalty to the crown.[10]

In verse seven the ballad maintains that God inspires the king

> To heal those evil Sores
> And them to Cure,
> By his most gracious hand
> And prayers pure;
> Though simple people say
> Doctors do as much:
> None but our lawful King
> Can cure with a touch,
> As plainly hath been seen
> Since he returned:
> Many hath cured been,
> Which long hath mourned.

The ballad states that the healings rely on prayer as well as the king's sacred touch, and that the ceremony is efficacious. The mild critique of the practice is that 'simple people' say that doctors can cure scrofula too: certainly people with scrofula could and did opt for medical, surgical or spiritual treatments.[11] It is interesting that 'simple people' implies that it was the non-educated who did not fully appreciate the king's thaumaturgic powers, in contrast to the presumptions of some of the secondary literature that maintain that belief in the royal touch can be explained by pre-Enlightenment credulity.[12] The verse also says that the king is the only lawful practitioner of tactile healing, thus discounting sectarian healers.

The ballad continues in verse eight with a further mention of the royal touch that informs us that the benevolent king has even healed some of those who were his enemies, just as Charles I had done during the 1640s:

> The poorest wretch that hath
> this Evil sure
> May have ease from the King,
> And perfect cure;
> His Grace is meek and wise,

---

[10] McShane, 'Rime and reason', 49.

[11] For an interpretation that seems to place the doctors as rivals to the king, mistakenly in my view, see Weber, 'The monarch's sacred body', 52.

[12] See pp. 7–8 above.

loving and civil,
And to his enemies
doth good for evil:
For some that are his foes
were by him healed.
His liberal hand to those
is not concealed;
He heals both poor and rich
by God's great power,
And his most gracious touch
doth them all cure.

The ninth and tenth verses then explain that the enemies of the monarchy are 'Infidels ... false Prophets ... [and] Quakers' who 'did spring up by toleration' during the Interregnum, after which the ballad concludes with praise for the new king. Although there is only presumptive evidence concerning the popularity of this ballad, it is intriguing to think of people singing about the king's healing powers and refuting the scepticism of some dissenters.

Turning to Bird's *Ostenta Carolina*, a succinct passage at the end contains his defence of the royal touch against four criticisms.[13] Some argued that because the royal touch did not heal everyone it differed from the healings performed by Christ and his disciples and so was not miraculous. Bird responded to this by saying that the thaumaturgic power given to kings was different from that given to Christ and his disciples, and might be expected to be less efficacious as the king was not the son of God. Bird then said that some sceptics objected that Christ and his disciples healed all sort of ailments, whereas the king only healed scrofula. Bird's defence was that the biblical healings were performed to fulfil prophesies, whereas the king's were not. A further line of scepticism maintained that the royal touch was problematic because the king of France performed it, and he was a Roman Catholic. Bird defended the English king, but not the French, by saying that even 'reprobates' could sometimes cast out devils.[14] Lastly, some sceptics said that the ritual was not effective because sometimes scrofula reappeared after it was meant to have been cured by the royal touch. This was the most difficult point for Bird to refute, which implies that it was the strongest of the criticisms. He argued weakly that it did not mean that the king's healings were 'different from the like miracles of old', although he allowed that sometimes a second touch was needed to cure scrofula that had newly reappeared. In the end, he had to concede that even if the royal touch did not cure everyone, at least it usually alleviated the condition. He also blamed the failure of royal therapeutics on the sinfulness of the person with scrofula, a unique and slightly bizarre claim as it was usual to think that they carried the

---

13 Bird, *Ostenta Carolina*, 89–91.
14 This will be discussed further at pp. 166–7 below.

collective weight of the sinful nation. This is revealing in terms of the pressure Bird must have felt that he was under. He concluded that 'this virtue given to our Kings is miraculous, although not to perfection'.

Bird provided no clues as to whether these were standard seventeenth-century criticisms of the royal touch, or whether the radicalism of the Interregnum and the topicality of the ritual during the early years of the Restoration gave rise to new sceptical arguments. It is likely that the latter was the case though, as none of these views had been addressed by Tooker in his defence of the ritual at the end of Elizabeth I's reign.

Adenochoiradelogia and the growth of scepticism during the 1670s and '80s

A key source on the different views on the royal touch held by the 1680s is John Browne's *Adenochoiradelogia* (1684). This book marks a watershed in the history of the royal touch in England. It contains the longest eye-witness account of the ceremony ever published, case studies arguing for the efficacy of royal therapeutics, and detailed information concerning the numbers of people who were touched. It also contains detailed medical information on scrofula, as well as a strong refutation of scepticism towards the ritual. Charles II was delighted with the book, finding it to his 'great Liking and Satisfaction'.[15]

The background to the book is that Browne was surgeon-in-ordinary to Charles II, meaning that he would have assisted Richard Wiseman, the serjeant surgeon, with his scrofula-related duties: both men would assess whether those who sought the king's touch really did have scrofula, and both would officiate at the ceremony. Browne was a well-educated man, a competent naval surgeon who had worked at St Thomas' Hospital, and he has the distinction of being the first medical practitioner to describe cirrhosis of the liver, in *Philosophical Transactions* in 1685.[16]

Adenochoiradelogia was the most important book on the royal touch of its day, so it is fitting that it was printed by the king's printer, Thomas Newcomb, and sold by Samuel Lowndes, a leading Restoration publisher.[17] The book is

---

[15] Becket, *Free and impartial enquiry*, 60. *Adenochoiradelogia* is a Greek neologism, 'Adeno' meaning 'glands', 'choir' meaning 'healing' and 'adelogia', meaning 'to do': it means, approximately, 'the healing of glands'.

[16] I. Lyle, 'Browne, John (1642–1702/3)', ODNB; 'The database of court officers, 1660–1839', directed by R. O. Bucholz, chamber list 4 at <http://www.luc.edu/history/fac_resources/bucholz/DCO/Database–Files/CHAMBER4.list.pdf>

[17] J. Dunton, *The life and errors of John Dunton, citizen of London*, London 1705, 290; H. R. Plomer and others, *A dictionary of the printers and booksellers who were at work in England, Scotland and Ireland from 1668 to 1725*, London 1922, 192, 136–7; I. Gadd, 'Newcomb, Thomas, the elder (1625x7–81)', ODNB.

a lengthy octavo, and the material aspects of the book as well as its structure, scope, priorities and tone mark it out as very different from the earlier apologies, *Ostenta Carolina* and *The excellency or handy work of the royal hand*. Browne's book is the English counterpart to *De mirabili strumas* (Paris 1609), the book on the French royal touch written by Andreas Laurentius (1558–1609), physician to Henri IV. This book also provides a detailed account of the history of the practice and its underlying principles, as seen from the French, Roman Catholic point of view. It praises Henri IV for using the royal touch to help bring peace to France after decades of civil war: some copies of the book have a fold-out engraving of Henri IV touching for scrofula bound into them.[18] Browne provided a list in his book of other works that he had read on the royal touch and on health more broadly, revealing that his chief influences were Laurentius and Tooker.[19] Perhaps partly because of this, the Plymouth surgeon James Yonge denounced Browne as a plagiarist, maintaining that Browne's treatment was taken straight from Tooker, Clowes and Wiseman.[20] Despite this unfair accusation, Browne's book sold well.

Adenochoiradelogia is divided into separate books, with separate titles (in Latin, though the text is in English). The first, *Adenographia*, discusses the human glands; the second, *Chaeradelogia*, discusses scrofula as a medical condition, including its symptoms and cures; the third, *Charisma basilicon*, addresses the royal touch. The contents of the first two books, as well as Browne's medical position at court, suggests that *Adenochoiradelogia* was aimed specifically at doctors and ministers, its detailed contents being intended to help them diagnose scrofula in their patients and parishioners. The improvement of provincial diagnoses would greatly ease Browne's task of assessing whether or not the large numbers of people who sought the king's touch really had scrofula.

What did Browne say about scrofula? Describing the symptoms as physical matter that invaded the glands, he stated that scrofula was one of England's 'particular Diseases' though it was not contagious as it was rare for all the members of a household to contract it. Contributory causes included cold and moist humours, poor nutrition, age (apparently people aged between forty-two and sixty were unlikely to develop it), heredity and damp environ-

---

[18] A. Laurentius (A. Du Laurens), *De mirabili strumas sanadi vi solis Galliae regibus Christianissimus divinitus concessa*, Paris 1609; Bloch, *The royal touch*, 211 (376); Brogan, 'Royal touch' (dissertation), 178; A. Finley-Crosswhite, 'Henri IV and the diseased body politic', in M. Gosman, A. MacDonald and A. Vanderjagt (eds), *Princes and princely culture, 1450–1650*, Leiden 2003, i.131–46; S. Wheeler, 'Medicine in art: Henry IV of France touching for scrofula, by Pierre Firens', *Journal of the History of Medicine and Allied Sciences* lviii/1 (2003), 79–81. The copy of *De mirabili strumas* at the Welcome Library includes the engraving (record no. 14317507). The engraving is available via Welcome Images, and is reproduced in Bloch, *The royal touch*, facing p. 149, and in *Les Rois thaumaturges*, as plate 3.

[19] Browne, *Adenochoiradelogia*, bk II, unnumbered page.

[20] J. Yonge, *Medicaster medicatus, or, A remedy for the itch of scribbling*, London 1685, a3v.

ments. The primary cause was unknown, though he speculated that it could be 'vicissitudes of Things, Sins of the people, ill Habits, or worse Constitutions'.[21] Elsewhere Browne said that sin caused illnesses, but surprisingly he only mentioned sin on six brief occasions in his book.[22] This marks a significant departure from the two books of the 1660s, both of which emphasised the causal relationship between sin and scrofula. Browne's focus on the natural causes of scrofula might seem to imply that by the 1680s the connection between sin and the body politic had lost its grip on contemporaries: yet not long after the publication of Browne's book England experienced the rise of Societies for the Reformation of Manners, and if anything an increase in educated concern for national perils which were thought to be caused by private vice.[23]

Browne did not explain his shift of emphasis but the reasons for it are likely to be that, firstly, Browne may have focused upon natural causes because he was a doctor. Of John Bird, T. A. and John Browne, it was Bird who emphasised the most that sin was the primary cause of scrofula, and he was a clergyman. This is not to say that only clergymen thought this way, but rather that Browne might have been one of those doctors who concentrated on natural causes rather than sin.[24] Secondly, by the 1680s Charles II was healing on a greater scale than any previous English monarch. Paradoxically this was problematic vis-a-vis the books by Bird and T. A., which argued that England was sinful and in need of a royal healer for the purpose of regeneration. If, after more than twenty years of the touching for scrofula, Charles II had not healed the nation, this implied that sin was still rife. This in turn meant either that the English were exceptionally sinful or that their king's touch was not particularly efficacious. The Popish Plot and the Exclusion Crisis can only have emphasised that the body politic was not in good health during the late 1670s. By the time that Browne published his book, Charles II had overcome his adversaries and was ruling without parliament,

---

[21] Browne, *Adenochoiradelogia*, bk I, 39, 42, 55–6; bk II, 34, 35–9, 44, 57; bk III, 1–2.

[22] Ibid. bk I, pp. 15, 18; bk III, pp. 13, 14, 100, 107.

[23] For the reformation of manners see M. M. Goldsmith, 'Public virtue and private vices', *Eighteenth-Century Studies* ix (1976), 477–510; T. C. Curtis and W. A. Speck, 'The Societies for the Reformation of Manners: a case study in the theory and practice of moral reform', *Literature & History* iii (1976), 45–64; R. B. Shoemaker, 'Reforming the city: the Reformation of Manners campaign in London, 1690–1738', in L. Davidson and others (eds), *Stilling the grumbling hive*, Stroud 1992, 99–120; J. Spurr, 'The Church, the societies and the moral revolution of 1688', in J. Walsh, C. Haydon and S. Taylor (eds.), *The Church of England, c. 1689–c. 1833: from toleration to Tractarianism*, Cambridge 1993, 127–42; J. Barry, "The Society for the Reformation of Manners, 1700–5', in J. Barry and K. Morgan (eds), *Reformation and revival in eighteenth-century Bristol*, Stroud 1994, 1–62; and S. Burt, 'The Societies for the Reformation of Manners: between John Locke and the devil in Augustan England', in R. D. Lund (ed.), *The margins of orthodoxy: heterodox writing and cultural response, 1660–1750*, Cambridge 1995, 149–69.

[24] See pp. 20–1 above.

but he followed Tory policies at the cost of alienating Whigs. It could be that Browne did not emphasise sin as the primary cause of scrofula because to do so would be the equivalent of saying that since 1660 the moral regeneration of England had failed. The nation was still as divided ideologically as it had been in the mid-century, the religious settlement had not worked, and the hopes of those such as Allen and Bird that the return of Charles II would usher in an age of godliness had not been realised. The difference between the intellectual climate of the 1680s and that of the 1660s could explain why by then apologists for the royal touch used different terms of reference.

Although Browne did not privilege sin within his book, he probably sought to counter-balance this by emphasising the biblical mandate for the royal touch: he went into greater detail about this subject than Bird, Allen or even Tooker. Unlike earlier authors, Browne quoted from the Old Testament as well as the New, citing Isaiah xlix.23, 'Kings shall be their nursing fathers, and Queens their nursing mothers'. He referred to Charles II as 'the great parent of our Health and Safety' and, like Bird, said that the king outdid his predecessors with his 'sanative faculty'.[25] Throughout his book, Browne asserted that the ultimate power to heal comes from God. He also defended the royal touch against its various critics.

Dissenters and 'superstition'

Browne denigrated dissenters for doubting the efficacy of the royal touch. They denied that it had any special powers, yet sometimes for pragmatic reasons they were touched, and according to Browne all were cured and some converted to the Church of England. This enabled Browne to take the moral high ground: the healing of these religious minorities and their subsequent conversion 'proved' that the Church of England was the true faith. The most extreme example connected to this was that of a sectarian who had five children all of whom had scrofula; the king cured one by his touch, the other four were not touched and died.[26]

Alternative criticisms made by dissenters, also discussed by Browne, were that although the royal touch worked, it was 'superstitious' or it worked by the power of suggestion.[27] Puritans usually believed that the Reformation had not gone far enough and so yearned for further reform of both society and the state Church; in the latter case by a reduction in ceremony and emphasis on the individual's direct relationship with God. For these minorities, too much ceremony was problematic because it was reminiscent of popery which was

---

[25] Browne, *Adenochoiradelogia*, 61, 76.
[26] Ibid. 169.
[27] Lloyd, *Wonders no miracles*, 13; Stubbe, *Miraculous conformist*, 9.

synonymous with 'superstition'. The problem with a 'superstitious' practice was that it offended their view of God and the correct way to worship him.

Browne described a nonconformist's wife who had scrofula. Her husband would not let her be touched by the king as the he thought 'it was a piece of Superstition, and that there was no more Virtue in the Kings Touch than in another mans'. Luckily for the woman, her husband had to make a long journey, so she took advantage of his absence to be touched by the king and was cured.[28] Browne used this narrative to bolster belief in the royal touch since the woman evidently had more faith than her husband and was rewarded with good health.

Beyond Browne, there are two brief mentions of this kind, although they are far less detailed. In 1660 Samuel Pepys noted that his friend, the surgeon Thomas Hollier (1609–90), came to dine with him and that they had a 'great discourse concerning the cure of the King's evil, which he doth deny altogether any effect at all'.[29] It is frustrating that Pepys did not explain why Hollier thought that the royal touch was not efficacious, but as the surgeon was a staunch Puritan it is possible that he believed it 'superstitious'.[30] An intriguing coda to this case that suggests that pragmatism overcame principle is that in the 1680s Browne reported that Hollier's son had scrofula that his father could not treat; so the son was touched by the king and cured.[31]

What may be a comparable case concerns one of the king's physicians, William Denton. On 21 November 1677 Denton wrote to his nephew Sir Ralph Verney that 'the king healed privately this day about six, whereof Lady Stewkely and Palmer were two. His healings are very uncertain, and everybody must take their fortune'.[32] Denton had been appointed court physician to Charles I in 1636; when the Stuarts were restored he became physician to Charles II and the duke of York and was made an honorary fellow of the Royal College of Physicians.[33] Denton participated in the royal touch ceremony between 1636 and the Civil War, and again once the Stuarts were restored, which makes his candid ambivalence concerning Charles II's healing powers all the more noteworthy. As well as being a respected physician, Denton was described by contemporaries as a staunch Protestant who published two polemical, anti-Roman Catholic tracts; it is therefore possible

---

[28] Browne, *Adenochoiradelogia*, 175–6, and at pp. 71, 101 for Browne denying that the ceremony was 'superstitious'.

[29] Pepys, *Diary*, i. 281, entry for 2 Nov. 1660.

[30] Ibid. x. 189; G. C. R. Morris, 'A portrait of Thomas Hollier, Pepys's surgeon', *Annals of the Royal College of Surgeons of England* lxi (1979), 224–9 at p. 226.

[31] Browne, *Adenochoiradelogia*, 178.

[32] HMC, *Seventh report*, 494: 21 Nov. 1677.

[33] Munk, *The roll of the Royal College of Physicians*, i. 327; A. Wood, *Athenae Oxonienses*, ed. Philip Bliss, London 1813–20, iv. 307–9.

that, like Hollier, he considered the royal touch 'superstitious'.[34] However, it should be noted that his comments suggest that he was ambivalent towards the ritual, whereas Hollier evidently denied that it had any power at all.

The problem for early modern people and for historians concerning the view that the royal touch was 'superstitious' is that the term is slippery: it is pejorative rather than analytical and so needs to be handled carefully.[35] The royal touch was the key manifestation of mystical monarchy and as such it appealed to many people for exactly the same reasons that made others worried that it was 'superstitious'. It was structured around prayers; the key moment of the ceremony was when each ill person received the healing touch of the divinely-appointed sovereign; each supplicant then received from the monarch a special commemorative gold medal that was inscribed with words and images that related to the health of the individual and of the nation, and to God's healing powers. Some of those who believed in the efficacy of royal therapeutics stressed the importance of the touch, others the prayers, others the wearing of the gold Angel. The problem with this was that too much deference to any one of these could be viewed critically as 'superstitious'. Indeed, apologists sometimes encouraged a 'superstitious' or magical view of proceedings, and especially of the king. T. A. wrote that 'when a man does that which another cannot do, we usually say *He conjures* ... [and] that Magic is laudable, and lawful, where there is not *Potentia in nocendo sed restituendo* [power to do harm but to restore or cure]'. T. A. then stated that Charles II 'is an Object for Love and Wonder to stand amazed at', noting that the correct way to receive the royal touch was kneeling as this denoted humility and reverence.[36]

The problem of 'superstition' can be further illuminated by examining two key concerns of the religious minorities, namely their objections to the liturgy and the touch-piece.[37] The liturgy was problematic because to credit the spoken word of prayer with any operative power blurred the boundary between religion and magic, and appeared to be Roman Catholic. This harks back to similar objections noted by Tooker and to those made by James VI and I;[38] and it helps to explain why some Protestants put their trust in providence rather than prayer.[39] Yet many people believed that the power of prayer could be extraordinary, hence the contemporary conviction that prayer and healing were symbiotic and that prayer could supplement natural remedies. The fact that many ministers were also physicians strengthened

---

[34] Munk, *The roll of the Royal College of Physicians*, i. 328; *Memoirs of the Verney family*, ii. 238.

[35] See pp. 70–1 above.

[36] T. A., *Excellency*, 28.

[37] Browne, *Adenochoiradelogia*, 71, 116.

[38] See pp. 63–4, 71–2 above, and Fuller, *Church history*, 145.

[39] Harley, 'Spiritual physic', 102; Shaw, *Miracles*, 40.

the connection between religion and medicine. In reality both Protestants and Catholics thought that God listened to prayers and so petitionary prayer was a common feature of early modern life.[40] If prayers were not answered then it was usual to think that the petitioner lacked faith.

Browne replied strongly to the charge that the liturgy was 'superstitious'. Prayers could not be condemned as 'Faith ... [came] by hearing the word of God', a quotation from Romans x.6. He insisted that the liturgy was 'the legitimate use of the Divine Word' as opposed to the illegitimate – popish or magical. He castigated the critics as people 'who cannot ... speak well of anybody or anything', who 'mock the Holy Spirit' and its 'Miracles, Scriptures, Sacraments and all other Ecclesiastical Ceremonies'.[41] Browne's response was far harsher than Tooker's nearly a century earlier: this suggests that such scepticism had grown stronger since the Elizabethan period.

Turning to the gold touch-pieces, it is clear that they were sometimes worn as amulets. The origins of this practice lay in the pre-Reformation Tudor liturgies which explicitly stated that the Angel must be worn until the person's scrofula had been cured. Thus the healing was believed to be wrought by the touch of the sovereign and the wearing of the Angel.[42] This caused problems after the Reformation because Protestants were not meant to believe that objects could have thaumaturgic properties. Yet the belief that scrofula would be healed if the Angel was worn persisted and appears to have been widespread.[43] Browne was ambivalent concerning this, mostly attacking the 'old received Opinion' that wearing an Angel cured scrofula, but sometimes recommending that ill people wear their medal as a curative practice. When arguing the former case he said it was the touch, not the gold, which was therapeutic, citing Charles I's healings that were brought about during the 1640s with silver coins or none at all.[44] To emphasise the sacrality of the monarch, Browne recounted the startling case of the Welsh prophet Arise Evans who tried to obtain the royal touch from Charles II as a cure for his fungous nose through his contact at court, the antiquarian Elias Ashmole. This was denied as Ashmole thought Evans unfit to approach the king. Undeterred, Evans knelt in front of Charles II during one of the king's morning walks in St James's Park: when the king gave him his hand to kiss, Evans rubbed it into his fungous nose and later said he was cured.[45]

---

[40] Thomas, *Religion and the decline of magic*, 124, 113–14; Shaw, *Miracles*, 123.

[41] Browne, *Adenochoiradelogia*, 116–17.

[42] See pp. 49–51 above.

[43] For an example of the persistence of this belief see van Wiquefort, *Relation*, 78.

[44] Browne, *Adenochoiradelogia*, 107–8. Richard Wiseman also discussed the status of the Angels, wondering whether people had found relief from scrofula by wearing other forms of gold: *Several chirugial treatises*, 241.

[45] Browne, *Adenochoiradelogia*, 162–4; cf. J. Aubrey, *Miscellanies upon the following subjects collected by John Aubrey Esq*, London 1696, 81; E. Ashmole, *Elias Ashmole: his*

Touch-pieces could be thought of as amulets for a number of reasons. The alchemical properties of gold are important, as are beliefs connected to the power of holy inscriptions. It is also worth remembering that touch-pieces were handled and bestowed by the monarch during a special ceremony, so charisma was important as well.[46] Furthermore, the touch-pieces were strikingly similar to sigils, metal objects cast from gold, iron or tin at astrologically favourable times which were inscribed with magical inscriptions and symbols and often worn around the neck or in a ring. Their purpose was to cure diseases and ailments, to provide protection, or to increase one's standing in the eyes of others.[47] As wearing gold was thought to induce someone to lead a less sinful life, and scrofula was associated with the sins of the nation, it is not surprising that touch-pieces were revered. John Aubrey even went so far as to suggest that it was the gold that cured scrofula rather than the king's touch.[48]

Many people wore their touch-pieces constantly.[49] In Dunstable, in 1682, one John Field was examined by the local JP because he was involved in the theft of two touch-pieces worn in bed by his master's two children. Another lodger, Richard Smith, had stolen the gold medals in the early hours of the morning, as well as some linen and two veal pies, and he offered Field one of the coins as a reward for keeping quiet about the theft. The JP's account is noteworthy because of its language: he wrote that Smith had 'actually taken [the touch-pieces] off the Childrens knecks where on they were put by his Majesty for Cure of the Evill'. This suggests that the JP, as well as the family that was robbed, thought that the Angels needed to be worn if the scrofula were to be cured. It also hints that the crime of theft was accompanied by the sacrilege of removing what the king had put on. Obviously, Smith could

autobiographical and historical notes, ed. C. H. Joster, Oxford 1967, ii. 778–9; T. N. Corns, 'Evans, Arise [Rhys, Rice], (*b. c.*1607, *d.* in or after 1660)', *ODNB*.

46 Browne, *Adenochoiradelogia*, 107. For amulets see Wallis Budge, *Amulets and superstition*; C. Bonner, 'Magical amulets', *Harvard Theological Review* xxxix/1 (1946), 25–54; Thomas, *Religion and the decline of magic*, 210, 227, 243, 275–6; S. Paine, *Amulets; sacred charms of power and protection*, Rochester, VT 2004; and J. Roper (ed.), *Charms and charming in Europe*, London 2004.

47 L. Kassell, 'The economy of magic in early modern England', in M. Pelling and S. Mandelbrote (eds), *The practice of reform in health, medicine and science, 1500–2000: essays for Charles Webster*, Aldershot 2005, 43–57. The term 'sigil' could also apply to the magical symbol on the object: F. Gettings, *Dictionary of occult, hermetic and alchemical sigils*, London 1981, 8–9.

48 Aubrey, *Observations*, in Buchanan Brown, *Three prose works*, 238. Cf. Pepys, *Diary*, i. 128, entry for 4 May 1660: Pepys sent his wife a gold coin when she was unwell.

49 Bedfordshire and Luton Archives, Bedford, HSA/1682 S/38 1682, HAS/1682 S/41 1682; Browne, *Adenochoiradelogia*, ch. x contains many accounts of people wearing their touch-pieces.

have sold the touch-pieces and indeed Browne lamented that it was some-times possible to buy them second-hand in 'Gold-Smiths shops'.[50]

And yet the fetishising of touch-pieces caused tensions for some Prot-estants, even allowing that theory and practice do not always mirror each other – especially when the stakes are high, as they are in health-related matters. This strain is evident in Browne's book. Although he emphasised that touch-pieces were mere 'tokens of Health', later on he described a number of people – including a student at Trinity College, Cambridge, a nobleman's daughter, and a maid – who were cured by the royal touch and wore their touch-pieces constantly. Each of them then lost their Angel and their scrofula returned until the medal was found and worn again, at which point the disease vanished.[51] These cases were described neutrally, without any reference to 'superstition'. Browne also described someone who did not find their lost Angel but instead was touched for a second time, thus acquiring a new one which achieved the same results.[52]

The inference in Browne's book is that the gold Angel played a crucial role in healing scrofula, and this is particularly evident in the most dramatic of these case studies. A father and son both had scrofula but only the father was touched by the king:

> The Father being distempered and ill, keeps the Gold about his own neck, which kept him in health, and gave him speedy ease and relief: The Son falling ill, he borrows his Fathers Gold from his neck, and puts it about his own, which likewise gave him ease and relief. The Father after this by leaving his Gold, had his Distemper seized him afresh, and then took the Gold again, and this made it as readily vanish. And thus by the intercourse or change of Gold from Father to Son, and from Son to Father, whoever of them kept the Gold, was defended against any new … appearance of his Distemper; and this was kept and maintained by them for many years together.[53]

On one occasion Browne even recommended that a woman with recurring scrofula wore her touch-piece at all times, a remedy which he said worked.[54] As one of the king's surgeons, Browne's official line was that the royal hand cured scrofula; but he evidently also believed in the curative properties of gold, even if he foregrounded it less in his book.

Browne also voiced inconsistent views concerning another belief that some contemporaries regarded as 'superstitious', namely that the royal touch was most efficacious at Easter, especially on Good Friday. Easter was the most popular time to be touched as it related to redemption, but Browne said

---

50 Browne, *Adenochoiradelogia*, 93.
51 Ibid. 107–8, 148–9, 167, 171, 174, 181, 184.
52 Ibid. 106.
53 Ibid. 138.
54 Ibid. 175.

that it was 'a sin' to suppose that God worked differently at different times of the year, and dismissed this belief. Yet elsewhere he recounted without criticism the tale of a blacksmith who was touched at Easter and received 'immediate benefit' but was not fully cured, so he returned each Easter to be touched again.[55] This is interesting not least because it contradicted government policy that sought to avoid people being touched more than once.

Having considered the liturgy and the gold touch-piece, a final aspect of the concerns about the 'superstition' that it engendered needs to be examined. For many Protestants 'superstition' was synonymous with Roman Catholicism. Bird also recorded that some people objected to the royal touch because it was performed by the French as well as the English monarchs.[56] The royal touch was a difficult issue for English Protestant apologists because it related to the broader debate concerning the cessation of miracles.[57] Protestant polemic maintained that Roman Catholic miracles were fraudulent or diabolical; but this did not stop miracles from occurring in Protestant countries. In England this was partly because miracles were 'Protestantised' in as much as they were shorn of intermediary figures and external trappings.[58] The problem with the royal touch was that it had both: an intercessor in the form of the king and the external trappings of the ceremony.

Obviously, Catholics used belief in miracles to validate the mass, the cult of saints and the Virgin Mary, reverence for images, and belief in the power of relics, all of which were denied by Protestants, albeit to varying degrees, as with relics.[59] Consequently the debate over miracles was part of an intense struggle to assert which type of Christianity was the true faith. This was a complicated issue, not least because if a Catholic miracle were not obviously fraudulent, Protestants attributed it to the devil even though they agreed with Catholics that the powers of the devil were superhuman rather than supernatural. This theory had its own problems because some Catholic miracles transcended the natural order (such as raising the dead) and therefore could not be attributed to the devil. This meant that occasionally Protestants allowed that there were rare instances when God permitted the devil to perform supernatural miracles in order to test the faithful.[60]

This illuminates Bird's defence of the royal touch against the charge that it was not only 'superstitious' but Catholic. He noted that the French king cured scrofula even though he belonged to a 'false Church', but said that the New Testament taught that 'at the last day, some reprobates should say

---

[55] Ibid. 106–7, 193–4.

[56] See p. 156 above.

[57] See p. 71 above.

[58] Walker, 'Cessation of miracles', 111; Shaw, *Miracles*, ch. ii.

[59] See p. 95 above.

[60] Walker, 'Cessation of miracles', 119, 114–15, 116–17. For the limitations of the devil's powers see also P. Dear, 'Miracles, experiments, and the ordinary course of nature', *Isis* lxxxi (1990), 663–83 at pp. 671–2.

unto our Saviour, *Have we not in thy Name cast out devils?*' thus implicitly connecting the royal touch with exorcism. Bird argued that the French king's ability to heal was a 'signe of things to come' and that Christ would soon judge those who performed miracles but were 'evil'.[61] Bird chose not to dismiss the French royal touch as diabolical, as this would have been too radical, but rather to set it in a millenarian context. Whether or not this convinced his readers is an open question.

In the 1680s Browne addressed the problem of the French Catholic royal touch, but he did not go so far as Bird because by then Charles II's heir was Roman Catholic and the English court had become very Francophile. Browne discussed Catholic miracles only once and contrasted the views of their protagonists with those of dissenters. Whereas Catholics were too eager to see miracles, dissenters denied the abundant evidence of their own eyes, a reference to their scepticism about the king's touch.[62]

The power of suggestion

Some modern accounts of the royal touch speculate that the cures were psychosomatic, the implication being that this was largely unrecognised by contemporaries.[63] This was not so. Some doctors and dissenters certainly thought that the royal touch worked by natural rather than supernatural means, in that the physical presence of the monarch stimulated the imaginations of the ill people, which then precipitated a cure.[64] In pre-modern Europe it was usual to think that faith was needed for treatments and medicine to work. It was also commonplace for early modern people to think that the imagination could affect the body, and so, for example, epidemics were thought to strike the fearful, and pregnant women were said to be able to affect the physical and emotional wellbeing of their unborn babies by their thoughts. Furthermore, theories of natural magic maintained that planetary influences affected the mind, the results of which included psychosomatic cures.[65]

Browne did not castigate those who thought that the royal touch worked by the power of suggestion because as a Christian and a doctor he allowed that the imagination, or faith, had an important role to play in the healing of diseases.[66] He even described how the positive effects of the power of sugges-

---

[61] Bird, *Ostenta Carolina*, 89–90.

[62] Browne, *Adenochoiradelogia*, 72–3.

[63] Block, *The royal touch*, 237–8 (419–21); Keay, *Magnificent monarch*.

[64] E. Chamberlayne, *Anglia notitia, or, The present state of England*, London 1670, 160–1; Lloyd, *Wonders no miracles*, 13; *An answer to a scoffing and lying libell*, 2.

[65] D. P. Walker, *Spiritual and demonic magic from Ficino to Campanella*, London 1958, 76–80, 149–50, 160–1, 200–1.

[66] Browne, *Adenochoiradelogia*, 35.

tion helped a doubter to see the light. A Quaker gunsmith from Winchester had scrofula and procured a ticket to be touched, but nevertheless said that 'his Faith was so small that he did not believe the Kings Touch could much help him, or that there was any Power or Virtue therein, but resolved notwithstanding to make use of his Favour'. However, on seeing the king the Quaker's 'Spirits immediately raised to a higher degree of Faith', and after he was touched Browne said that he was cured and converted to the Church of England.[67]

Browne wrote a vivid commentary on the moment when a sick person was touched by the king, emphasising how close proximity to the monarch could stimulate the imagination (or 'fancy') which then played a part in the healing:

> Thus when a poor Creature who never saw ... the King, shall behold his Princely and Royal Hand with a charitable confidence and touch to chase away his troublesome and loathsome Swellings; to see a Hand so humble, of an Arm so high, shew such condescention; of a King so great to stroak the Sores of so mean, and low, and despicable a Subject; to see Him who sits in his Royal Chair, vouchsafe his Presence and helping Hand, where many or most of his Subjects would both stop their Nostrils, and shut their Eyes at, as scorning to come near them, this may well raise and enlarge the Patients fancy, summoning his Spirits to assist Nature for the encountring this Disease with the utmost might.[68]

However, there was a problem with attributing cures to the patients' imaginations because, as with privileging the gold over the touch, it lessened the mystical role of the king. This was why in the passage above Browne said that the imagination assisted with the cure rather than producing it on its own. If too much stress were placed on the role of the imagination then the apologists had an answer, namely that many young infants were touched by the monarch and healed and yet they could not be sensitive to their environment in the manner that this explanation required.[69]

At the end of the Elizabethan period Tooker had denied that the imagination was powerful enough to work miracles and in the 1660s T.A. agreed in even stronger terms as he had to refute the sectarian healers who had proliferated in the 1640s and 1650s.[70] He insisted that the cures wrought by seventh sons and other healers 'must either be miraculous, or wholly attributed to the Imagination of the Patients'. They were not miraculous as it was 'not lawful for ordinary persons to assume so great a power'; nor was the power of suggestion a sufficient explanation because it was stronger in

---

[67] Ibid. 172–3; for a comment concerning the widespread view that faith was needed for the royal touch to work see p. 189.

[68] Ibid. 70. See also Fuller, *Church history*, 145.

[69] Heylyn, *Examen historicum*, 47; Chamberlayne, *Anglia notitia*, 160.

[70] For Tooker see p. 63 above.

some people than others and so it could 'deceive sense' and 'obscure Reason'. Unsurprisingly, T. A. concluded that the so-called healings of seventh sons were fraudulent. Yet the royal touch was different to the radical healers and T. A. was careful not to rule out the need for faith if the former were to work. Faith was essential for healing, as was prayer: 'Prayers have wings for flying, without fear of falling' while 'the Sick man's confidence, oft-times speeds beyond all other remedies.'[71]

The physical reality of scrofula

Scrofula can sometimes go into remission of its own accord. Marc Bloch in particular averred that scrofula has the ability to relapse naturally as an explanation for belief in royal therapeutics (he dismissed the possibility that the imagination could work a cure), and this view remains popular within secondary works.[72] Implicit in this view is the assumption that modern science knows that scrofula can relapse whereas early modern people did not. Just as with the power of suggestion, this is not in fact the case. Some unidentified critics of royal therapeutics argued that the cures which seemed to be wrought by the royal hand were really nothing more than the coincidence of this happening shortly after supplicants had been touched by the monarch.[73] This represents outright disbelief, whereas those who thought that the ritual was 'superstitious' or that the cures were psychosomatic allowed that healings happened but questioned what brought them about.

When Browne discussed the physical reality of scrofula he wrote that it was particularly difficult for doctors to treat because of its ability to relapse naturally, and his case studies at the end of his book contain numerous references to the process of relapse.[74] Bird and T. A. were also aware of this: Bird said that the royal touch was sometimes criticised as it did not always produce a permanent cure which shows an awareness of scrofula's ability to reappear after it was supposedly cured;[75] T. A. similarly stated that both children and adults who had scrofula often experienced its 'spontaneous cessation' which he attributed to 'Nature ... The Lady physician of all Diseases'.[76] Thus the appearance and disappearance of scrofula could be attributed to the royal hand, or to whether the person who had been touched wore their gold Angel, or to natural causes.

71 T. A., *Excellency*, 4, 6, 27.

72 Bloch, *The royal touch*, 242 (428); Thomas, *Religion and the decline of magic*, 205; Keay, *Magnificent monarch*, 113; Crawfurd, *The King's evil*, 25.

73 *Ostenta Carolina*, 90.

74 Browne, *Adenochoiradelogia*, bk II, p, 83; bk III, pp. 131, 140, 144, 162, 167, 175, 178, 181.

75 Bird, *Ostenta Carolina*, 89.

76 T. A., *Excellency*, 11–12.

All of this brings into sharp relief the question of just how miraculous was the royal touch? Orthodox Protestants tended to be cautious about current-day miracles because they were difficult to define. Browne expressed the hope that the royal touch 'may not come short of an English Miracle'; presumably by 'English' he meant Protestant.[77] He also said that, because scrofula was made by God, it should be 'thus cured by the hand of his Vicegerent' which 'doth not come much beneath one [a miracle]'.[78] The author and Fellow of the Royal Society Edward Chamberlayne also considered that if the royal touch was not miraculous it was 'super-excellent'.[79]

Seventeenth-century Europeans understood a miracle to be a spontaneous intervention by God that over-ruled or suspended the usual course of nature: in order to detect when this happened it was therefore necessary to know how nature operated, and especially what its limitations were.[80] The problem of which contemporaries were aware was that, since the laws of nature were not fully understood, there was sometimes doubt concerning the status of a supposed miracle. There were two specific problems with the royal touch with regard to this. First, scrofula did not obey regular laws: sometimes it went into remission of its own accord, sometimes it remained chronic, sometimes it was cured by medicine, sometimes it was fatal, and sometimes the royal touch worked, but not always. The capriciousness of scrofula meant that there was no regular, natural pattern against which a miraculous cure by the royal touch could be defined. Secondly, the fact that scrofula was sometimes cured or alleviated by medicine was problematic in itself because miracles were meant to be beyond the order of nature.

The emergence of the new science during the Restoration privileged observation and experimentation rather than *a priori* assumptions about nature. The boundaries of the natural world were extended due to scientific enquiry, so that those of the preter- and supernatural shrunk. As nature became more fully understood, some phenomena that had been thought to be miraculous – such as comets -- were reclassified as natural.[81] At the same time contemporaries were aware that uneducated people often attributed supernatural causes to things that they did not understand, which could tarnish the notion of the miraculous for the educated.[82] None of this boded well for miracles, yet Protestants did not claim that God no longer inter-vened in human affairs as this denied his omnipotence and was too close

---

[77] Browne, *Adenochoiradelogia*, 102.

[78] Ibid. 71–2.

[79] Chamberlayne, *Anglia notitia*, 160.

[80] Dear, 'Miracles, experiments, and the ordinary course of nature', 672–4, 683; Walsham, 'Miracles in post-Reformation England', 273–306.

[81] S. Shaffer, 'Newton's comets and the transformation of astrology', in P. Curry (ed.), *Astrology, science and society: historical essays*, Wolfeboro, NH 1987, 219–43; J. Henry, *The scientific revolution and the origins of modern science*, 2nd edn, London 2002, ch. iv.

[82] Clark, *Thinking with demons*, 177.

to atheism. Consequently, in theory some miracles could be reclassified as a providence or a special providence, events that God had planned in advance. Yet in reality the new demarcations between *miracula* and *miranda* were blurred because of the subjectivity involved in differentiating between them.[83]

Biblical miracles produced immediate cures, but it was obviously not the case that between 1660 and 1688 well over 100,000 people were cured of their scrofula at the very moment that Charles II or James II touched them. Yet the ritual had to produce some sort of results, or why bother to keep practising it? It is worth reiterating that the royal touch was not expected to cure everyone and those who remained ill might be thought to need a second touch, or to be lacking in faith; but at the very least, it was hoped that the rite would alleviate people's scrofula, even if it did not heal it. This might not have been as problematic for contemporaries as it initially appears because an incremental improvement could signify God's blessing whilst miracles that brought about physical transformations had always been rare. As Martin Luther put it in a sermon of 1535, there were two types of miracles, those of faith that produced a deeper sense of God's purpose and those of the body that brought about physical alterations, the latter having always been more rare than the former.[84]

In the case of scrofula, matters were convoluted because the royal touch was described as producing a range of results, from the very rare cases of an immediate cure, to the more usual slower improvement in people's conditions, to not working at all. Commentators were well aware of this range, even if they did not all always address it directly. Browne might have boasted that 'near half the Nation' had been touched and healed by Charles II, who had cured more people in any one year than the doctors had since 1660, but this was hyperbole. Richard Wiseman was more realistic. In his treatise of 1676 he claimed to have witnessed 'many hundreds of cures', yet he had been serjeant surgeon for four years, a period during which the king had touched almost 18,000 sufferers.[85] At the end of *Adenochoiradelogia* Browne put forward eighty-six case studies that testified to the efficacy of the royal touch;[86] but his book was published in 1684, by which time the king had touched almost 100,000 people, so his eighty-six cases need to be viewed with this in mind.

Browne's examples are extremely useful, however. The fact that he needed to provide proof of the efficacy of royal therapeutics hints at a climate of scepticism in some quarters, while the case studies themselves contain details

---

[83] Walsham, 'Miracles in post-Reformation England', 285–6.

[84] Walker, 'Cessation of miracles', 111–12; Walsham, 'Miracles in post-Reformation England', 286.

[85] Browne, *Adenochoiradelogia*, 105–6; Wiseman, *Several chirugial treatises*, 240.

[86] Browne, *Adenochoiradelogia*, 127–96.

of people's circumstances and conditions, a reflection of the new intellectual culture of observation and enquiry. A small number of cases suggest an immediate cure but the bulk of his evidence suggests a slower improvement, the first signs of which were usually apparent about two weeks after people were touched.

The fast, dramatic, cures were surely the most useful in bolstering faith in the ritual, and sometimes aligned it with biblical miracles. They make vivid reading. When one young girl who was blind with scrofula was touched by Charles II, the film that covered her eyes broke and her sight returned. The daughter of one Mr Harbins of Winchester was blind with scrofula: she was touched, but later that same day her sight had returned to the extent that when she saw a Maypole on the Strand she asked her mother 'what that long pole was for'?[87] Cases such as these two probably reminded people of the four blind men healed by Christ.[88] Two women travelled from Breda and Virginia to be touched, both of whom experienced a dramatic improvement in their condition as soon as they were touched, with a full recovery following within a fortnight or so. Slightly less immediate but still remarkable was the case of a 'very poor Country woman' who was so incapacitated that she was 'brought in a Chair' to be touched; the next day she could walk 'about the room' and within two days was 'perfectly recovered'. Similarly, a man who had had scrofula since 1648 was touched in 1662 and said that he was 'very much at ease' within 'two or three days' and was cured within a fortnight.[89]

Yet it is the slower improvements in people's health that are more characteristic of Browne's cases; sometimes we are also told that these people have not relapsed. One Mr Edwards from Curry Rivel, Somersetshire, had scrofulous sores on his face which caused him to be blind; in 1660 he came to London and was touched, and within six weeks his sores had gone and his sight returned. Marmaduke Ling of North Petherton, Somersetshire, had particularly florid scrofula on his face: he was touched, with an improvement noticeable within fourteen days, a full recovery within six weeks. Two years later he had still not relapsed. A Berkshire woman blind with scrofula regained partial sight within 'less than fourteen days' after she was touched, and continued to improve. Sir Roger Hasnet, serjeant-at-arms to the king, told Browne that a six-year-old girl was touched for the second time: an improvement was noticeable within two hours, a full recovery within fourteen days. One Dorothy Philips was touched, after which she travelled to Leicestershire, returning to London one month later 'very well and cured'. Another woman who had been blind for four months due to scrofula was touched, regaining her sight 'within a month'. Browne told of a man with

---

[87] Ibid. 168, 192–3; see also p. 186.

[88] Mark viii.22–6, Mark x.46–52, Matt. xx.29–34, Matt. ix.27–31, Luke xviii.35–43, John ix.1–12.

[89] Browne, *Adenochoiradelogia*, 194–5, 186–7, 190.

particularly acute scrofula who was touched by Charles II at Windsor, and within fourteen days 'he was discharged from his Swellings'.[90]

The notion that the ritual produced miraculous cures was also undermined by the fact that scrofula was sometimes cured or alleviated by medicine and not just the royal touch. The discussion of this issue seems to have become more intense by the 1680s because Browne refuted this view far more strongly than Bird had in 1661. Bird argued that Christ healed all diseases in order to fulfil prophecies, whereas this was not expected of the king.[91] Browne wrote defensively that Christ and his disciples sometimes healed people with curable diseases such as paralysis, yet this did not mean that they had not performed a miracle. Thus, for Browne, it did not matter that scrofula was sometimes alleviated or cured by medicine. He also stated that Charles II did not consult with his surgeons before he touched the sick, implying that the king touched people regardless of the severity of their scrofula or any previous treatments that they had undertaken.[92]

Turning directly to the issue of whether the royal touch was miraculous, Browne said that although the age of miracles was thought to be over, God gave the English monarchs their 'sanative gift' in order to keep the faith alive; but he was adamant that only God performed miracles, stating that man was the 'Organ and Instrument' and God was the 'chief Agent and Master of the Operation'.[93] He further explained that:

> The true Rule therefore of Miracles is this, If God gives the power of doing good to anyone, let him prosecute the same and prosper in the action. These being given according to the will which can and will do what he pleaseth: In former times … this Gift was bestowed on Pious and Religious Men, of which sort in those times were great plenty to be found. But our succeeding Ages have much lessened in the number thereof.[94]

Thus for the orthodox the royal touch signified goodness in an increasingly irreligious age. This was why Browne wrote that the gift was given to the king, who was also the governor of the Church.[95]

Doubt among the learned: John Aubrey's ambivalent commentary

The Restoration antiquarian and biographer John Aubrey made three important comments on the royal touch. These are intriguing because they shed

---

[90] Ibid. 161–2, 174, 181, 167, 171, 172, 170. For other people described as not having relapsed see pp. 166, 182.

[91] See p. 156 above.

[92] Browne, *Adenochoiradelogia*, 2–3, 34.

[93] Ibid. 62, 18, 21.

[94] Ibid. 56–7.

[95] Ibid.

light on how it was debated in prestigious intellectual circles. Although Fuller and Browne noted in general terms that there was 'still much controversie kept up amongst the Learned',[96] Aubrey provides detail. Aubrey was uncertain about the efficacy of the royal touch, but it aroused his intellectual curiosity because he was interested in history, medicine, popular customs and belief, and supernatural phenomenon.[97]

First, there is Aubrey's suggestion that the ceremony was only superficially religious in character. In a manuscript he noted that "Tis true (indeed) there are prayers read at the touching, but neither the King minds them nor the chaplains.' However, when Aubrey published his remarks in his *Miscellanies* (1696) he added the word 'perhaps' so that his comment read 'but perhaps neither the King minds them nor the chaplains', thus slightly modifying his scepticism.[98] Consequently, there are problems with taking Aubrey on trust, appealing though this is to modern commentators.[99] His is the only eyewitness commentary to suggest that the ceremony was only ostensibly religious. In fact, as the records make very clear, the ceremony was highly religious in character. It was structured around a liturgy and the two printed images depict the chaplains praying in prominent positions next to the king; the sovereign re-enacted Christ's healing ministry; and the rite was often performed in cathedrals and chapels. Foreign eyewitnesses such as the Italian savant Lorenzo Magalotti emphasised the religious nature of the ceremony even though he was a Roman Catholic who witnessed the royal touch performed in a non-palatial house in Newmarket. He wrote that the prayer book was kept on a table on a cushion, and the chaplains wore their surplices and read the liturgy with a 'great appearance of devotion'.[100] All of this militates against Aubrey's point of view.

Why did Aubrey hold the view that he did? The answer is that although he took for granted a religious outlook he was highly anti-clerical: he thought it was rare to find 'Humility and Charity' among the clergy. He was also anti-ceremonial and his religious outlook was tolerant, 'rational' and irenic, rather than traditional. He shared these values with contemporaries such as Thomas Hobbes, William Petty and Sir Thomas Browne.[101] By the standards of the day, Aubrey had a secular attitude towards life. The suggestion is that

96 Ibid. 70; Fuller, *Church history*, 145.

97 M. Hunter, *John Aubrey and the realm of learning*, New York 1975, 47–56, 103 n. 5, 132–47, 209–15.

98 J. Aubrey, *Remaines of Gentilisme and Judaism*, ed. James Britten, London 1881, 241, and *Miscellanies upon the following subjects collected by John Aubrey Esq*, London 1696, 98. The manuscript source is Royal Society, MS RS 92, fos 361–2; a copy of Aubrey's *The natural history of Wiltshire*, Bodl. Lib., MSS Aubrey 1, 2; a further transcript appears in J. Aubrey, *The natural history of Wiltshire*, ed. John Britten, London 1847, 120.

99 Keith Thomas has taken Aubrey on trust: *Religion and the decline of magic*, 194.

100 Magalotti, *Travels of Lorenzo the Third*, 215.

101 Hunter, *Aubrey*, 33, 56–8, 220.

Aubrey projected his own anti-clerical, anti-ceremonialist views onto the royal touch which explains why his comments are at odds with those of other contemporary observers.

The second of Aubrey's comments relates to the way in which the efficacy of the royal touch was debated in learned circles. Aubrey wrote that 'the Curing of the Kings-evil by the Touch of the King, does much puzzle our Philosophers: For whether our Kings were of the House of York, or Lancaster, it did the Cure for the most part'.[102] This speaks for itself, including the remark at the end that the ceremony did not heal everyone. It indicates that although apologists argued that the royal touch worked by virtue of hereditary powers they created a problem for themselves because the obvious sceptical retort was to mention the disruptions to the direct line of succession during the Wars of the Roses.

The third comment highlights the incompatibility of the royal touch with the new mechanical philosophy, which maintained that the universe was a great machine made up of matter in motion. One philosopher whom Aubrey specified was the doctor and cleric Ralph Bathurst, 'no Superstitious Man', who protested to Aubrey that 'the Curing of the Kings Evill by the touch of the King does puzzle his Philosophie'.[103] Aubrey and Bathurst were lifelong friends who met at Trinity College, Oxford, during the 1630s. Bathurst was a doctor of medicine, one of the original members of the Oxford Experimental Philosophy Club that was a precursor of the Royal Society. In 1663 he became chaplain to Charles II and a Fellow of the Royal Society, the following year President of Trinity, and in 1670 dean of Wells.[104]

Aubrey's brief mention of Bathurst's sceptical view of the royal touch is interesting for a number of reasons. As chaplain to the king, Bathurst would have gained first-hand experience of the ceremony and he was known to be extremely loyal to the Stuarts. Unlike Aubrey, Bathurst was not opposed to religious ceremonies: he planned to write a history of them extolling their usefulness, though this does not seem to survive. It also appears from the little surviving evidence that we have, namely Bathurst's sermons, that he did believe in the possibility of healing by touch as he preached that 'Christ cures our sins with as much ease as he once did our sickness: a word of his mouth, a touch of his hand, nay the hem of his garment will do the work.'[105] Bathurst thus believed that Christ cured the sick miraculously, whatever his views on the continuing possibility of miracles of a similar kind.

---

[102] Aubrey, *Miscellanies*, in *Three prose works*, 79.

[103] Idem, *Natural history of Wiltshire*, 120.

[104] T. Warton, *The life and literary remains of Ralph Bathurst*, Oxford 1761, 61, 152–3, 204; M. Steggle, 'Bathurst, Ralph (1619/20–1704)', ODNB; Hunter, *The Royal Society and its Fellows*, 164.

[105] Steggle, 'Bathurst, Ralph'; Warton, *Literary remains*, 56, 223. This history does not appear to have been written.

As Aubrey pointed out, Bathurst was at a loss to explain the efficacy of the royal touch because of his 'Philosophie'. He had been an adherent of the new Cartesian philosophy since his time as a young scholar at Oxford.[106] He was also an admirer of Hobbes, especially his book *Human nature* (1650).[107] Yet in 1663 Bathurst joined the Royal Society, which had recently been involved in a public dispute between Hobbes and Boyle in which Boyle championed empirical findings against Hobbes's *a priori* theories.[108] Though many Fellows of the Royal Society were sympathetic to mechanical explanations, they were ambivalent about the derivable forms of mechanism associated with Hobbes and Descartes, insisting that such ideas should be subjected to empirical testing. Their systems also allowed for occult qualities in nature which Cartesians and Hobbesians rejected, while they were also sympathetic to the idea of supernatural intervention in the natural world – as seen in miracles – which they believed could also be empirically tested.[109] Bathurst appears to have been a stricter mechanist than many of his Royal Society peers: Aubrey tells us that he laughed at astrology, and his comment on Bathurst's difficulty in explaining the royal touch according to his view of nature makes sense in this context.[110]

Aubrey was interested enough in Bathurst's point of view to record it, but he was not a strict mechanist like his friend. Aubrey believed in many supernatural phenomena, even if not the efficacy of the royal touch as described by its apologists. Indeed, he offered a reductionist reading of it, reflecting his mixed world view that was partly secular, partly occultist.[111] Because Aubrey thought that gold could cure ulcers, he suggested that those who originally devised the royal touch ceremony did so because they too were aware of this. Aubrey emphasised the importance of the gold in the healing ceremony: he stated that the gold was very pure, and the touch-pieces were made at times that were astrologically propitious.[112] This suggests that Aubrey thought of the touch-pieces as sigils, although no evidence has so far come to light to support his astrological claim. For Aubrey it appears that it was the gold rather than the king's touch that had the potential to heal scrofula because

---

[106] R. G. Frank, Jr, *Harvey and the Oxford physiologists: scientific ideas and social interaction*, Los Angeles 1980, 107.

[107] T. Hobbes, *Human nature*, London 1650; Warton, *Literary remains*, 49; Frank, *Harvey and the Oxford physiologists*, 107.

[108] S. Shapin and S. Shaffer, *Leviathan and the air pump: Hobbes, Boyle and the experimental life*, Princeton 1995, ch. iv; Hunter, *Boyle: between God and science*, 135–8.

[109] Hunter, *Science and society*,37; Henry, *Scientific revolution*, 74–5; M. Hunter, 'Boyle et la surnaturel', in M. Dennehy and C. Ramond (eds), *La Philosophie naturelle de Robert Boyle*, Paris 2009, 213–36.

[110] Hunter, *John Aubrey*, 144, 198. For the complexities of the Royal Society and its attitudes to magic see Hunter, 'The Royal Society and the decline of magic', 103–19.

[111] For Aubrey's worldview see Hunter, *Aubrey*, 198.

[112] Aubrey, *Observations*, in Buchanan Brown, *Three prose works*, 238.

he believed more strongly in its occult properties than in the sacred touch of the king. It is frustrating that Aubrey said nothing on the French royal touch though, as this ceremony did not involve the gift of gold, supplicants being given a small amount of money by the king just as in medieval England.

So, Aubrey's ambivalence towards the royal touch was due to his disdain for orthodox Christianity and its ceremonies. He did not deny that sometimes the royal touch cured scrofula, but rather than adhering to the customary explanation of this he attributed it to the occult properties of gold. Bathurst, on the other hand, was less opposed to ceremonies, probably because they were useful for the practice of religion, but as a strict Cartesian he could not believe in miraculous healings and so was more sceptical of the royal touch than Aubrey.

Wit and ridicule

Aside from religious minorities, doctors and intellectuals who were influenced by occult or mechanical philosophies, Browne informs us that the royal touch was assailed daily by people who mocked it:

> Others by spleen, disdain, ridicule, and private injury, will needs put a blind upon this most excellent Operation ... to what an Age of Incredulity are we arrived at, where resolution, spleen and injury, shall confirm a Mans opposition to the very light of Reason and Truth itself?[113]

Browne does not spell out to whom he is referring or what their criticisms were, but in all likelihood the culprits were the wits, the self-confident, sceptical young men who frequented the coffee houses and the royal court, personified by John Wilmot, second earl of Rochester, and playwrights like William Wycherly.[114] The wits were also known as 'scoffers' as they mocked religious orthodoxy, while sometimes living debauched lives. *The character of a coffee-house* (1673), an anonymous pamphlet that describes the 'town wit', mentions how such men rejected belief in magic: 'talk of witches and you tickle him; speak of spirits, and he tells you, he knows none better than those of wine'.[115] The rejection of spiritual healing must have gone hand-in-hand with that of magic, although it is unfortunate that there is no direct evidence

---

[113] Browne, *Adenochoiradelogia*, 114.

[114] For the wits see J. H. Wilson, *The court wits of the Restoration*, Princeton 1948; *The court wits of the Restoration: an introduction*, London 1967; and *Court satires of the Restoration*, Columbus 1976; S. I. Mintz, *The hunting of Leviathan*, Cambridge 1962, ch. vii; and J. Spurr, *England in the 1670s: this masquerading age*, Oxford 2000, 91–3, 102–10. T. A. and Bird made no mention of the royal touch being ridiculed because their books date from the early years of the Restoration, when the culture of wit was less established.

[115] *The character of a coffee-house with the symptomes of a town-wit*, London 1673, 5.

of this. However, as with religious minorities, sometimes the wits did access the royal touch, with pragmatism overcoming principle.

The roots of the culture of wit lay in the 1640s and 1650s when authority was questioned on an unprecedented scale, and religious extremism led some to indifference, both circumstances which helped to generate a culture of scepticism.[116] The key intellectual influence on the wits was Thomas Hobbes, and to a lesser extent Descartes and Machiavelli. Hobbes wrote in *Leviathan* (1651) that it was better to trust one's senses, experiences and 'naturall Reason' than to accept received wisdom; he was critical of the authority of the Bible and revealed religion, and cynical about priests.[117] This alternative philosophy was intoxicating for the young wits as it provided a strong sense of liberation from orthodox Christian doctrine. This is proof that during the Restoration thankfully not everyone was preoccupied with sin and redemption; indeed, the wits can be seen as a reaction to this: the royal touch was ridiculed by the wits as part of their attack on orthodoxy.

The wits found favour at the royal court because, in some respects, Charles II had a similar world view to theirs.[118] Although the wits are often thought to personify their age, the sarcasm and flippancy of fashionable literature and conversation caused great anxiety because for the mainstream this reflected an increase in apostasy, blasphemy and atheism.[119] It was generally thought that the immoral life of libertines resulted in the denial of religion,[120] which led to the body politic being in poor health.

The trial of Sir Charles Sedley in 1663 particularly outraged many contemporaries. Sedley admitted to getting drunk with two others at the Cock Tavern on Bow Street and then 'showing himself naked on a balcony, and throwing down bottles (pissed in) *vi et armis* among the people'.[121] Pepys recorded hearsay that Sedley had also mocked the Bible, preached a mountebank sermon, performed lewd poses and 'took a glass of wine and washed his prick in it and then drank it off; and then took another and drank the king's health'. This caused a riot, and enraged many Puritans. Sedley was fined £500 and imprisoned and Pepys wrote that the judge said that it was because of 'such wicked wretches' as Sedley that 'God's anger and judgements' hung over the country.[122]

---

116   Hunter, *Science and society*, 168.

117   T. Hobbes, *Leviathan*, ed. C. B. Macpherson, 409–10.

118   Mintz, *Hunting of Leviathan*, 142.

119   Spurr, *Restoration Church of England*, 238. For the fear of atheism and the culture of anxiety see also Hunter, *Science and society*, ch. vii.

120   Mintz, *Hunting of Leviathan*, 134.

121   J. Keble (ed.), *Reports in the Court of King's Bench from the XII to the XXX year of the reign of Charles II*, London 1685, i. 168; Wilson, *Court wits*, 41–2; H. Love, 'Sedley, Sir Charles, fifth baronet (*bap.* 1639, *d.* 1701)', *ODNB*.

122   Pepys, *Diary*, iv. 209, entry for 1 July 1663.

On the other hand, despite being notorious sceptics and libertines, it is wrong to assume that all wits discounted the royal touch completely, as is illustrated by a revealing letter written by Rochester to his wife Anne in 1672 concerning the ill health of their twenty-month-old son Charles.[123] In the letter Rochester mentioned the royal touch, which might have seemed an ideal target for his biting wit, his extreme scepticism surely being incompatible with sacral monarchy and orthodox Christianity. According to Gilbert Burnet, the theologian who attended Rochester during the earl's last illness in 1680 and effected his conversion, Rochester had previously conceptualised God as a 'vast power' who worked through nature with 'none of the attributes of Goodness and Justice we ascribe to the Deity'. Rochester rejected the idea of a providential God and thought that religious ceremonies were invented by priests in order to subjugate the masses; he dismissed the efficacy of prayer and thought that miracles were really conjuring tricks that demonstrated the credulity of the people.[124]

In fact, Rochester thought that his ill son had scrofula, and wrote to his wife to explain that he was arranging for the boy to 'come up to London this weeke to bee touch't' by the king.[125] It is unfortunate that Rochester's extant correspondence and works reveals nothing of what he thought about the royal touch, but his willingness to have his son touched is telling with regard to the strength of the tradition that surrounded the ritual. It suggests that Rochester probably adopted a pragmatic attitude towards the possible effectiveness of the royal touch because doctors often struggled to cure scrofula and procedures to remove tumours were gruesome even by the standards of the day. As the king was godfather to the young Charles, it might also have been politic to have the boy touched: many aristocratic free-thinkers held orthodox political views and Rochester probably recognised when outward conformity was required. Free-thinkers and wits were not republicans and anti-monarchists[126]

The suitability of Charles II for the role of healer

Although it is not known on what grounds the wits mocked the royal touch, they probably would have criticised it for all the reasons so far examined. A further issue that surely cannot have escaped them is that of the suitability of Charles II for the role of healer. How could a king who was notorious

[123] *The letters of John Wilmot, earl of Rochester*, ed. J. Treglow, Oxford 1980, 82–3.
[124] G. Burnet, *Some passages of the life and death of John, earl of Rochester who died the 26th of July, 1680*, London 1680, 22, 52, 53, 72–3.
[125] *Letters of John Wilmot*, 83.
[126] Wilson, *Court wits*, 47–66; Ellenzweig, *Fringes of belief*, especially the introduction. Rochester's son Charles did not have scrofula but died at the age of ten in 1681, a year after his father, probably of congenital syphilis.

for his many mistresses and his decadent court, and who befriended rakes such as Rochester, claim to heal by his sacred touch? Surprisingly, from our point of view, the royal touch was not satirised in this way in text or image during the Restoration; but this suggests censorship and self-censorship at least with regard to published satire. Disillusion with the Charles's court and government was certainly noticeable by 1670, yet it did nothing to lessen the demand for the king's touch.

The free-thinker John Toland commented on the apparent contradiction of the dissipated Charles II practising the royal touch. Looking back on the Restoration from 1699 he wrote that 'if I did persuade my self that King Charles the Second (who is said to have cur'd very many) was a Saint, it should be the greatest Miracle I could believe'.[127] Humorous though this observation is, Toland was an anti-clerical, secular thinker writing during the reign of William III, who did not practice thaumaturgic healing. Toland had no truck with revealed religion, priestcraft or 'modern superstition', views he elucidated in his *Christianity not mysterious* (1696). He idealised the natural, uncorrupted worship of the ancients, especially the Egyptians who had originally eschewed idolatry and 'superstition' and aspired to a true worship of God through nature.[128] Thus Toland's radical views on religion were incompatible with the Christian underpinnings of the royal touch.

Toland's scepticism is not surprising because he was a deist, but his views on Charles II are significant. A defence of the king was offered by William Baron in his *Regicides no saints nor martyrs* (1700). He said that the gift of healing was given by God to the office of king, which was 'inseparable' from its 'character' and hence could not be lost by 'any irregularities of life, that [the Old Testament king] David himself was not free from'. He explained that neither '*Edward the Confessor's* Superstition nor *Charles the Second's* no *Saintship*, could obstruct that Salvation which in this sence *God may be said to give unto Kings*'.[129] Thus for Baron neither the Catholicism of Edward the Confessor (and by implication James II), nor Charles II's sex life could affect the royal gift of healing.

No other late Stuart commentator appears to have discussed this issue in print, which is surprising. On the other hand more people were touched for scrofula during the Restoration than at any other time in English history, despite one king being very sexually adventurous and the other Roman Catholic. This is difficult to account for, though suggestions may be put forward. The first point to bear in mind is that this apparent contradiction is evidence of the difference between early modern and modern mindsets. Although some of Charles II's contemporaries were scandalised by his virility, between the Restoration and the twenty-first century stands nineteenth-

---

[127] J. Toland, *Amyntor, or, A defence of Milton's life*, London 1699, 103.

[128] Champion, *Pillars of priestcraft shaken*, 148–52.

[129] W. Baron, *Regicides no saints nor martyrs*, London 1700, 129–30.

century prudery which can skew twenty-first-century views of late Stuart norms and values. Secondly, for some people deference to the crown was not undermined by any 'short comings' of an individual monarch. This related to the groundswell of popular royalism that began in 1660, itself partly a product of the trauma of the Civil Wars and especially the regicide. The trauma was so intense that the demand for royal therapeutics was not lessened by the circumstances of individual kings. The reason for this is that the practice of healing by touch was associated with the office of king rather than the person of the king, as Baron stated, and Charles II's contemporaries were evidently able to differentiate between his sacred touch and his sexual touch. This is why the proclivities of an individual ruler did not always affect the popularity or perceived efficacy of the royal touch as much as might be expected.

Although the office of king had a sacral aspect, this was not the same as expecting the king to be saintly in person. Yet the office of king demanded decorum, and when occasion demanded Charles II could drop his sceptical, licentious ways and assume the role of king effectively, which is exactly what he did when called upon to touch the sick. Before the ceremony he would have taken communion and might have fasted, and so was purified in preparation for his therapeutic role. Once the full apparatus of the ceremony was in place, it is possible that even those who had concerns about the king's morality would be impressed by the spectacle of him touching hundreds of sick people, flanked by clergy and courtiers. It is possible to argue that this was the cynical Charles doing whatever was required to keep his throne; but on the other hand there was far more to him than the myth of the 'Merry Monarch'. His listened attentively to sermons and would criticise them if he disagreed with them, and he punished courtiers if their louche behaviour was too disrespectful.[130] It is frustrating that England's most prolific royal healer has left us no statement of his own views on the royal touch, but his willingness to perform the ceremony on so vast a scale and his delight in Browne's book suggests strongly that he was committed to thaumaturgic kingship. No doubt he could reconcile his ability to enjoy life with his public duties: he told Gilbert Burnet that he did not think that 'God would damn a man for a little pleasure' and Burnet wrote that the king thought that 'to be wicked and design mischief is the only thing that God hates ... he was sure that he was not guilty of that'.[131]

Ambivalent and sceptical attitudes towards the royal touch caused apologists great anxiety because of what was at stake: the thaumaturgic powers of the king rested on the belief that God intervened in life. This was why Browne described those who doubted the power of the royal touch as

---

[130] J. Miller, *Charles II*, London 1991, 3; R. Hutton, *Charles II: king of England, Scotland and Ireland*, Oxford 1989, 452–3.

[131] G. Burnet, *Supplement to the 'History of my own time'*, ed. H. C. Foxcroft, Oxford 1902, 50.

atheists. Indeed, the unprecedented enthusiasm for the royal touch during the Restoration could itself represent a reaction to the developments that were summed up as atheism because to deny the royal touch was to deny the presence of spiritual agency in the world. To deeply religious people, this would be attributed to the devil. Browne makes this point succinctly on four occasions in his book. He likened the sceptics to 'Pagans' and 'Infidels' and warned against false healers whose powers, such as they were, came from the devil.[132] This is a reminder that in the second half of the seventeenth century the orthodox believed in the real presence of the devil, and that the binary system of philosophy described by Stuart Clark with particular reference to the Renaissance remained equally potent.[133]

The ambivalent and sceptical views expressed towards the royal touch during the Restoration fit into a wider culture of dissent, doubt and wit at this time. As such they are another reminder of the need to analyse the royal touch from below in any attempt to approach the historical reality. The rationale and practice of the ceremony was contested, not least because people had different views on the key apparatus of the ceremony which included the role of the king. That the rite did not cure or alleviate everyone's scrofula fuelled the debate concerning its status. Yet none of this decreased the demand for the royal touch, which helps to explain why the dispute was not concluded to anyone's satisfaction.

---

[132] Browne, *Adenochoiradelogia*, 11, 54, 113, 117.
[133] See p. 72 above.

6

The Royal Touch and the Early English Enlightenment, 1689–1750

This chapter examines the changing fortunes of the royal touch during the reigns of William III, who did not practise it, and Anne, who revived and reformed it. In England the ceremony ceased to be performed once and for all in 1714, with the succession of the Hanoverian George I, although the Jacobite Pretenders on the continent continued to practise the rite. This explains why the debate concerning the ceremony's efficacy continued until the mid-eighteenth century. The Whig interpretation of the royal touch during its last stage, as exemplified by Lord Macaulay who referred to the ceremony as a 'mummery', maintained that William's decision not to touch the sick was a sound consequence of his acquiring the crown by parliament rather than divine right. The ceremony belonged to a pre-Enlightenment world in which 'superstition' reigned, it was maintained, and as such it was inevitably consigned to the dustbin during the Age of Reason.[1] From this viewpoint, Anne's revival of royal therapeutics has to be seen as anachronistic, or ignored.[2] These teleologies have long distorted the history of the royal touch during the early English Enlightenment.

By placing the royal touch within its political and religious contexts, this chapter argues that William's abandonment of the royal touch was not inevitable and Anne's revival was popular. This fits with the assertion of the previous chapters that the rite was a central feature of English culture throughout the early modern period. The present analysis supports recent scholarship that stresses the continuation of belief in the supernatural during the early Enlightenment. The circumstances under which William made his decision will be examined, together with the character of his kingship, and the reactions to his repudiation of his scrofula-related duties. Likewise

---

[1] For 'mummery' see T. B. Macaulay, *The history of England from the accession of James II*, London 1848–55, repr. London 1898, iv. 244–8 at p. 244. This view is echoed in Crawfurd, *The king's evil*, 138–41; Farquhar, 'Royal charities, III', 118–20; and Bloch, *The royal touch*, 219, 406–7 (390–1).

[2] Bloch, *The royal touch*, 219–20 (390–1); Thomas, *Religion and the decline of magic*, 193; E. Gregg, *Queen Anne*, London 1980, repr. 2001, 148. The two exceptions that do justice to Anne's thaumaturgic practices are R. Bucholz, *The Augustan court: Queen Anne and the decline of court culture*, Stanford, CA, 1993, 210–12, 223–4, and H. Smith, '"Last of all the heavenly birth": Queen Anne and sacral queenship', *History of Parliament* xxviii/1 (2009), 137–49.

the motives for Anne's revival will be analysed, as will her reform of the liturgy, and the scale on which she touched. The queen's reinstatement of royal therapeutics stimulated a new debate, which will be assessed; this will include teasing out the extent to which support for the royal touch was party-political. The decision of the Hanoverians to abandon the royal touch was not an inevitable result of 'enlightenment' but instead a calculated political act. Belief in the efficacy of the royal hand continued beyond 1714, which helps to explain why the debate was rehearsed well into the mid-century.

William III and 'superstition'

James II was ousted by a coalition of a number of English parliamentarians and his son-in-law the Dutch Calvinist William III, in the Glorious Revolution of November 1688. In recent decades our understanding of this revolution has been revised, with James no longer cast as the bogeyman of the late seventeenth century. Whereas the Whig interpretation depicted him as a failed absolutist who could not coerce his subjects into becoming Roman Catholic, recent scholarship stresses that he sought religious toleration by making alliances with dissenters and repealing punitive legislation against Roman Catholics and nonconformists. But he alienated too many within the political nation, men who were loyal to the Church of England and suspicious of his motives.[3] The tipping point was the birth of his son in 1688, who was baptised as a Roman Catholic, and who supplanted James's Protestant daughters in the line of succession. James's successor William was a Dutch Calvinist who refused to touch for scrofula, as he thought it might be 'superstitious', in other words, Roman Catholic. This meant that royal healings ceased in England just as they had during the Interregnum.

William's decision became apparent on 7 April 1689, Maundy Thursday, the first occasion on which he was expected to touch for scrofula and wash the feet of the poor. People had made their way to William at Hampton Court but the new king refused to participate in these ceremonies. William and Mary were not crowned until 11 April,[4] which suggests that those who wanted to be touched thought a *de facto* king could carry out the rite just as well as an anointed one. Later that month the *Paris Gazette* reported on events in London at Easter:

> On the 7th ... [of April], the Prince of Orange dined with Lord Newport. Following time honoured practice, he should on that day have performed the ceremonies of touching the sick and washing the feet of the many poor

---

[3] For a stimulating new account of James II's reign see Sowerby, *Making toleration*.

[4] L. G. Schwoerer, 'The coronation of William and Mary, April 11, 1689', in L. G. Schwoerer (ed.), *The revolution of 1688–89: changing perspectives*, Cambridge 1992, 107–30.

people as legitimate kings [of England] have always done. But he [William III] announced that he believed that these ceremonies were not far removed from superstition: and he only gave orders that alms should be distributed to the poor in keeping with the custom.[5]

In this instance the fact that people arrived at court expecting to be touched suggests that the new government had not announced William's decision via a proclamation, and indeed no such notice has come to light. Presumably no declaration was made because it would have been unpopular given the great appeal of the royal touch during the Restoration. A suggestive clue to this effect is found in the parish register kept at Kempston, in Bedfordshire, in which the vicar entered the names of those to whom he granted certificates between 1684 and 1688, after which he entered the years 1689, 1690, 1691 and 1692, but no names appear under any of them (see Figure 14).[6] Had the government announced that the king would not touch, the vicar would presumably not have entered these years, and by 1693 he had given up as the next entry is for 1704.

However, the situation with William is not quite straightforward, as it seems that he did touch for scrofula on a single occasion. William Whiston (1667–1752), who succeeded Isaac Newton as Lucasian Professor of Mathematics at Cambridge in 1702 until he was ejected in 1710 for heresy, looked back on William's reign from the mid-eighteenth century:

> I have very lately been informed that King William was prevailed upon once to touch for the king's evil; praying God to heal the patient and grant him more wisdom at the same time; which implied he had no great Faith in the Operation. Yet the patient was cured notwithstanding.[7]

Whiston thought that miracles were a result of God's special providence and in his *Memoirs* he discussed the royal touch favourably alongside anointing the sick, which he maintained could also sometimes be efficacious. It is frustrating that Whiston did not provide any information concerning his source for William III, but on balance the account seems plausible. It is yet another example of a monarch being solicited to touch the sick and acquiescing, in this case a monarch whose official policy was not to do so; it is also hard to see why Whiston would have included mention of it if he had doubted its reliability.

Turning to the context for William's overall decision not to touch: religion was an important component. The bulk of his supporters were Whigs, whilst non-jurors and Tories were sympathetic to James II and thought that

[5] *Paris Gazette*, 23 Apr. 1689. See also 'Mr T., L. B.' [Guillaume De Lamberty], *Memoires de la derniére revolution d'Angleterre*, La Haye 1702, ii. 216–17.

[6] Kempston, Bedfordshire, register book, 1680–1721, P60/1/ 9, unfoliated.

[7] W. Whiston, *Memoirs of the life and writings of William Whiston*, M.A., London 1753, i. 377.

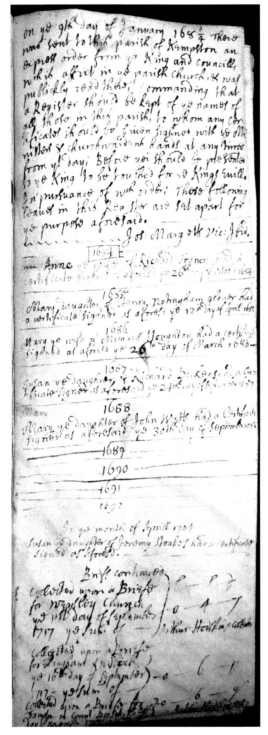

Figure 14. Register book for the parish of Kempston, 1680–1721.

the hereditary line of succession should not have been broken.[8] But although William's supporters could not claim that he ruled by hereditary divine right, they made much of his 'providential divine right'.[9] They argued that, like Henry VII, William had been chosen by God to rule and had saved the country from tyranny. Once William was king, he could have touched for scrofula, citing the precedent of Henry VII; or, like James VI and I, he could have performed the rite but emphasised the power of prayer. He chose to do neither of these.

Like James VI and I, when William became king of England he had already ruled a country with no tradition of sacral monarchy, having been Prince of Orange and the Dutch Stadholder since 1672. Both kings were Calvinists, and William presumably thought that the age of miracles had passed. But unlike his Scottish predecessor William did not change his mind and touch for scrofula. Marc Bloch suggested that William was more resolute than James VI, or that the increase in ambivalence and scepticism towards royal therapeutics during the Restoration made such views less heterodox than had hitherto been the case.[10] The former seems more likely than the latter – despite the rise of scepticism during the Restoration, such views do not appear to have been mainstream. The key to understanding William's decision is his dislike of what he saw as the excess of ceremony in the Anglican Church. He had been unhappy with his wife Mary Stuart's Anglican worship when they both lived in The Hague prior to 1688, and once king of England he sometimes made disparaging remarks concerning Anglican rituals, even though he was head of the English Church.[11] It was probably for this reason that Daniel Defoe stated bluntly that William did not believe that he could cure scrofula by touch.[12]

The decision not to touch the sick was made notwithstanding the fact that William and Mary were pious and the ethos of their reign was one of godly renewal after the oppression of James II. They sought to reform the court and the country at large by sermons, legislative changes, and especially national fasts and thanksgivings. A fast was a day of abstinence and prayer that sought to avert divine judgement, such as the one held every 30 January to commemorate the execution of Charles I, whereas a thanksgiving was a day of joyous celebration that marked God's blessing, such as the one held

[8] For the Glorious Revolution see J. Miller, *The Glorious Revolution*, London 1983; W. A. Speck, *Reluctant revolutionaries: Englishmen and the revolution of 1688*, Oxford 1988; E. Cruikshanks, *The Glorious Revolution*, Basingstoke 2000; J. Hoppit, *A land of liberty? England, 1689–1727*, Oxford 2000; G. De Krey, *Restoration and revolution in Britain*, Basingstoke 2007; and S. Pincus, *1688: the first modern revolution*, London 2009.

[9] J. P. Kenyon, *Revolution principles: the politics of party, 1689–1720*, Cambridge 1977, 5–21.

[10] Bloch, *The royal touch*, 219 (390).

[11] T. Claydon, *William III*, Harlow 2002, 99.

[12] See p. 202 below.

every 5 November to mark England's delivery from the Gunpowder Plot. The evidence suggests that the government's drive to make the country more godly was popular, and it appears that the 1690s were the most intense period of national piety and humiliation since the 1640s; alongside this, groups of individuals who were concerned about morality set up their own Societies for the Reformation of Manners.[13] The royal touch could easily have played a part in this programme had the king not thought it 'superstitious'. Since they were joint sovereigns, Mary could have touched for scrofula as she had been anointed on the hands, but she deferred to William in matters of politics.[14]

A number of other issues are germane to William's refusal to touch for scrofula, the first of which is his expectation of medicine. He was a military man, preoccupied with fighting Louis XIV in a series of European wars; as such, William had little time for doctors who followed the traditional path of trying to restore the health of their patients by altering their whole constitutions. William needed men to be fit for service, so he preferred doctors who prescribed remedies that worked quickly on everyone who had the same problem, regardless of their constitutions.[15] Seen in this light, William might have viewed the royal touch with suspicion as it was said to work only on some people, usually producing an incremental improvement.

Also connected to his military preoccupations, William was on campaign between March and October of most years, meaning that he was usually absent at Easter and Michaelmas, the two key times for royal healings. When he was in England his court was far less accessible than those of his two immediate predecessors as he did not like crowds, and he avoided central London whenever possible because the air exacerbated his asthma; he was therefore unlikely to want to hold large, urban healing ceremonies. It is also worth noting that although William had a lavish coronation, his style of kingship was for the most part distant and withdrawn and he seems to have been an unskilled public performer.[16]

William's decision not to touch for scrofula was perhaps reinforced by the fact that James II continued to touch in exile until his death in 1701.[17] According to Voltaire, James first 'touched the sick at the little English convent' in Paris soon after he arrived in France in 1688, while after James's death the bishop of Autun claimed to have been miraculously cured of his

[13] T. Claydon, *William III and the godly revolution*, Cambridge 1996, 91, 94–5, 100–10.

[14] Legg, *English coronation records*, 328; Claydon, *William III*, 48.

[15] H. J. Cook, 'Living in revolutionary times: medical change under William and Mary', in B. T. Moran (ed.), *Patronage and institutions: science, technology and medicine at the European court, 1500–1750*, Rochester, NY 1991, 111–35 at pp. 118–19.

[16] Claydon, *William III*, 36, 100, and *Godly revolution*, 93; W. Troost, *William III: the stadholder-king*, trans. J. C. Grayson, Aldershot 2005, 215.

[17] For the court in exile see E. Corp, *A court in exile: the Stuarts in France, 1689–1718*, Cambridge 2004.

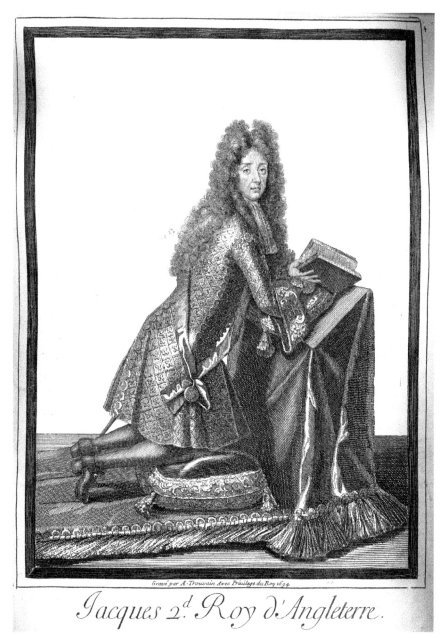

Gravé par A. Trouvain Avec Priuilege du Roy 1694.

Jacques 2.ᵈ Roy d'Angleterre.

Figure 15. James II at prayer.

long term dacryocystitis (an infection of the nasolacrimal sac that causes the eyes to appear red and swollen) after saying a mass for the dead king's soul.[18] James cultivated an image of himself as a pious king in exile, as can be seen in the printed image of him entitled 'Jacques 2. Roy d'Angleterre', published in Paris in 1694 (see Figure 15), and his thaumaturgic practices underwrote this.[19]

Given the great popularity of the royal touch during the Restoration, the paucity of extant commentaries on William's cessation of the practice is puzzling. Evidently the Dutch king's refusal to touch for scrofula did not mean that it was acceptable to criticise the ceremony in print. There must have been uncertainty, too, as to whether Anne would resume the rite when she succeeded. The little evidence that survives suggests, not surprisingly, that people held different views on William's decision.

In 1691 the royal touch was discussed briefly in the *Athenian Gazette*, edited by the bookseller John Dunton. This was a new form of publication: readers were invited to send their queries on any subject to the Athenian Society, an anonymous club of self-styled learned men who met at Smith's Coffee House and who would answer the questions.[20] The question concerning the royal touch was 'What are we to think of the Kings of England, who by their touch only cured the Evil?'[21] The answer was that in fact God wrought the healings, after which Dunton supplied a list of healers from the ancient world and from Catholic Europe. The message was that miraculous healings were not part of contemporary Protestant England. Dunton had Nonconformist connections and was a Whig propagandist for the Williamite government, so he was unlikely to lament the passing of the royal touch which was associated with the exiled James II.[22]

By contrast William's decision was bemoaned on humanitarian grounds by the Oxford scholar and non-juror Thomas Smith. Writing to his friend the mathematician Edward Bernard in March 1690, he stated that

> I am sorry to heare, that one of the Young Gentlemen is so indisposed [with scrofula]. It seemes that there is not that releife now for persons affected, as there was before this revolution: for it is lookd upon now as meere superstition and an effect of popery to pretend to the healing faculty and virtue: and accordingly there will not bee, at least there has not been yet, any attempt

---

[18] Voltaire, *The age of Louis XIV*, trans. M. P. Pollack, London 1926, 141.

[19] For James's healings in exile see Crawfurd, *The king's evil*, 138; Farquhar, 'Royal charities, III', 114–6; and Bloch, *The royal touch*, 221 (392–3).

[20] H. Berry, *Gender, society and print culture in late-Stuart England*, Aldershot 2003, and 'Dunton John (1659–1732)', ODNB.

[21] *Athenian Gazette* ii/24, 1691.

[22] N. H. Keeble, *The literary culture of nonconformity*, Leicester 1987, 124–6; Berry, *Gender, society and print culture*, 16, 27.

upon that part of Regality, which our Monarchs have claimed from the times of St Edward.[23]

The reference to the 'effect of popery' implies that the ceremony was associated with the exiled James II. Smith then went on to discuss medicine that was available to treat scrofula. Comparing this evidence with Dunton's it is tempting to conclude that the Whigs were sceptical while the Tories upheld royal thaumaturgy. There might be some truth in this as High Church Tories were predisposed towards sacral monarchy; but it is an oversimplification. Some of the duke of Monmouth's supporters, for example, who were Whigs, claimed that he touched for scrofula, and during Anne's reign belief and ambivalence were found on both sides of the political divide.

Queen Anne: revival and further reform of the royal touch

Anne succeeded William III on 8 March 1702. She was crowned on St George's day, 23 April, in a ceremony that included the anointing of her hands, and she first touched for scrofula in private in November that year.[24] Anne's historical reputation has been rehabilitated since the late 1960s: she is no longer thought of as the unintelligent woman who was dominated by female favourites, but rather as a competent politician who upheld the authority of the monarchy.[25] Her actions *vis-à-vis* the royal touch supports the scholarly reassessment of the queen.

Anne did not touch for scrofula during the first eight months of her reign, probably partly because it took time to prepare for the reintroduction of the ceremony after a hiatus of thirteen years, and partly because she would not have been expected to touch during the summer. Why did she revive the practice? She was a Stuart, an Anglican, and a queen regnant, so custom dictated that she touch for scrofula. Like Henry VII and James VI and I, she might have used it to legitimise her rule. When Anne succeeded in 1702, James II was dead while his son appears not have touched for scrofula until 1709, meaning that until then Anne had no Stuart rival to her thaumaturgic role.

The only eighteenth-century discussion of Anne's motives for her revival is that of the historian John Oldmixon who privileges party-political reasons, a view that is not fully convincing. By way of background, it should be noted that at the time of Anne's succession the Tories dominated high office and sought to undermine the principle of parliamentary monarchy in favour of

---

[23] T. Smith to E. Bernard, 1 Mar 1690, Bodl. Lib., MS Smith 57, p. 123.

[24] Gregg, *Queen Anne*, 154; J. R. Planché, *Regal records, or, A chronicle of the coronations of queens regnant of England*, London 1838, 123; *Flying Post*, 26 Nov. 1702.

[25] G. Holmes, *British politics in the age of Anne*, London 1987; Bucholz, *Augustan court*; Gregg, *Queen Anne*; Smith, 'Queen Anne and sacral queenship'.

heredity and divine right. This was helped by the publication of Clarendon's *History of the rebellion* between 1702 and 1704, which promulgated obedience to the crown, in addition to which the government published a genealogy of Anne that stretched back in an unbroken line to Edward the Confessor. Oldmixon claimed that, no doubt with the Confessor's supposed thauma-turgic practices in mind, 'some Wise ones of the Party put the Queen upon curing the King's Evil'.[26] Oldmixon's party-political reading is not entirely convincing because he wrote his account thirty-three years after Anne's succession, and had been a polemical Whig pamphleteer since 1710.[27] He was thus writing during the period of Whig supremacy when the Hanover-ians did not touch for scrofula, and he used the ceremony to emphasise that the Tories were on the losing side.

Party politics cannot fully illuminate Anne's motives, but further light can be shone on them by considering her religion and her ideas concerning her own sovereignty. Anne was devout and her religious proclivities were towards the High Church, which emphasised loyalty to the Stuarts, cere-mony and the sacral role of the monarch.[28] Anne revived the royal touch because she was committed to performing royal ceremony; as such, she rein-stated many other court rituals and public ceremonies that had lapsed during the previous reign such as progresses and public thanksgivings for military victories. This was because, like Charles II and James II, she understood the value of combining splendour with hospitality and benevolence.[29] Indeed, Anne was an expert in the ceremonial aspect of life at court. In the words of Jonathan Swift, who probably got his information from the queen's physi-cian John Arbuthnot and her favourite Abigail Masham, 'this princess was so exact an observer of forms, that she seemed to have made it her study'.[30] Anne had grown up seeing both her uncle and father touch for scrofula on a very large scale, and she liked to follow precedent in matters of court life. She evidently used their courts as the model for royal ceremony because so much of it had lapsed during her predecessor's reign.

Anne's reign was marked by bitter party politics, yet as queen she desired peace and unity, largely due to her Christian piety. This helps to explain one

---

[26] J. Oldmixon, *The history of England during the reigns of King William and Queen Mary, Queen Anne, King George I*, London 1735, 301–2; E. Hyde, *The history of the rebellion and Civil Wars in England*, London 1702–4. See also Farquhar, 'Royal charities, IV', 141–2, and Bloch, *The royal touch* 219 (390).

[27] P. Rogers, 'Oldmixon, John (1672/3–1742)', *ODNB*.

[28] Gregg, *Queen Anne*, 145.

[29] Bucholz, *Augustan court*, 203.

[30] Jonathan Swift, 'Memoirs relating to that change which happened in the queen's ministry in the year 1710', in *The prose works of Jonathan Swift: historical and political tracts – English*, ed. T. Scott, London 1901, 5. 367; R. Bucholz, '"Nothing but ceremony": Queen Anne and the limitations of royal ritual', *JBS* xxx/3 (1991), 288–323 at pp. 289–90; Bucholz, *Augustan court*, 203.

of her key models of sovereignty, the 'nursing mother' or *mater familias*. At Anne's request John Sharp, the archbishop of York who was her favourite preacher and who would become her Lord High Almoner and close adviser, preached her coronation sermon on Isaiah xlix.23, 'Kings shall be thy nursing fathers, and queens thy nursing mothers.' This verse had been described as an important part of the biblical mandate for the royal touch by John Browne in the 1680s.[31] Anne was referred to as the nation's 'nursing mother' in numerous sermons, poems and addresses, and she was sometimes addressed as a second Elizabeth.[32] This was taking things too far because as the mother of eighteen children Anne could not be another Virgin Queen, nor could she match Elizabeth's political acumen; but Anne's maternalism was beyond doubt.[33] Anne did not succeed in healing party-political divisions but she did her utmost to remain above them; and she presided over the Union of England and Scotland. Viewed in this context, the royal touch allowed Anne to act the part of the caring mother of the nation who touched the sick, regardless of their religion or nationality, in much the same way as had her predecessors. In one of Anne's many letters to her favourite, Sarah Churchill, the queen mentioned the royal touch in a way that implies a maternal streak: writing in the spring of 1704 she said that she intended to 'touch as many poor people as I can before the hott weather coms'.[34]

One further issue that arises in connection with Anne's motives for reviving the royal touch is her view on divine right, an ideology to which she gave considerable thought. Strange as it may initially seem, it does not appear that Anne wanted to be associated with this ideology, although a little ambivalence on her part is detectable. She was the driving force behind the publication of a sermon preached by the High Church bishop of Exeter, Offspring Blackall, *The divine institution of magistracy* (1708), which emphasised that the queen ruled by divine right and attacked the notions of popular and contractual kingship, and by implication, the revolution of 1688.[35] But the sermon also made clear that Anne was accountable to God, and so bore a great responsibility to rule justly. Against Anne's partiality to this sermon has to be weighed strong evidence that suggests that she distanced herself from divine right. She participated actively in the Glorious Revolution, which torpedoed the principles of divine right and primogeniture. She rejected the legitimacy of James II's son, the so-called 'warming pan baby'; once William III had landed she deserted her father, and her husband deserted James's army; once James had fled to France, Anne accepted the

---

[31] See p. 160 above.

[32] Sharpe, *Rebranding rule*, 349–50, 347.

[33] Bucholz, '"Nothing but ceremony"', 292–4, and *Augustan court*, 205–6, 209, 222, 345 n. 43.

[34] Queen Anne to Sarah Churchill, Kensington, 29 Apr. 1706, in *The letters and diplomatic instructions of Queen Anne*, ed. Beatrice Curtis Brown, London 1935, 185.

[35] Kenyon, *Revolution principles*, 120.

Revolutionary Settlement and appeared in public with her ladies, all dressed in orange to broadcast their political sympathies.[36] Further antipathy to divine right can be detected in Anne's response to the Sacheverell case. On 5 November 1709 Henry Sacheverell, a High Church clergyman, preached his notorious sermon that maintained that the Church was in danger from nonconformity, while asserting divine right monarchy. The sermon was a thinly veiled attack on government, the Revolution Settlement, and the Hanoverian succession. Sacheverell was impeached and tried in the spring: he was suspended for three years and his sermons burned. Anne told Gilbert Burnet, the bishop of Salisbury, that 'the sermon was bad and he deserved well to be punished for it'.[37] Eight months later when she read a loyal address from the City of London, congratulating her on her new Tory administration, the duke of Shrewsbury reported that 'she immediately took exception' to the statement within it that 'her right was Divine'. The queen told the duke that 'having thought often of it, she could by no means like it, and thought it so unfit to be given to anybody that she wished it might be left out'. She insisted that the text was amended so that her right to rule was 'indefeasible' rather than 'divine'.[38]

By touching the sick, Anne would appear to be advocating divine right monarchy, yet that does not fit well with her views on it. In order to try to solve this conundrum it needs to be borne in mind that although she was Tory by inclination, she was a moderate Tory, and although she was High Church, she was tolerant of dissent.[39] One reason that she shied away from divine right ideology was doubtless because it was associated with the bigotry of the High Church. Another was that it was allied with Jacobitism: Anne was no Jacobite, and favoured the Hanoverian succession.[40]

Anne's caution concerning divine right fits with her reform of the royal touch liturgy. Her revival of royal therapeutics marked a return to the sole use of the Anglican liturgy after James II's partial use of a Roman Catholic one, but she altered the rubric in three ways. The most radical of these reveals a noticeable restraint concerning the miraculous status of the practice and relates to the key moment of the ceremony when the sovereign touched the sick person's scrofulous sores. Since at least Henry VII's time the custom had been that the chaplain read out Christ's words to his disciples after the Resurrection 'They shall lay their hands on the sick and they shall recover' (Mark xvi.18). Although this verse was read once early on

---

[36] Gregg, *Queen Anne*, 68.

[37] G. Burnet, *Bishop Burnet's history of his own time: with notes by the earls of Dartmouth and Hardwicke, Speaker Onslow and Dean Swift: to which are added other annotations*, Cambridge 1833, v. 446.

[38] HMC, *Calendar of manuscripts of the marquis of Bath at Longleat, Wilts.*, London 1908, i. 199.

[39] Sharpe, *Rebranding rule*, 349–50, 558.

[40] E. Gregg, 'Was Queen Anne a Jacobite?', *History* lvii/191(1972), 358–75.

in Anne's liturgy, thereafter it was not recited when the queen touched a sick person. Instead, the chaplain prayed 'God give a blessing to this work: and grant that these sick persons, on whom the queen lays her hands, may recover, through Jesus Christ our Lord.'[41] The phrase 'may recover' is far more tentative than the earlier verse and must have been a more realistic reflection of the ceremony's efficacy (it must have been usual to hope that the ceremony would produce an improvement in people's condition, rather than an immediate full recovery). This greater caution concerning miracles was also evident in a change made to the French rubric after Louis XV's coronation in 1722. Traditionally the French king's chaplain had said that 'The king touches you, God heals you' each time the king touched a sick person, but this was changed to 'The king touches you, may God heal you'.[42]

In keeping with this remarkable change, the second alteration to the liturgy is that most of the scriptural passages have been removed but more prayers added, meaning that further emphasis is placed on the importance of prayer for recovery. This stress on prayer and supplication meant that people appealed to God for healing. It also guarded against anyone assuming that the ceremony had an automatic efficacy.

The third reform concerned the Angels. The images of the ship of state and St Michael slaying the devil and the legend 'Soli Deo Gloria' remained intact but what changed was that Anne gave each person their medal immediately after she had touched them. Hitherto the procedure had been for people to queue up once to be touched, and then queue again to receive their medal. The liturgy reads:

> Then shall the infirm Persons, one by one, be presented to the Queen upon their Knees, and as every one is presented, and while the Queen laying Her Hands upon them, and putting the Gold about their Necks [the Chaplain shall recite the prayer].[43]

This new procedure is depicted in a pack of playing-cards in the British Museum, on one side of which are engraved scenes from the reign of Queen Anne.[44] On the nine of hearts is an image of 'Her Majesty touching for the Evil', produced by Robert Spofforth (see Figure 16).

---

[41] *Book of Common Prayer*, London 1707 (BL shelfmark 3405.c.15); Crawfurd, *The king's evil*, 149. For details of the many editions of the Book of Common Prayer from Anne's reign that contain her liturgy see MacDonald Ross, 'The royal touch', 434.

[42] Bloch, *The royal touch*, 225 (399).

[43] *Book of Common Prayer* etc; Crawfurd, *The king's evil*, 149.

[44] 'A complete pack of 52 playing-cards: reign of queen Anne', BM, Schreiber E.64, 90.00 mm x 59.00 mm. See J. R. S. Whiting, *A handful of history*, Dursley, Glos., 1978, 125. The pack is unusual in that, in addition to the normal card suit numbers, the cards are also numbered in a chronological sequence that cuts across the suits. The scene depicting the royal touch is number 14 out of 52 which supports other evidence that indicates that Anne started touching fairly soon after she became queen.

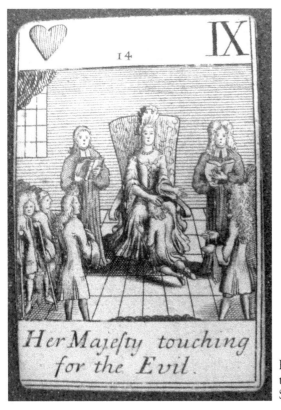

Her Majesty touching for the Evil.

Figure 16. Queen Anne touching for scrofula, BM Schreiber E.64.

The depiction shows Anne touching the head of a boy who kneels in front of her; to the left are the people waiting to be touched, including a man on crutches, together with a man whose dress and position suggests that he is a surgeon. On either side of Anne are the chaplains who are reading the new liturgy from prayer books. Anne is shown touching the boy's head with her right hand, while she holds out her left to receive an Angel threaded on a ribbon from a man standing to her right. The image contains a number of other clues as to how Anne's ceremony was further simplified when compared to the Restoration rite: the queen is shown seated on an armchair rather than on a throne under a canopy of state; she is not shown with her court in attendance; and there is no ornate ewer for her to wash her hands at the end of the ritual. No evidence has yet come to light that explains why these changes were made; but Anne was often very ill due to her numerous miscarriages, her gout and her rheumatism, meaning that she could not walk easily; it is therefore possible that the changes were introduced in order to speed up the ceremony and so lessen the strain on the queen.[45] Thus they

---

[45] For Anne's poor health see Gregg, *Queen Anne*, index at p. 472.

196

are testament to Anne's commitment to the royal touch despite her own poor health.

A further piece of evidence illustrating Anne's commitment is a lode-stone that belonged to the queen. She held this in her hand whilst touching the sick because the act was painful to her due to the gout in her hands.[46] Lodestones were the palatal teeth of the fossil fish Lepidotus, and had been worn since the Middle Ages as amulets that were thought to ease the pain of childbirth.[47] By the early seventeenth century their magnetic properties were recognised and it was thought that they could ease the pain of gout.[48]

Although Anne's personal beliefs concerning the royal touch are not known, the evidence suggests that, like her Stuart predecessors, she was committed to her therapeutic duties. Despite her poor health she conducted regular healing ceremonies even though she must have been exhausted by them and sometimes even had to be carried to them in a sedan chair because she could not walk.[49] Just before Anne died in 1714, Mary Lovett née Verney, the second daughter of the Tory MP Sir John Verney, reported that 'the Queen disorders herself by preparing herself to touch, [so] that noe one about her cares that she should do it; for she fasts the day before and abstains severall days, which they think does her hurt'.[50] This is the sole mention in the early modern period of a monarch fasting before touching the sick, giving a powerful sense of the need for purification. As Anne was a traditionalist, it is possible that her predecessors also prepared for the royal touch in this manner.

The evident popularity of Anne's reformed healing liturgy is discernible from the scale and frequency of her ceremonies. It is true that she did not touch such vast numbers as Charles II or James II, but she did administer on a scale similar to Charles I. Though this suggests that during Anne's reign the strong association of medicine and politics had become weaker since the Restoration as the likelihood of another civil war receded, it reminds us that health and medicine were still underpinned by religion and so royal thera-peutics remained central to English culture. As soon as it became known that Anne would touch for scrofula she found herself in a position similar

---

[46] This lodestone was bequeathed to John Rooper, Anne's Deputy Cofferer, and remained in his family until the early twentieth century when it was bought by the Wellcome Collection; it is now kept at the Science Museum, London (object number A506).

[47] E. Ettlinger, 'Documents of British superstition in Oxford', Folklore liv/1 (1943), 227–49 at pp. 233–4.

[48] Ibid. 234; Evans, Magical jewels of the Middle Ages and Renaissance, 112, 151; Farquhar, 'Royal charities, IV', 150. For the use of magnets in eighteenth-century healings see Porter, The greatest benefit to mankind, 285–6.

[49] Bucholz, Augustan court, 223; The Wentworth papers, 1705–1739: selected from the private and family correspondence of Thomas Wentworth, Lord Raby, created in 1711 earl of Strafford, ed. James J. Cartwright, London 1883, 325.

[50] M. Lovett to Lord Fermanagh, 8 Mar. 1714, in Verney letters of the eighteenth century from the MSS at Claydon House, ed. M. M. Verney, London 1930, i. 356.

to that of Charles II in 1660, with 'great multitudes' of sick people flocking to London, having been denied the royal touch for more than a decade.[51] In March 1703 John Sharp wrote to William Lloyd, bishop of Worcester, that there were 'several thousands of people' in London 'come up out of the country waiting for Her Healing [at Easter] ... some of them ready to perish'.[52]

The popularity of Anne's healing touch meant that she faced the same problem as her Stuart predecessors, namely, that of crowd control. In the twenty-eight years between 1660 and 1688 the crown issued at least thirty-six notices in the press seeking to regulate the royal touch; during Anne's reign of twelve years at least thirty-eight notices were published, the bulk in the *London Gazette*, which was the government's mouthpiece. These often served more than one purpose. Between November 1702 and March 1703 three notices were issued alerting the public to the reintroduction of royal healings.[53] Thereafter, fourteen notices announced the commencement of seasonal healings, and fifteen that the healing season had finished.[54] Sixteen notices sought to regulate the ritual process. As in the previous century, people were told to provide a certificate from their vicar confirming that they had scrofula and had not been touched before; in addition, a new procedure was introduced: henceforth tickets for the ceremony were issued by the surgeons at the newly-built Guards' Chamber, adjacent to the Banqueting House, rather than at the surgeon's house in Covent Garden.[55] All types of notices appeared throughout the reign: in retrospect it is a telling comment on the popularity of the ritual, as well as the difficulties in organising it, that as late as February 1714 the crown was still having to insist that people obtained a certificate from the clergy.

What of the scale of Anne's ceremonies? At first Anne touched relatively small numbers of people – twenty on one occasion in December 1702 – but this soon increased.[56] The annalist Narcissus Luttrell noted that Anne

---

[51] *London Gazette*, 18 Mar. 1703.

[52] J. Sharp, archbishop of York, to W. Lloyd, bishop of Worcester, 31 Mar. 1703, transcribed in B. C. Browne, 'Letter copied by G. E. Lloyd Baker, 24 August 1888 from the letter in his possession at Hardwicke Court, Gloucester', *EHR* v/17 (1890), 120–4 at p. 122.

[53] *Post*, 26 Nov. 1702; *Flying Post*, 17 Dec. 1702; *English Post*, 19–22 Mar. 1703.

[54] Ceremonies were announced in the *London Gazette*, 29 Mar. 1703; 1 Nov. 1705; 31 Oct., 4, 7 Nov. 1706; 23 Feb. 1710; 26, 28 Feb. 1712; 28 Feb., 7 Mar. 1713; 16, 20 Feb., 23 Mar. 1714; and in the *Evening Post*, 5 Mar. 1713. The ending of the healing season and cancellations were announced in the *London Gazette*, 15, 24, 28 May 1704; 31 May, 17 Dec, 1705; 29 Apr., 2, 6 May, 16 Dec. 1706; 1, 5 Apr. 1708; 23, 25 June 1709; 25 Apr. 1710; 17 Apr. 1712.

[55] *London Gazette*, 11, 18 Mar. 1703; *London Gazette*, 24, 28, 31 May, 1 Nov. 1705; 31 Oct., 4, 7 Nov. 1706; 23 Feb. 1710; 26, 28 Feb. 1712; 28 Feb., 7 Mar.1713; 16, 20 Feb. 1714.

[56] *Flying Post*, 17 Dec. 1702.

touched 100 people at each Easter healing in April 1703 and that by 1705 this had increased to 200.[57] In 1713, when she was ill, she still touched 150 'poor people' at one healing even though she had to be carried to the ceremony in a sedan chair.[58]

Although extensive Treasury records exist for Anne's reign, the only mentions of sums spent on touch-pieces are not very specific, recording simply that the annual budget for the 'Privy Purse and Healing Medals' was £20,000 between 1702 and 1711, and £26,000 from 1711 to 1714.[59] On the other hand, records from the Mint reveal that 12,347 touch-pieces were produced between 1703 and 1707 and between 1711 and 1714, at intervals that adhere to the healing calendar.[60] Though the records are patchy in places the suggestion is that on average Anne touched 1,372 people each year.

However, the Marlborough papers contain a number of documents that suggest that Anne may have touched on a slightly larger scale. Sarah Churchill was Keeper of the Privy Purse for Anne between 1702 and 1711, so was responsible for ordering touch-pieces and paying for them, and ensuring that they were delivered to the queen. They were made at the Mint and then delivered by the goldsmith John Coggs at intervals that also adhere to the healing calendar.[61] The extant documentation reveals that between 16 May 1706 and 11 June 1707 Churchill took delivery of 2,073 Angels on sixteen occasions, of which 1,794 were 'sent on to her Majesty'. The rest may have been surplus to requirements or sent to people with contacts at court who requested an Angel to wear, presumably as an amulet. Of the 1,794 Angels, only twenty-seven were sent back unused to the Privy Purse, which suggests that Anne probably touched 1,767 people during the period recorded. The records reveal that she held nine large public ceremonies – five at St James' Palace, one each at Windsor, Newmarket and Kensington, and one at an unspecified location – at which a total of 1,508 people were touched, meaning that the average attendance at each large ceremony was 168 people. In addition, 259 people were touched at smaller ceremonies.[62]

[57] Luttrell, *Brief historical relation*, v. 285, 288, 518.

[58] *Wentworth papers, 1705–1739*, 325.

[59] *Calendar of treasury papers preserved in Her Majesty's Public Record Office*, prepared by J. Redington, London 1868–97, iii [1702–7], 30, 219, 419; iv [1708–14], 43, 371, 434.

[60] Woolf, 'The sovereign remedy' (1980 for 1979), 119.

[61] Records of Angels requested and received from Mr Coggs, and of Angels sent to Queen Anne, 16 May 1706–1 June 1707, Marlborough papers, BL, MS Add. 61420, transcribed in Brogan, 'Royal touch' (dissertation), appendix 4. See also HMC, *Eighth report: manuscripts of the duke of Marlborough at Blenheim, County Oxford*, London 1907–9, i. 15.

[62] BL, MS Add. 61420.

These may well have been private, held for people with connections at court.[63]

It is likely that the touch-pieces were delivered on the morning of the ceremony; if so, all but two of the public ceremonies were held on a Saturday, which was a departure from the Restoration practice of holding the ceremony on Fridays or Sundays.[64] The rituals at St James's were sometimes held in the courtyard rather than the chapel, another innovation.[65] This was probably due to Anne's wish to avoid the heat and the pungent odour associated with crowds of diseased people, and the Banqueting House appealed for the same reason. In 1706 Anne wrote to Sarah Churchill that the ceremony now took place 'in the Banqueting House, which I like very well, that being a very cool room, and the doing of it there keeps my own house sweet and free from crowds'.[66]

The Augustan debate

Anne's revival of the royal touch stimulated a new debate concerning its efficacy. In November 1704 the renowned dissenter and author Daniel Defoe published two letters concerning the royal touch in the third supplement to his *Review*. This was a widely-read journal that appeared three times a week, discussing subjects such as current events, history and morality, sometimes in a satirical and humorous vein. Its supplements were inspired by publications like the *Athenian Gazette* as they contained questions sent in by the public that were answered by a committee from the 'Scandal club', which in reality was Defoe. The discussion of the royal touch strongly suggests that, not surprisingly, it continued to be debated in coffee houses and other social spaces, the *Review* being read in public places.[67] The first letter concerning the ceremony was written by a correspondent who had been advised by a friend to 'go to the Queen for a touch' but who had 'not a Belief, that it can be of any Service to my Case'.[68] The writer continued by speculating that

[63] For small ceremonies see *The London diaries of William Nicolson, bishop of Carlisle, 1702–18*, ed. C. Jones and G. Holmes, Oxford 1985, 300.

[64] *A handbook of dates for students of English history*, ed. C. R. Cheney and M. Jones, Cambridge 2000, 111, 151.

[65] Luttrell, *A brief historical relation*, v. 518, Tuesday 8 May 1705.

[66] Queen Anne to Sarah Churchill, Kensington, 29 Apr. 1706, *Letters of Queen Anne*, 185.

[67] P. Backscheider, *Daniel Defoe: his life*, London 1989, 151, 153; M. E. Novak, *Daniel Defoe: master of fictions*, Oxford 2001, 213–20; P. R. Backscheider, 'Defoe, Daniel (1660?–1731)', *ODNB*. For a brief allusion to the royal touch being debated see also Jeremy Collier, *An ecclesiastical history of Great Britain*, London 1708–14, i. 226.

[68] D. Defoe, *A supplement to the advice from the Scandal Club*, No. 3, London 1704, 15, in *Defoe's Review*, ed. A. W. Secord, New York 1938, i, facsimile bk 3.

the cure might be miraculous or might be due to the 'force of a spell', which Defoe humorously elucidated in a marginal note as consisting of 'serious Words used in a Charm, [such] as those of the Bishops'. As a dissenter, Defoe rejected High Church practices and hierarchies, here conflating a prayer read by a bishop with a spell. The writer then requested information concerning the origins and efficacy of the royal touch. The second letter was less sceptical of it, and also asked about the ceremony's origins – but in addition it asked whether a deposed king could heal by touch, an allusion to the therapeutic practices of the exiled Stuarts.

Defoe replied that the royal touch could cure scrofula, but not always, maintaining that the origins of the ceremony remained 'very much in the Dark'. He explained the efficacy of the ceremony primarily in terms of the occult properties of the gold in the Angel, which was then supported by the faith both of the princes who touched and that of their supplicants. Defoe stated that the gold contained a quality that was antithetical to the ' Malignant Nature' of scrofula; and he stressed that there was 'never any person ... Cur'd by the Royal Touch, whose Faith rejected the Method as a Cure, and firmly believ'd it would do them no good'.[69] Defoe therefore maintained that the practice worked by natural as opposed to supernatural means, but his thoughts were not original. His privileging of the gold as the healing agent is reminiscent of the dissenters of the Restoration, the antiquarian John Aubrey, and the numerous people who were touched who thought that their cure depended on wearing their touch-piece constantly – a belief that even John Browne sometimes endorsed. Defoe's emphasis on faith or the power of the imagination is also unsurprising as the idea that the mind could influence recovery was an early modern commonplace.[70]

Defoe ignored the power of prayer and of the sacred touch in his explanation of how royal thaumaturgics worked, presumably because as a dissenter he thought that these could lend themselves to 'superstition', whereas in his view the gold contained natural healing properties. Defoe did believe in the supernatural, in providence, and in an interventionist God, but he was careful to distance himself from those who quickly ascribed anything strange to the supernatural, as this seemed to him too credulous.[71]

Turning to the contentious issue of whether a deposed English king could heal by touch, and by implication whether this was the mark of a legitimate sovereign, Defoe offered a brief yet conciliatory answer that implied that the healing power belonged to the office rather than the person of the monarch. He suggested that thaumaturgic powers could not be 'in this or that particular Royal Family' because 'the advocates for this Cure, carry back its Original to *Edward the Confessor*'. As the hereditary line of succession

---

[69] Ibid. 16.

[70] See pp. 167–9 above.

[71] R. M. Baine, *Daniel Defoe and the supernatural*, Athens, GA 1969; Novak, *Defoe*, 272.

had been broken on many occasions, Defoe said that the power to heal must instead reside in 'some *Addenda* to the *English* Crown' but that it was too difficult to make a 'Philosophical Demonstration' proving this to be the case. He concluded that William III had not touched for scrofula as he doubted his ability to cure by such means.[72]

Defoe was a Whig and a dissenter who in 1704 had been imprisoned and pilloried for his part in the crisis over occasional conformity, the practice of dissenters who wanted to hold public office taking Anglican communion in order to do so. He might therefore have been expected to be more wholly sceptical of the royal touch. But after his release Defoe worked for Robert Harley, earl of Oxford, who thought that Defoe was better employed in the government's service, and the *Review* often promulgated official policies; Defoe was also loyal to the queen.[73] On the other hand, Defoe rejected hereditary divine right monarchy and mystical kingship; he thought that the power of the crown should be balanced by that of the House of Commons and the House of Lords, concluding that the monarch had the same sort of power as the mayor of a town, albeit on a larger scale.[74] This 'secular' view of monarchical power must also help to explain his naturalistic interpretation of the royal touch. However, what is noteworthy about Defoe's commentary is that he published his ambivalent point of view on the royal touch, possibly the first of its kind expressed first-hand in print. This is telling with regard to how the debate must have moved on since the Restoration and the reign of William III.

Defoe toed a middle line with regard to royal therapeutics, avoiding both apologetic and scepticism. This alerts us to the importance of not presuming overly simplistic party-political divisions concerning belief in the royal touch. Obviously the ideology of High Church Tories lent itself to belief in it, so it is not surprising that Jonathan Swift sought to procure a ticket to one of Anne's healings for the son of a friend who had scrofula.[75] But even here it is necessary to tread carefully as is revealed by the case of Anne's sergeant surgeon Charles Bernard, a High Church Tory. According to Oldmixon, Bernard made the royal touch

> the Subject of his Raillery all his Life-time, till he became Body Surgeon at Court, and found it a good Perquisite, [and] solv'd all Difficulties by telling

---

[72] Defoe, *Supplement*, 16.

[73] Backscheider, *Defoe*, 84–99, 133–4; Novak, *Defoe*, 135–6, 195–6, 200–1, 414–17; K. Clark, *Daniel Defoe: the whole frame of nature, time and providence*, Basingstoke 2007, 34–50.

[74] D. Defoe, *Reflections upon the late, great revolution in England*, London 1689, 36–40, and *Jure divino*, London 1706; M. Shonhorn, *Defoe's politics: parliament, power, kingship and Robinson Crusoe*, Cambridge 1991, 9–20, 89–140.

[75] J. Swift, *Journal to Stella*, ed. H. Williams, Oxford 1948, i. 263–4, letter of 22 May 1711.

his Companions with a Fleer; *really one could not have thought it, if one had not seen it.*[76]

Bernard was the leading surgeon of his day: elected Fellow of the Royal Society in 1696, he became sergeant surgeon to Anne in November 1702, around the time that she started to touch for scrofula.[77] His change of heart could have been nothing more than a political expedient as his explanatory remark was accompanied by a 'fleer' (or jeer). The tone of the passage suggests that having scorned royal therapeutics for many years, he now feigned a 'change of mind' in equally sarcastic terms. However, the issue is even more complex because the apothecary John Badger wrote that although Bernard laughed at the rite amongst his 'intimate friends' he 'seriously affirmed' to Badger that the ceremony cured cases of scrofula that medicine could not.[78] Either Bernard was truly conflicted concerning royal therapeutics or he was disingenuous in public. Whichever the case, it is not what one expects of a High Church Tory.

If High Church Tories could mock the royal touch it is also true that not all Whigs were secular-minded sceptics. Most Whigs were Anglicans and many defended the Glorious Revolution in providential terms. As Mistress of the Privy Purse, the arch-Whig Sarah Churchill was responsible for ordering touch-pieces: the records also reveal that she procured a touch-piece for someone on her estates at Woodstock who presumably had scrofula.[79] This does not automatically mean that she believed in the efficacy of the royal hand; like Defoe she might have had more faith in the healing properties of gold. But it does imply that she was willing to use her connections with the queen to try to alleviate someone's scrofula.

The Hanoverian succession and Jacobitism

Anne died in 1714 and her successor George I was a Lutheran who, like William III, decided not to touch for scrofula, but who also made no formal declaration to this effect.[80] Indeed, there appears to be no official explanation for his decision. However, George had certain things in common with William. On becoming king of England George had already ruled Hanover

---

[76] Oldmixon, *History of England*, 302; cf. D. Turner, *The art of surgery*, London 1722, i. 159.

[77] Ian Lyle, 'Bernard, Charles (*bap.* 1652, *d.* 1710)', ODNB; Bucholz and Sainty, *Officials of the royal household, 1660–1837*, i. 48.

[78] J. Badger, *A collection of remarkable cures of the king's evil, perfected by the royal touch, collected from the writings of many eminent physicians and surgeons and learned men*, London 1748, 24–5.

[79] BL, MS Add. 61420.

[80] R. Harron, *George I: elector and king*, London 1978, 165.

since 1698, a duchy with no tradition of sacral monarchy; and he was a Lutheran, so might have thought that the age of miracles had passed. On the other hand, the royal touch had been reformed throughout the Tudor and Stuart age in order to make it more Protestant, the recent changes instigated by Anne emphasising the role of prayer and supplication to an unprecedented degree. Surely George I could have touched for scrofula by continuing this emphasis on prayer? One issue that is clear, however, is that George did not make his decision because belief in royal therapeutics had experienced a mass decline. He inherited a situation where the crown appears to have touched some 1,300 people a year, meaning that the rite was as popular in 1714 as it had been for much of the seventeenth century.

The most likely explanation for George I's decision is that he did not think that he possessed thaumaturgic powers. At the same time the royal touch had taken a new political turn, in that it was now associated with Jacobitism.[81] This may even have been encouraged by George himself. There is one source that suggests this, although it is not the most reliable evidence. Writing in the early nineteenth century, the historian Robert Chambers said that he had been informed by 'an ancient non-jurant still alive' that as soon as the new king arrived in England he was asked by an English gentleman to touch his child for scrofula but declined 'peevishly', instead referring the case to the Pretender. Unlike William III, George did not dismiss the ceremony as 'superstitious'; indeed, by referring the gentleman to the Pretender, George seems to be saying that the exiled prince might be able to cure scrofula, whereas he could not, implying that the power to do so was hereditary to the Stuarts. This might explain why the German king declined his suppliant with obvious irritation. The gentleman obeyed George: he took his child to the Pretender, who performed the rite with apparent success, resulting in the man becoming a Jacobite.[82] On the other hand, when a sick Whig gentlewoman tried to obtain George I's touch partly to undermine the Jacobite claims, a compromise was made whereby she was allowed to kiss the king's hand rather than have him ceremoniously touch her, which she did for two minutes. Whether she recovered or not is not recorded.[83]

The Hanoverian succession gave the royal touch a new political dimension. Jacobites said that the Hanoverians would not perform the ceremony as they did not want to risk it not working, which would reveal that they were not legitimate sovereigns.[84] It is not surprising that the royal touch was especially associated with the Stuarts due to the huge numbers of people who had been touched by them since 1603 and especially since 1660, and the

---

[81] P. K. Monod, *Jacobitism and the English people, 1688–1788*, Cambridge 1989, 127–32; Shaw, *Miracles*, 71.

[82] R. Chambers, *History of the rebellion in Scotland in 1745, 1746*, Edinburgh 1827, i. 183.

[83] J. Doran, *London in the Jacobite times*, London 1877, i. 345.

[84] Chambers, *History of the rebellion*, i. 183.

fact that the exiled James II had performed the ceremony while William III had not. After James's death in 1701, his son, styled James VIII and III and known as 'the Old Pretender', regularly touched for scrofula in Paris, Italy and Spain, probably beginning in 1709.[85] James III used the Catholic liturgy of James II and dispensed silver touch-pieces when he could afford to have them minted, even collecting Stuart touch-pieces himself.[86] The iconography of the medals remained the same as during the Restoration, although the ship of state is different. Whereas it had previously been depicted in full sail to infer the healthy monarchical state, James II changed this once he was in exile to a new image which continued to appear on all Jacobite touch-pieces.[87] The Jacobite ship has limp sails and is shown sailing away from the viewer from left to right (*see* Plates 8, 9 and Figure 17), surely an allusion to exile and political disempowerment. Yet James III's ceremonies were popular, and both Catholic and Protestant supplicants travelled to him from all parts of Britain and Europe. Evidently this means that a hereditary claim to thaumaturgy meant more to his 'patients' than the coronation and anointing. When in Italy James touched on the last Thursday of every month, in his Chapel Royal, and probably held impromptu ceremonies too: he wrote that 'the evil … is very common here, so that I often touch people for it, and always have medals by me for that use'.[88]

But things were very different because this was the touch of an exiled claimant to the throne. Whereas in England one of the functions of the royal touch had been to help assert monarchical authority, it was now used by a displaced pretender to try to discredit the incumbent sovereign. And whereas apologists in England had claimed that by healing the individual the monarch ministered to the body politic, no such claim could be made by the exiled Stuarts. Indeed, political uses aside, it seems that the exiled Stuarts touched for scrofula primarily as an act of compassion.

In England, reactions to Jacobite thaumaturgy varied. Samuel Johnson (1709–84) had been touched by Anne as a baby in 1711, and, even though he was plagued by ill health throughout his life, he seems to have worn his touch-piece constantly, partly as a charm, partly as a memento of his childhood, his mother and the Stuarts. Johnson remembered Anne as a 'lady in diamonds, [with] a long black hood'.[89] He was the most famous person to have been touched by an English sovereign, but this did not stop his friend

[85] Farquhar, 'Royal charities, IV', 161–3.

[86] Autobiographical narrative of an English student at the English College, Lisbon, around the year 1718, Wellcome Library, MS 6083/5; N. Woolf, *The medallic record of the Jacobite movement*, London 1988, 39, 50, 76.

[87] Woolf, *Medallic record*, 39.

[88] E. Corp, *The Stuarts in Italy: a royal court in permanent exile*, Cambridge 2011, 182 n. 61, 318.

[89] J. Boswell, *Boswell's life of Johnson*, ed. G. Birkbeck Hill, Oxford 1974, i. 11–12; S. Johnson, *Diaries, prayers and annals*, ed. E. L. McAdam, London 1958, 8–9; R. McKeith,

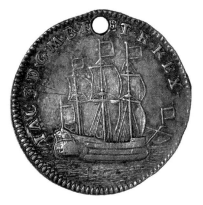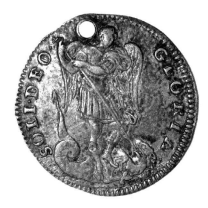

Figure 17. A touch-piece of James Stuart, the Old Pretender, styled James VIII and III. 20mm. diameter.

James Boswell from teasing him about it. Boswell joked that although John-son's mother had made the three-day journey from Lichfield to London with her infant son, she 'had not carried him far enough; she should have taken him to ROME'.[90] This could refer to Catholic thaumaturgy associated with shrines and relics, or, more likely, it denoted the healing practices of the Jacobite Pretender, whose principal residence was Rome.

The aftermath

The debate concerning the royal touch, and by implication the legitimacy or otherwise of the English sovereign, continued into the middle of the eight-eenth century and the best understanding of what was at stake can be gained from the debate between the surgeon William Becket (1684–1738), a Whig, and Daniel Turner (1667–1741), surgeon and licentiate to the Royal College of Physicians, a High Church Tory.

Becket and Turner's disagreement was stimulated by an anonymous pamphlet that was published in London in 1721 which made much of the fact that the exiled 'Old Pretender' had successfully touched for scrofula.[91]

'Samuel Johnson's childhood illnesses and the king's evil', *Medical History* x/4 (1966), 386–99.

[90] J. Boswell, *The life of Samuel Johnson*, ed. J. Canning, London 1991, 7; Pat Rogers, 'Johnson, Samuel, 1709–84', *ODNB*. Johnson's touch-piece is now in the British Museum (CM M8007) as is discussed in N. Guthrie, 'Johnson's touch-piece and the "charge of fame": personal and public aspects of the medal in eighteenth-century Britain', in J. C. D. Clark and H. Erskine-Hill (eds), *The politics of Samuel Johnson*, London 2012, 90–111.

[91] *A letter from a gentleman at Rome to his friend in London, giving some very surprising cures in the kings evil*, London 1721. The pamphlet did not mention the Pretender by name.

This was Jacobite propaganda, used to discredit the Hanoverian succession. Becket responded to it in 1722 with *A free and impartial inquiry into the antiquity and efficacy of touching for the cure of the kings evil*, printed by John Peele, a 'very considerable bookseller'.[92] The book consists of two letters, the first addressed to Dr John George Steigertahl, physician to George I, Honorary Fellow of the Royal College of Physicians, and a Fellow of the Royal Society. This discusses the royal touch and argues that when it worked it was due solely to the power of suggestion, which could be explained mechanistically. Thus Becket did not deny that the royal touch sometimes worked, but he reframed it from a supernatural to a natural phenomenon, in keeping with the new intellectual trends of his day. The second letter, addressed to the physician and collector Sir Hans Sloane, who had been President of the Royal College of Physicians since 1719, argued that all charms worked psychosomatically. It then further examined the royal touch, concluding that its apologists were biased flatterers.

Becket's work contains three new elements that distance it from earlier apologetic works, which are partly explained by his being a founding member of the London Society of Antiquaries and a Fellow of the Royal Society. He claimed impartiality; he was interested in archival work and refused to take earlier authors on trust;[93] and he processed data connected to scrofula to support his interpretation.

Becket's archival work produced three original contributions to the history of the royal touch that greatly undermined its perceived antiquity and efficacy. He examined royal accounts, concluding that Edward I, not Edward the Confessor, was the first English king to touch for scrofula. He also read the contemporary chronicles of the Confessor's life, noting that they did not mention him performing the ceremony: Becket said that the supposed miraculous cures had been invented later by priests.[94] Becket then delivered a devastating blow, stating that the London Bills of Mortality revealed that during periods when kings did not touch for scrofula people with the condition sought medical aid, which explained why the mortality rate was lower then than at times when the royal touch was available. As he put it:

> More people have died of this disease in those Reigns when our Kings did touch, than when they did not, as appears by the Bills of Mortality: for when our Kings did not touch, the People sought out for early Helps for their Maladies, whereby great Numbers were cured; whereas when our Kings did touch,

---

[92] Plomer and others *Dictionary*, 234. Becket was assisted with his book by fellow antiquarian John Anstiss the Elder.

[93] Becket's interest in source material is evident in that he appended various liturgies and proclamations at the end of his book.

[94] Becket, *Enquiry*, 11–13, 19.

they depended so much upon its Efficacy, that they neglected all other means till their Cases became … incurable.[95]

In fact, a close reading of the Bills does not fully support Becket's assertion. The Bills reveal that the average annual number of deaths from scrofula during the Interregnum was twenty-four; during the Restoration it rose to sixty-six; during William III's reign it climbed to seventy-eight; it remained close to this at seventy-six during Anne's reign; and then from 1714 until 1722 it dropped to fifty-nine. The problem with Becket's interpretation is three-fold. First, the sharp increase from the Interregnum to the Restoration was more likely due to 1660 being the first year in which data from Westminster was included in the Bills, which seems to point to a higher incidence of scrofula in that part of London as compared to others.[96] Second, the annual totals increased during the 1690s, in contradiction to Becket's assertion. Third, people who were ill with scrofula tended to access a range of treatments, meaning that his dichotomous model of either the royal touch or medical aid is not especially helpful. However, the annual totals did drop after 1714, although only to a rate just below that of the Restoration. This must be significant, not least because the population of London rose from around 200,000 in 1660 to some 700,000 by 1750, but further work is needed on this phenomenon if its meaning is to be understood.

Becket's other ideas concernng the royal touch were less original. He argued that it was not miraculous, as, if it worked, it did so by degrees and not immediately; he also noted that whereas Christ had healed many illnesses, English monarchs only addressed themselves to those ill with scrofula. He suggested the power to heal could not be hereditary as the line of succession had been broken so often. In terms of what actually wrought cures, he said it could not be the ceremony (and by implication the prayers) as this had been changed many times over the years; nor could it be the gold, as Charles I had often had none to distribute during the 1640s.[97]

Becket concluded that when the royal touch worked it was due to the power of the imagination, which had been stimulated by contact with the monarch. This was nothing new, and compared to his comments on both Edward the Confessor and the Bills of Mortality it is anti-climactic. But Becket gave this theory a mechanistic explanation in keeping with the prevalent scientific ideas of the day that privileged matter in motion. People with scrofula, he said, had 'impoverish'd' blood' and were 'languid'.

---

[95] Ibid. 25.

[96] Before 1660 the bills covered the ninety-seven parishes within the City walls, the sixteen parishes outside the walls, and the twelve out-parishes in Middlesex and Surrey. In 1660 the five parishes of Westminster were included: V. Harding 'The population of London, 1550–1700: a review of the published evidence', *London Journal* xv (1990), 111–28.

[97] Becket, *Enquiry*, 26–8.

When they were touched, this stimulated their imagination, which increased their blood flow and filled it with their 'Animal spirit'; this unblocked the trapped scrofulous matter in their 'Canals' or glands. The healings were not miraculous but worked by the 'Mechanical Powers of Matter and Motion'.[98] This reflected the idea that had become fashionable during the Restoration: that medical phenomena could be explained mechanically; it was popular, not least with Fellows of The College of Physicians, as it allowed them to continue prescribing traditional medicine while appearing to be at the cutting edge of the new science.[99]

Turner responded to Becket later in 1722, in his surgical text book that contained 110 case studies for surgeons.[100] This was printed and sold by Charles Rivington, the leading theological publisher in London.[101] In the section on scrofula, Turner did his best to refute Becket but struggled to address some of his opponent's key points. The debate highlights one of the main intellectual problems of the day: the new science emphasised that God worked through the predictable rules of nature, giving less attention to special providences and miracles, but at the same time it was deemed essential to refute atheist materialism and views differed as to how far extraordinary occurrences should be emphasised for this purpose.[102] Thus Becket offered a natural, mechanical explanation of the efficacy of the royal touch that stripped it of its mystery, while Turner remained convinced that God was omnipotent.

Turner's short response to Becket began with his own claim to disinterested analysis, suggesting an apology was now unfashionable, possibly because it would seem too Jacobite. Turner did not attack Becket's conclusion concerning the psychosomatic aspect of the royal touch as being unoriginal. This is probably because Turner upheld the early modern belief that the imagination could affect physical health, having published a tract on

[98]   Ibid. 35–8.

[99]   T. M. Brown, 'The College of Physicians and the acceptance of iatromechanism in England, 1665–1695', *Bulletin of the History of Medicine* xliv/1 (1970), 12–30, esp. p. 29. For the continuation of this into the eighteenth century see T. M. Brown, 'Medicine in the shadow of *Principia*', *Journal of the History of Ideas* xlviii/4 (1987), 629–48; A. Guerrini, 'Isaac Newton, George Cheyne and the "Principia Medicinae"', in R. French and A. Wear (eds), *The medical revolution of the 17th century*, Cambridge 1989, 222–45, and 'Newtonianism, medicine and religion', in Grell and Cunningham, *Religio medici*, 293–312.

[100]   Turner, *Art of surgery*; Munk, *Roll*, ii. 35–7; P. K. Wilson, 'Daniel Turner and the art of surgery in eighteenth-century London', *Journal of the Royal Society of Medicine* lxxxvii (1994), 781–85, and 'Turner, Daniel (1667–1741)', ODNB.

[101]   Plomer and others, *Dictionary*, 182–3; B. Laning Fitzpatrick, 'Rivington family (per. c.1710–c.1960)', ODNB.

[102]   Hunter, *Science and society*, ch. vii; J. Gascoigne, '"The wisdom of the Egyptians" and the secularisation of history in the age of Newton', in S. Gaukroger (ed.), *The uses of antiquity*, Boston 1991, 171–212; Henry, *Scientific revolution*, 87–8.

this with regard to pregnancy in 1714.[103] In his view, even if the royal touch worked by psychosomatics, it did no harm but 'possibly much good'. Why then was it out of favour? The answer was because of the 'present Indulgence of *Free-Thinking*, above what we enjoy'd in former Times'. Moreover, free-thinking was accompanied by '*Free-Speaking*, and *Free-Acting*'. Turner lamented that his age had not benefited from any of this intellectual change as people had '*talk'd* away our *common Christianity*, as well as *Morality*; and I think we may give Instances of our having *acted* more inhumanly, than any of our Ancestors, when *Free-Thinking* was less in Fashion'.[104] These remarks were probably also aimed at Becket: when concluding that the royal touch was not supernatural, he had stated that 'happy is it for us now, that our minds are free from these Incumberences; an unrestrained Freedom of Thought, and a right Method of Reasoning, are become the happy Characters of this Age'.[105] Becket's claim that free-thinking was a central feature of the 1720s is remarkable considering that his book was published a mere nine years after the notorious *Discourse of freethinking* (1713), written by the deist Anthony Collins.[106] In this book Collins defined free-thinking as the right to judge all propositions on probability and on evidence; he castigated the clergy for having so many different opinions on matters of religion, the inference being that much religion was false. This caused a furore: the book was burned by the public hangman and dozens of replies were printed in Britain and on the Continent.[107]

Turner took the view that cures wrought by the royal hand might be psychological, or due to the power of prayer or the sacred touch, but that it was not for him to determine which, thus revealing his wish to leave God inscrutable. Turning to Becket's objection that fewer people died of scrofula when kings did not touch, Turner argued that at times when 'poor *strumous* Patient[s]' were denied the royal touch, God lessened the amount of scrofula that was in England.[108] He did not comment on any of Becket's other critical points; the impression is that Becket won this dispute.

Evidently by the 1720s it was safe to publish a sceptical interpretation of the royal touch which suggests that opinions that were once fairly marginal were becoming mainstream. The groundwork for this shift began in the 1690s. Up until then one reason why it must have been difficult openly to criticise the royal touch was that it was so central to Stuart sovereignty –

103 D. Turner, *De morbis cutaneis: a treatise of diseases incident to the skin*, London 1714.

104 Idem, *Art of surgery*, i. 161–2, 164–5.

105 Becket, *Enquiry*, 62.

106 A. Collins, *A discourse of freethinking*, London 1713.

107 On Collins see J. O' Higgins, *Anthony Collins: the man and his works*, The Hague 1970; W. Hudson, *The English deists: studies in early Enlightenment*, London 2009; and J. R. Wigelsworth, *Deism in Enlightenment England: theology, politics, and Newtonian public science*, Manchester 2009.

108 Turner, *Art of surgery*, i. 160.

the Stuart kings touched on a vast scale. But when William III refused to participate it is likely that he gave credence to doubt concerning royal thaumaturgy – even though this did not mean that it was acceptable to criticise royal therapeutics in print, deference to the monarchy still being important. At the same time, James II's continued practice of the rite in exile began its association with Jacobitism. Aside from politics, the 1690s experienced an important intellectual shift. Since the middle of the seventeenth century the new science had been a research activity, with the mechanical philosophy available for study by undergraduates; but during the 1690s a noticeable change in the public role of science began, in that the educated public began to accept that this was the way to understand the natural world.[109]

The mechanical philosophy was dualistic: it explained the physical world by emphasising secondary causes, but offered no account of the spiritual realm. This in itself questioned the notion of exchange between the two spheres. A consequence of this was caution concerning miracles, which helps to explain why Anne's liturgy was drastically revised to reflect this. The English tradition of mechanical philosophy culminated in the early eighteenth century with Newtoniansim, which dominated intellectual life and induced an overridingly naturalistic interpretation of the world. All of this highlights the radical intellectual change that occurred in the period under discussion. Yet the different interpretations of the workings of nature and the place of God in the world that existed at this point were debated: although mechanists emphasised secondary causes, this was controversial as others like Turner wanted God to remain involved in human affairs.[110]

A further point that is noteworthy in this context is the changing views of medical practitioners. Throughout the early modern period doctors had recommended the royal touch, often as a last resort when medicine failed to work. Obviously this had to cease once George I became king, but nevertheless during the eighteenth century doctors abandoned their belief in royal therapeutics – or at least they no longer published apologies for it. The picture becomes clear if the men at the heart of the debate of the 1720s

---

[109] M. Hunter, 'Science and the English public', in M. Hamilton-Phillips and R. P. Maccubbin (eds), *The age of William III and Mary II: power, politics and patronage, 1688–1702*, Williamsburg 1989, 165–70 at p. 168; L. R. Stewart, *The rise of public science: rhetoric, technology and natural philosophy in Newtonian Britain, 1660–1750*, Cambridge 1992.

[110] For the eighteenth-century controversy concerning non-mechanical forces in nature see P. M. Heiman (later Harman), '"Nature is a perpetual worker": Newton's aether and 18th-century natural philosophy', *Ambix* xx (1973), 1–25; P. M. Harman, *The culture of nature in Britain*, New Haven–London 2009, ch. viii; S. Schaffer, 'Natural philosophy and public spectacle in the 18th century', *History of Science* xxi (1983), 1–43; S. Schaffer, 'The consuming flame: electrical showmen and Tory mystics in the world of goods', in J. Brewer and R. Porter (eds), *Consumption and the world of goods*, London 1993, 489–526; and O. P. Grell and A. Cunningham (eds), *Medicine and religion in Enlightenment Europe*, Aldershot 2007.

are considered. All four were medical practitioners who cared for the sick (Becket and Turner were both surgeons, and Becket dedicated his book to two eminent physicians, John Steigertahl and Hans Sloane), so for them the debate concerning whether or not scrofula really was cured by the royal touch was not an abstract one. Sloane was the most eminent practitioner of the four, and he was known for his compassion, being a governor of most of London's hospitals. From 1712 he was physician extraordinary to Anne and attended her on her death bed.[111] Both Sloane and Steigertahl attended George I as royal physicians, so had he touched for scrofula it is likely that they would have had a role in the ceremony.

Sloane did not believe in magic, and by implication spiritual healing, attributing belief in it to disorders of the mind, in a reductionist manner.[112] He was not an innovator – in his medical practice he was cautiously progressive.[113] There is no sense in Becket's book that he is trying to convince his dedicatees to take up a new point of view concerning the power of suggestion: his prose is calm and balanced. Thus it appears that Becket's dedication to Sloane could represent what was now the mainstream view amongst medical professionals: that cures wrought by the royal touch were really caused by the power of suggestion. During the sixteenth and seventeenth centuries this idea appears to have been articulated orally, possibly with some restraint, perhaps by a relatively small number of doctors, but by the 1720s it might have become the majority view of such men.[114] Doctors in early modern England had a similar professional standing to lawyers and clergymen, so their view on psychosomatics and the royal touch might have represented a new orthodoxy within the educated classes.[115]

A symptom of such dismissive views of the royal touch is seen in the fact that the material culture of the royal touch began to be of interest to eighteenth-century antiquarians and collectors, one of the earliest examples of whom was Sloane. He collected a silver touch-piece and the lozenges that were burned to perfume and cleanse rooms in which the monarch touched, as well as certificates verifying that supplicants did have scrofula.[116] Collec-

[111] A. MacGregor, 'The life, character and concerns of Sir Hans Sloane', in A. MacGregor (ed.), *Sir Hans Sloane: collector, scientist, antiquary, founding father of the British Museum*, London 1994, 11–44 at p. 15.

[112] *Magic and mental disorder: Sir Hans Sloane's memoir of John Beaumont*, ed. M. Hunter (Robert Boyle Project, 2011).

[113] MacGregor, 'Sloane', 15.

[114] For doctors' thoughts on the royal touch and the power of suggestion before 1700 see pp. 167–9 above.

[115] G. S. Holmes, *Augustan England: professions, state and society, 1680–1730*, London 1982.

[116] M. Archibald, 'Coins and medals', and A. MacGregor, 'Medieval and late antiquities', in MacGregor, *Sir Hans Sloane*, 150–66 at p. 163; certificate for the king's evil from Wymondham, Staffs., n.d. and certificate from Dr Thomas Edgar recommending

tions such as his were to prove invaluable to the nineteenth-century historians who wrote the earliest histories of the ceremony.

However, none of these changes mean that belief in royal therapeutics was extinguished as is evident from the final flurry of texts that was published in the mid-eighteenth century. It is unfortunate that little is known of the authors of these tracts, but none the less they are revealing in two significant ways. First, they have a stronger political connotation than the works from the 1720s, due to the Jacobite rebellion of 1745 during which Charles Edward Stuart had touched an eight-year-old girl for scrofula at Holyrood House in Edinburgh.[117] Secondly, the texts may reflect two different attitudes towards the Enlightenment. The interpretation of the Whigs and their heirs is that the Enlightenment privileged science, reason and the rejection of the supernatural and that these principles were pervasive, leading to the creation of the modern world.[118] By contrast, revisionist scholars stress that the Enlightenment was more limited and piecemeal, with religion and the supernatural continuing to play an important role in eighteenth-century life.[119] The mid-century debate on the royal touch reveals that both points of view flourished.

In 1748 *A Dissertation upon superstition in natural things* was published, to which was appended *Occasional thoughts on the power of curing the king's-evil ascribed to the kings of England*. The author of the *Dissertation* was Samuel Werenfels (1657–1740), Professor of Divinity at Basel. His tract was translated by an unknown scholar, and it was he, not Werenfels, who wrote on the royal touch.[120] The anonymous author was stimulated to write by the recent commotion involving the historian Thomas Carte, a Jacobite and Tory, who mentioned in a footnote in the first volume of his *History of England* (1747) a startling case of scrofula being healed earlier in the century by the Old Pretender. A Bristol labourer called Christopher Lovel had for many years had been very ill with scrofula that had resisted all medical treatments. As a last resort in 1716 he went to the Old Pretender at Avignon, who touched him: the rite was so efficacious that Lovel was completely cured by the time that he reached Bristol, resulting in his case becoming well known. Carte was taken to see Lovel by the eminent Bristol physician Dr Lane, who had failed to cure the labourer, and was impressed. The historian concluded that

---

Catherine Dinnish of Colchester, 1676, BL, MS Sloane 206 B fos 61, 62; pass for Anne Story and her daughter, MS 2723, fo. 57.

[117] For the Holyrood House ceremony see Chambers, *Rebellion*, i. 183–5.

[118] An excellent account from this point of view is R. Porter, *Enlightenment: Britain and the creation of the modern world*, London 2000.

[119] Jonathan Clark puts forward a convincing revisionist case: *English society, 1688–1832: ideology, social structure and political practice during the ancient regime*, Cambridge 1985.

[120] Cf. Weber, *Paper bullets*, 87, and Shaw, *Miracles*, 70, both of whom cite Werenfels as the author. In the preface to the *Dissertation* the translator explains that he is the author of the second tract: *Dissertation*, A2.

even if the healing 'is not to be deemed miraculous, it at least deserved the character given it by Dr Lane, of being one of the most wonderful events that has ever happened'.[121]

Carte's publication caused a storm: numerous Whigs wrote in to the press denouncing him. One writer from Bristol claimed that Carte had only told half the story, and that the Pretender's doctors had tended to Lovel after he was touched, which, alongside the change of air and diet during his journey to Europe, explained his cure. More drastically, the correspondent reported that Lovel had quickly relapsed, and died travelling to the Pretender for a second time.[122] The affair ended badly for Carte, despite his trying to appease the hostility by declaring that he only mentioned Lovel to indicate that unction was not a necessary prerequisite for royal thaumaturgy: the aldermen of London who had financed Carte's book withdrew their funding.[123] The Carte affair reveals a party political division concerning the royal touch, while the fact that it created a storm reveals that, despite the ceremony not having been practised in England for forty-three years, it was still politically sensitive, linked as it was to the issue of legitimate sovereignty. The initial report that maintained that the Pretender's touch was so powerful that it quickly cured a case of extremely bad scrofula inferred that the prince was the true king of Britain.

Returning to *Occasional thoughts on the power of curing the king's-evil*: the author denied that the royal touch worked, rehearsing the usual objections. The source of the healing power was not ceremonial – it could not be the sign of cross as this had been abandoned since James I's reign, nor could it be the wearing of the Angel as Charles I had apparently cured people even when he had no gold to distribute. This meant that the ability to heal resided in the monarch's hands, but how to explain this? The anointing could not be the source as the Pretender had touched Lovell despite not being crowned (there is no mention of legitimate monarchs touching before their coronations). The author then observed that the ceremony did not produce miraculous cures, because it did not heal people immediately and permanently.[124] Turning to current events, he pointed out that the royal touch was now an object of scorn, and reinforced its association with the disempowered Stuarts. He referred to the declarations issued by Charles Edward Stuart during the 1745 uprising, which did not mention the royal

---

[121] T. Carte, *A general history of England*, London 1747–55, i. 291–2. See also J. Nichols, *Literary anecdotes of the eighteenth century*, London 1812–16, ii. 494–504; Crawford, *The king's evil*, 155–7; Bloch, *The royal touch*, 221 (393–4); and Clark, *English society*, 160–1.

[122] Letter to the *General Evening Post*, 14–16 Jan. 1748, reproduced in Whiston, *Memoirs*, 360–3.

[123] See Carte's letter to the *General Evening Post*, 20–23 Feb. 1748, repr. in Whiston, *Memoirs*, 363–6, and S. Handley, 'Carte, Thomas (*bap.* 1686, *d.* 1754)', *ODNB*.

[124] *Occasional thoughts on the power of curing the king's-evil ascribed to the kings of England*, London 1748, 50–1, 65.

touch: this was because the 'Faction cannot well stand the Ridicule of one of their own best reasons'. In a key passage the author implicitly contrasted the exiled Stuarts with William III and George I, insisting that the latter did not touch the sick 'from a true Greatness of Mind' and a 'generous Detestation of Fraud and Imposture'.[125]

Yet, in the same year, 1748, a defence of the royal touch was published that was more vigorous than Turner's. *A collection of remarkable cures of the king's evil, perfected by the royal touch*, was the work of the apothecary and Cambridge graduate John Badger.[126] According to Badger, the royal touch was a victim of 'the Prejudices of the present Age', that is, fashionable free-thinking.[127] To counter this, he presented the longevity and efficacy of the royal touch as a 'matter of fact'.[128] This echoed debates associated with the new science, whereby a consensus was reached on the basis of 'matters of fact' which could be experimentally demonstrated and corporately agreed, and to which hypothesis and speculation were tangential.[129] The royal touch was 'experimentally demonstrated' by both its long history and its cures, and Badger discussed both, re-publishing many of Browne's case studies from the last part of *Adenochoiradelogia* as well as the annual totals of people touched by Charles II. The rite had 'corporate agreement' from its eminent apologists: Badger cited Fortesque, Tooker, Clowes, Laurentius, Wiseman, Browne, and Turner, maintaining that it was ridiculous to say that they had all been wrong. The last three were 'learned and skilful Surgeons; and their Writings have ever been approved and received by the experienced Surgeons of their Age'. Added to which, 'Archbishops, Bishops, clergy, Nobility, Gentry, Physicians, Surgeons, and the Mighty Multitude of People, which came from far and near to receive the Benefit of the Touch' all believed in its efficacy.[130] Badger concluded that the power of the royal touch lay with God, so was beyond man's understanding, and he quoted Cicero in order to demolish the sceptics: 'truth always had so much power, that it could not be subverted by any schemes, or any man's clever trick or device; and although it might obtain no patron or defender in trials, it nevertheless defends itself'.[131]

---

[125] Ibid. 68. David Hume made the same point: *The history of England, from the invasion of Julius Cæsar to the abdication of James the Second, 1688*, London 1754–61, repr. Boston 1856, i. 138.

[126] T. D. Whitet, 'John Badger, Apothecaryite', *Pharmaceutical Historian*, iii/1 (1973), 2–4.

[127] J. Badger, *A collection of remarkable cures of the king's evil, perfected by the royal touch, collected from the writings of many eminent physicians and surgeons and learned men*, London 1748, 2.

[128] Ibid. 25, 63.

[129] Shapin and Schaffer, *Leviathan and the air pump*; Michael Hunter, 'Scientific change: its setting and stimuli', in B. Coward (ed), *A companion to Stuart Britain*, Malden, MA 2003, repr. Chichester 2009, 214–29 at p. 220.

[130] Badger, *Remarkable cures*, 63–4.

[131] Ibid. 64.

A further point concerning the mid-century tracts is their attitude towards Roman Catholicism. The critical authors all provided more general denigrations of Catholicism which reinforced their anti-Jacobitism and suggested an anti-magical outlook on life, a view that was becoming increasingly common during the Enlightenment. The Whig letter-writer who attacked Carte insisted that belief in the royal touch had been 'long exploded by men of sense and existed nowhere but in the brains of Popish enthusiasts, and credulous bigots'.[132] The author of *Occasional thoughts* remarked on the royal touch that 'We must be falling into the Dregs of time, and sinking into the Follies of a fabulous Age if so idle a Tale can obtain a general Credit … If we give it a kind Reception, we cannot refuse the same … To all the Absurdities and Superstitions of Popery.'[133]

By contrast, the Jacobites championed the royal touch and so were associated with belief in the supernatural. The most extreme example of this dates from 1751, when the Jacobite press tried to take revenge for the hurt done to Carte by reporting that one David West, a Birmingham iron-box maker, was cured of his scrofula on Restoration day 1749, after an encounter with an apparition, the 'most comely' stranger that he had ever beheld. This was code for Charles Edward Stuart, whose beauty was such that it enabled him to disguise himself as a woman whilst escaping to Europe after the failed uprising of 1745. The stranger recited Latin prayers which included a borrowing from the French royal touch ceremony, 'I touch, but God healeth', after which he laid his hands on West and instructed him to keep the matter secret for a year.[134] Although there was no precedent for an apparition of a living prince curing scrofula, and no doubt the episode was an 'outrageous fable', nevertheless it elicited a hostile response in the press.[135] 'If a man will … believe in *One Miracle*, he may as well in *One Thousand*, and so may swallow all the Miracles of the Romish Church', wrote another outraged Whig Bristolian, proving again how politically and religiously sensitive the royal touch remained in some quarters.[136]

The mid-century debate was just as inconclusive as that of the Restoration or the early eighteenth century. Defenders of the royal touch still cited its endurance and efficacy, and argued that God was omnipresent and omnipotent, whilst sceptics drew on the many changes to the practice and the disruptions to the direct line of succession, and foregrounded the rite's ineffectiveness. With hindsight we know that the defenders would lose the battle: over time generational change meant that the protagonists of the

132 Whiston, *Memoirs*, 361.
133 *Occurrences*, 73.
134 *Adam's Weekly Courant*, 16 July 1751; *True Briton* ii/9, 21 Aug. 1751, 198–201; *London Evening Post*, 17 Aug. 1751.
135 For 'outrageous fable' see Monod, *Jacobitism*, 130.
136 *Bristol Weekly Intelligencer*, 31 Aug. 1751.

royal touch were replaced by people for whom it was historical, incompatible with Enlightenment values, or continental and Roman Catholic. But the outcome of the debate was far from clear throughout much of the eighteenth century. After 1714 people still wore touch-pieces, they bequeathed them to those who needed them, and they travelled in large numbers to Europe to be touched by the Jacobite Pretenders.[137] Indeed, the last Pretender, Henry Benedict Stuart, cardinal of York, regularly touched the sick until his death in 1807: had he provided an heir, the practice might have continued.[138] The liturgy for the royal touch remained in certain editions of the English Book of Common Prayer until 1732 and in the Latin version until 1759: although George I repudiated the rite, it seems to have been uncertain whether this was a precedent or a decision personal to him.[139] In fact, the cessation of the royal touch owes more to an accident of biology than to the Enlightenment. In other words, had Anne's son the duke of Gloucester survived and inherited the throne in 1714, the royal touch would surely have continued to be performed by the Stuarts in England throughout the eighteenth century just as it was in France.

[137] Farquhar, 'Royal charities, IV',160; Bloch, The royal touch, 222–3 (395–7); Thomas, Religion and the decline of magic, 193–4; Corp, Stuarts in Italy, 182, 193, 318–19.

[138] For the cardinal of York's touch-pieces see Crawfurd, The king's evil, 159; Farquhar, 'Royal charities, IV', 175–80; and Woolf, 'Sovereign remedy, II', 100–5.

[139] For the survival of the liturgy see MacDonald Ross, 'Royal touch', 435.

Conclusion

This book has argued that the royal touch was a central feature of early modern England, a juncture at which politics, medicine and religion met. It has concentrated on the ways in which the crown used the ceremony to assert its authority, as well as the great public demand for royal therapeutics and the associated problems that this brought with it. The full range of views on the royal touch has been assessed, from belief to uncertainty to outright denial that it worked. The ceremony has been analysed within the context of early modern views on the authority of the monarch and on the connection between the physical and supernatural worlds, as well as the expectations that people had of medicine and health care.

In theory the royal touch provided the opportunity for the monarch to display the ultimate charismatic power, the ability to heal by touch, just as Christ had done. However, the royal touch was not just a tool for the crown to project its authority. After all, three monarchs could have used it to their advantage immediately after becoming king, but did not: James VI and I expressed his doubts publicly in 1603 before changing his mind, while William III and George I both refused to practise it. Before the autumn of 1603 James did not believe that he could heal by touch, partly because as a Calvinist he thought that the age of miracles was over; William and George shared his scepticism but did not change their minds. This was even though the royal touch was not expected to heal everyone immediately. Although people who were touched by the sovereign no doubt prayed for an immediate and full cure, in reality people's expectations were different. The benefit of the royal touch was often described as being an improvement in someone's condition in the weeks following the ceremony. This was acceptable to many, partly because miracles that wrought physical change had always been rare, and partly because of the expectations people had of medicine in pre-modern Europe. Doctors were expected to provide consolation and pain management, a complete cure being exceptional.

The ceremony was subjected to numerous changes throughout the Tudor and Stuart age, largely to make it more Protestant in character. From this a number of insights may be derived. Sceptical attitudes towards royal thaumaturgy were not restricted to heterodox or marginal groups such as freethinkers or religious minorities. Such views certainly existed in those circles; but it is also clear that the first Stuart king of England was initially doubtful about the royal touch. Less obvious, but just as pertinent, is the fact that all the monarchs who reformed the ceremony must have had certain reservations about it – why else did they change it? Fear of 'superstition' often drove these reforms, thus exposing anxieties concerning Roman Catholicism or magic. The reforms were evidently popular as the numbers who sought the royal touch increased greatly between 1530 and 1688. The drive to reform is also telling in regard to the crown's commitment to minister to those of its subjects who were ill with scrofula. It might have been easier to suppress the ceremony, but this was not what happened.

There seems to have been a pattern between the Civil War and the Glorious Revolution whereby the numbers who sought the royal touch increased during times of political crisis. Sick people appear to have voted with their feet, seeking out royal therapeutics as a way of showing loyalty to the crown, and to God, during traumatic times. This reinforces the view that the privation and trauma of the Civil War was widespread, and that for the bulk of the population the trial and execution of Charles I was a step too far. During the political crises of the Restoration the legacy of the 1640s meant that there were severe anxieties that '1642 has come again', not least because the Whigs and Tories seemed to be re-enacting the political divisions of the war. The royal touch was an antidote to this, a view that highlights the pacific and benevolent nature of the ceremony. The rite was a healing practice that was performed in imitation of Christ, who forgave people's sins as he healed them. Just as recovery from disease was synony-mous with the triumph of good over evil, so the king's touch could symbolise forgiveness and peace, concepts which presumably were especially attractive during a political emergency. Thus various monarchs touched people who might have been considered their foes. Elizabeth I touched Roman Catholics, Charles I touched parliamentarians, Charles II touched those who had sided against the crown during the 1640s, or who were likely to have done so, and James II touched Protestants. Similarly, people turned to the monarch for relief even if they disagreed with the sovereign's religion or politics. While there was no doubt an element of pragmatism involved in this – people were ill and wanted a cure – what is especially interesting is that the royal touch appeared at times to collapse political and religious divisions. If we are searching for the origins of pluralism, we have glimpses of it at these healing ceremonies that temporarily brought together people from different, sometimes opposing, groups.

The survival of the royal touch beyond the Tudor Reformations and the regicide into the early eighteenth century is revealing in terms of the devel-opment of an English Protestant culture. Current scholarship rejects or qual-ifies the old Weberian model of 'disenchantment' leading to secularisation and progress; the continuity of pre-Reformation ideas and practices has been stressed, with reform appearing more piecemeal and gradual. Some points can be made in connection with royal therapeutics that support this view.[1] First, although the Reformation dispensed with numerous saints' days and

---

[1]   Here I am working alongside the astute observations of Alexandra Walsham, 'The Reformation and "the disenchantment of the world" reassessed', HJ li/2 (2008), 497–528, esp. pp. 513–15.

holy days, it is worth stating that it did not de-mystify the concept of time. Instead, to a certain extent it replaced special Catholic days with Protestant holy days and patriotic anniversaries. The proper keeping of the Sabbath was important. Current events provided the impetus for the development of new commemorations, most notably deliverance from 'popish' foes – new memorials included those that marked the accession of Elizabeth I every 17 November, and the Gunpowder Plot of 5 November 1605 – while the regicide was atoned for every 30 January. Viewed in this way, the seasonal healing calendar of the royal touch played a significant part in the Protestant year. Key times for the royal touch were Easter and Michaelmas, tying the ceremony to Christ's passion and the harvest.

Secondly, although Protestants abolished much Catholic ceremony, denying its automatic efficacy in favour of personal virtue, self-confidence and soul-searching, adherents of the new religion retained and developed their own forms of ritual. Prayer, humiliation and fasting were used to appease God during disasters or times of communal anxieties, while rogation-tide processions and Puritan rites of exorcism were widely practised. Monarchs were crowned and anointed very much according to the old ways. The royal touch fitted into this culture of Protestant rites, being reformed many times between the 1530s and the reign of Queen Anne to ensure that it really was no longer Roman Catholic.

Thirdly, although Protestants rejected the Catholic idea of intermediary figures and objects, claiming instead that salvation came through faith, prayer or predestination, official Churches still maintained a hierarchy of clergy, while sects often centred on charismatic leaders who had their own disciples, such as the Quaker George Fox. Similarly, relics were collected and treasured, such as those of the Marian martyrs. Officially, these people and objects possessed no special supernatural powers, but in practice slippage occurred. This is the context in which the Protestant royal touch flourished. The sovereign could act the part of Christ during the royal touch (and on Maundy Thursday, when he or she washed the feet of the poor), while at the same time proceedings emphasised the importance of prayer, faith and supplication. The gold Angel given to each sick person was meant to commemorate the ceremony, but sometimes was worn as an amulet. This is not entirely surprising given the occult properties of gold, and the words and images engraved on the medal which were chosen because they emphasised that the ceremony was a spiritual form of healing. All of this attests to the 'messiness' of aspects of reformed theology and practices, and of lay belief as well. On the one hand, the appeal of the royal touch increased as it was 'Protestantised'; on the other, supplicants sometimes wore their Angel as a charm.

The royal touch ceased to be practised in 1714, but George I was still a personal monarch who reigned as well as ruled. Through the eighteenth century the character of the English monarchy would change, becoming less sacral and less ostentatious, a process that culminated with the image of

George III as 'Farmer George' tending his livestock. In Europe, the model for Enlightened monarchy was similarly shorn of its sacral elements, though the difference was that pioneers such as Frederick the Great and Joseph II drove bureaucratic reform as the self-styled 'first servants of the state'.[2] By contrast, the French Bourbons continued to touch the sick until the Revolution that began in 1789; the ceremony was then revived on one occasion by Charles X in 1825, as part of his coronation, though it appears that enthusiasm for it was modest.[3] In England during the eighteenth century the gap created by the cessation of royal therapeutics was filled by other forms of charitable benevolence. This began in 1704 with Queen Anne's Bounty, a fund to augment the incomes of poorer clergy, and reached its apogee in 1897 with the establishment of The Prince of Wales' Hospital Fund.[4] Later renamed The King's Fund, this raised money to finance the voluntary hospitals of London, the only places in the capital that provided healthcare for the poor. Thus royal therapeutics was transformed into royal charity, with The King's Fund occupying an important role in the hands-on provision of medical aid during the first half of the twentieth-century until the arrival of the National Health Service in 1948.

What is remarkable is that, even as medicine became secularised and the charismatic aspects of monarchy declined, the British crown continued with its Royal Maundy service, held each Maundy Thursday. Indeed, this ceremony is still conducted every year because the sovereign is head of the Church of England. The service is similar to the royal touch ceremony in that it is structured around verses from the New Testament, especially minted coins are distributed, and both rites are a re-enactment of a significant aspect of Christ's life. Just before the Last Supper, Jesus washed the feet of his disciples and gave the commandment to love one another. However, William III was the last monarch to wash the feet of the poor during the Royal Maundy ceremony. No doubt Anne was too infirm to kneel down for very long, and the Hanoverians eschewed such charismatic re-enactments.

The Order of Service for Royal Maundy is structured around two short passages. The first, John xiii.34–5: 'A new command I give you: Love one another. As I have loved you, so you must love one another. By this everyone will know that you are my disciples, if you love one another'; and the second, the passages from Matt. xxv in which Jesus explains the need to care for the vulnerable (the same text that provided the medieval belief that Christ might be present within crowds of sick people). The sovereign then distrib-

---

[2] T. C. W. Blanning, *The culture of power and the power of culture: old regime Europe, 1660–1789*, Oxford 2002.

[3] R. A. Jackson, *Vive le Roi! A history of the French coronation from Charles V to Charles X*, London 1984, 198.

[4] Gregg, *Queen Anne*, 179; F. K. Prochaska, *Philanthropy and the hospitals of London: the King's Fund, 1897–1990*, Oxford 1992; Porter, *Greatest benefit*, ch. xiii, 'Public medicine' provides the context for these nineteenth-century changes.

utes Maundy pennies to people who regularly attend Anglican service; these are non-circulating coins, the only British coins that still contain silver, and they are highly collectable. Their recipients are chosen for doing good works, the number equalling the monarch's age. The ceremony finishes with prayers and hymns.[5] This, then, along with the coronation, is the last remnant of sacral monarchy, and although it receives little attention in the modern world, it shows that the charismatic aspect of sovereignty still exists in our scientific age.

[5]   B. Robinson, *The Royal Maundy*, London 1977, and *Silver pennies and linen towels: the story of Royal Maundy*, London 1992; P. Wright, *The story of royal Maundy*, London 1990.

Bibliography

Unpublished primary sources

Aylesbury, Centre for Buckinghamshire Studies
PR 4/1/3 Register of burials in woollen, 1678–1717, for the parish of Amersham
PR 25/1/2 Register of births, deaths and marriages, 1695–1749, and burials, 1678–1715, for the parish of Great Brickhill
PR 72/1/2 Eton parish register, 1653–1715
PR 95/1/4 Register of baptisms, 1669–1741, marriages, 1670–1740, burials, 1669–1740, for the parish of Hardwick with Weedon
PR 220/1/2 Register of baptisms, 1695–1729, marriages, 1695–1728, 1730–53, burials, 1695–1753 for the parish of Wavendon
PR 230/1/1 Register of baptisms, 1653–88, marriages, 1653–92, burials, 1653–88, for the parish of Whitchurch

Bedford, Bedfordshire and Luton Archives and Records Service
HSA/1682 S/38 Deposition: Mary, wife of William Eames, Dunstable, 26 June 1682
HAS/1682 S/41 Deposition: John Field. 16 June 1682
HAS 1688/S/18 Presentment for theft of 'touching gold'
P31/1/3 1678–1702 Register of burials in woollen, 1678–1704, and baptisms and marriages, 1699–1702, for the parish of Maulden
P60/1/ 9 Register book for the parish of Kempston, 1680–1721
P72/28/14 Recipe for the cure of scrofula, 1808
R3 /75 Letter from [Septimus] Turton to John Temple, 23 Dec. 1740

Cambridge, Cambridge University Library
MS Add. 44, item 9 Patrick papers, transcription of Mary Tudor's cramp ring liturgy
MS Ec.3.59 *La Estoire de Seint Ædward le roi*
MS Mm. 1.51 Transcription of Mary Tudor's cramp ring liturgy

Cambridge, St John's College Library
MS Cam. L. 13 Transcription of Mary Tudor's cramp ring liturgy

Chelmsford, Essex Record Office
D/DP/F273/36 [Derentwater correspondence] Statement of Jo Vane, 23 Apr. 1719
D/DTw /F4/1/4 Almanac, 1757
D/P177/1/2 Register of marriages and burials, 1678–1809, for the parish of St Runwald, Colchester
D/P178/1/3 Register of burials, 1678–1782, for the parish of St Peter's, Colchester
DDE1/Z6 Miscellaneous papers, 1743–1857

DP/10/8 Overseer's book, 1659–1743, for the parish of All Saints', Greater Chestefield

DP/134/1/2 Register of baptisms, 1653–1762, marriages, 1654–1773, and burials, 1654–77, 1707–73, for the parish of St Mary the Virgin, Kelvedon

Chichester, West Sussex Record Office
Par 94/7/7 [includes an injunction from the bishop of Chichester about an order in council relating to touching for the king's evil, 12 Feb. 1684]

Par 149/1/1/1, fo. 184 Petworth parish composite register, 1559–1794

Par 192/1/1/1 Tangmere parish composite register, 1540–1776

Chippenham, Wiltshire and Swindon History Centre
500/1 Ramsbury parish register, 1678–1722

1901/2 Register, 1653–99, for the parish of St Edmund's, Salisbury

Dorchester, Dorset History Centre
PE /WSD/RG4/1 Winterbourne Stickland burials register, 1678–1750

PE/YETRE1/1 Yetminster parish records, 1677–1711

Durham County Record Office
EP/Du.SO 175t St Oswald, Durham, parish records, 1672–86

Edinburgh, The National Library of Scotland
MSS Advocates 15.2.17, fo. 23 Sir James Balfour's notes connected to Charles I's state visit to Edinburgh, 1633

Gloucester, Gloucestershire Archives
D688/1 Overseers' accounts, 1655–69, for the parish of Thornbury

P33IN1/1 Records, 1630–1742, fo. 22, for the parish of Bagendon

P154/9IN1/4 Records, 1656–93, for the parish of St John the Baptist

Hertford, Hertfordshire Archives
DP53/8/1 Parish records, parish memoranda, 1643–1770, for the parish of St Mary's, Hitchin

DP55/1/1 Register of baptisms, marriages and burials, 1538–1724, for the parish of Great Hormead

DP56/1/1Register of baptisms, marriages and burials, 1588–1686, for the parish of Little Hormead

DP85/1/1 Register of baptisms, marriages and burials, 1653–1715, for the parish of Rickmansworth

DP117/1/12 Register of burials in woollen, 1678–1713, for the parish of Watford

DP119/8/1 Vestry minute book, 1658–1731, for the parish of Welwyn

Kendal, Kendal Archive Centre
WPR/91/1/ Register, 1570–1687, for the parish of Grasmere

WSMB/K/1/5 Kendal chamberlain's accounts, 1661–2

Kew, The National Archives
C47/4/1/1 Household accounts for Edward I
E101/415/3 Account book of John Heron, 1500–3, treasurer of the chamber to Henry VII
E101/426/1 Account book of Sir William Paget, controller of the household, 1547–8
E407/85/1 Record of the numbers touched for the evil on various occasions, 1669–85
Exchequer accounts 388, 5 [Edward III], 409, 9, [Henry VI], 413, 9 [Henry VII]
LC5/133 Lord Chamberlain's department: miscellaneous records: warrant books: 'Declaration concerning the healing of the evill sett up at court gate', 1635
LC5/140, pp. 493–4 Lord Chamberlain's department: miscellaneous records: warrant books: 'Orders for chyrurgeons at healings', 1674
LC5/141, p. 33 Lord Chamberlain's department: miscellaneous records: warrant books: 'Chyrurgeons concerning healings' 1674
LC5/144, p. 195 Lord Chamberlain's department: miscellaneous records: warrant books: 'Orders for healings', 1682
LC5/2, p. 55 Lord Chamberlain's department: miscellaneous records: master of ceremonies: extracts from the notebooks of Sir John Cottrell, senior and junior, description of the duchess of Modena, Prince Renaldo etc viewing the royal touch ceremony incognito, 1673
LC5/200 Lord Chamberlain's department: miscellaneous records: order from Charles I to his apothecary, 1627
PC2/70 Privy Council: registers, Charles II: handwritten draft of the proclamation dated 9 Jan. 1684 concerning the king's evil
PRO31/9/87, fos 362–3 Rome Archives, ser. 1, general series from Vatican and other sources
PRO31/9/88 Rome Archives, ser. 1, general series from Vatican and other sources
SP78/180, fos 196r–197v Secretaries of State: state papers foreign, France: Robinson to Delafaye, the ceremony of 'touching for the evil' delayed by Louis XV's confessor, 1724

Lichfield, Lichfield Record Office
D20/1/2 Register, 1677–1754, for the parish of St Mary's, Lichfield
D35 Baliff's accounts, 1657–1707

Lincoln, Lincolnshire Archives
Par/1/1 General register, 1559–1707, for the parish of Irnham, fo. 31
Par/1/2 General register, 1653–1740, for Wootton
Par/1/4A Rough register 1683–1769, for the parish of St Botolph, Boston

London, British Library
MS Add. 9951 Daily account of Edward II, 8 July 1320–7 July 1321
MS Add. 21480 Household-book of Henry VII, as kept by John Heron, Treasurer of the Chamber, 1499–1505
MS Add. 22587, fo. 4 James I's 'extempore speech at the first touching of a diseased child of the king's evil', 1603
MS Add. 35182 Henry VIII's exchequer accounts

MS Add. 35183 Exchequer accounts: declaration for the year ending Michaelmas, 38 Hen. VIII. [1546, includes Edward VI's cramp ring expenditure]

MS Add. 35184 Edward VI's exchequer accounts

MS Add. 61420 Marlborough papers: records of Angels requested and received from Mr Coggs, and of Angels sent to Queen Anne, 16 May 1706–1 June 1707

MS Cotton Nero C VIII Edward III treasury receipts

MS Egerton 806, fos 59r–60r Number of people touched Apr.– Nov. 1668

MS Royal 16 G VI *Les Grandes Chroniques de France*

MS Sloane 206 B, fo. 61 Certificate for the king's evil from Wymondham, Staffs., n.d.

MS Sloane 206 B, fo. 62 Certificate from Dr Thomas Edgar recommending Catherine Dinnish of Colchester, 1676; in Latin

MS Sloane 2723 fo. 57 Pass for Anne Story and her daughter to travel from Carlisle to London to be touched by Charles II, 25 June 1681

London, British Museum

MS Schreiber E.64 'A complete pack of fifty-two playing-cards: reign of Queen Anne'

1849, 0315.31 *The manner of his majesties curing the disease called the kings–evill*, London 1679

London, House of Lords Records Office

HL/PO/JO/10/1/143 House of Lords, journal office, main papers, 1509–1700

London, London Metropolitan Archive

DRO/029/001 Composite register for the parish of St Mary, Hendon Church End, Hendon, 1653–1744

DRO/1/A/1/1 Register of baptisms, marriages and burials, 1568–1706/7, for the parish of St Martin, West Drayton

P78/NIC/3/1–4 Composite register, 1638–1735, for the parish of St Nicholas, Deptford, Deptford Green, Greenwich

P95TRI1/66 Register, 1678–1702, for the parish of Holy Trinity Church, Clapham, Lambeth

P97/MRY/2 Register of burials, 1680–Apr. 1694, for the parish of St Mary Magdalene, Church Street, Woolwich, Greenwich

London, Royal Society

MS RS92 John Aubrey, *Memoires of naturall remarques in the county of Wilts, to which are annexed observabes of the same kind in the county of Surrey and Flynt–shire*, 6 June 1685

Treasury of Receipt, miscellaneous books, 203 [Edward III]

London, Society of Antiquaries

James VI and I's liturgy, *The offices or prayers to be used at the ceremony of touching for the king's evil* (1618?), Lemon Collection, broadside 161

London, Wellcome Library
MS 5251 Document recording the numbers touched by James II on each of thirty-two occasions, 8 Jan.–20 June 1686
MS 6083/5 Autobiographical narrative of an English student at the English College, Lisbon, around the year 1718
WF/M/I/DM/02, Black-and-white photograph of a float 'Queen Elizabeth I cures a sufferer from king's evil', possibly from the 1953 coronation

London, Westminster Abbey
MS 7 Mary Tudor's missal

Maidstone, Kent History and Library Centre
P99/12 /1 Overseers accounts, 1599–1835, for the parish of Cowden
P193/1/1 General register, 1671–1810, for the parish of Horton Kirby
P241/5/21 Parish chest accounts, 1667–1727, for the parish of All Saints, Maidstone
P241/12/11 Overseers accounts for the parish of All Saints, Maidstone: vouchers, 1678–1723
P371/12/1/6 Parish chest accounts, 1670–1806, for the parish of Tonbridge
P406/1/2 Register of burials in woollen, 1678–1812, for the parish of St George, Wrotham

Norwich, Norfolk Record Office
MC 2577/2/24, 984X7 Antiquarian jottings by Goddard Johnson relating to Norwich ... payments for individuals to be touched for the king's evil, 1845–7

Oxford, Ashmolean Museum
MS Sutherland 114 (229) *The manner of his majesties curing the disease called the kings-evill*

Oxford, Bodleian Library
MS Aubrey A1 John Aubrey, *The natural history of Wiltshire*, pt I
MS Firth b.16 (1) *The manner of his majesties curing the disease called the kings–evill*
MS Rawlinson A 194, fos 247v–248r Letter from Samuel Pepys to James Pearce, 18 May 1681
MS Smith 47 Letter from E. Bernard to T. Smith, 4 Sept. 1687

Oxford, Oxfordshire History Centre
PAR 16/1/R1/2 Register of baptisms, marriages and burials, 1653–97, for the parish of Bampton, fo. 3b
PAR 265/1/R1/1 Register of baptisms, marriages and burials, 1568–1713, for the parish of Swyncombe, fo. 19
PAR 276/1/R1/3 Register of baptisms, marriages and burials, 1638–1697, for the parish of Wardington, fo. 37

Preston, Lancashire Archives
DDKE/HMC/434 Letter from Sir Thomas Preston to Roger Kenyon, London: cannot travel as his daughter is ill of the hen-pox, 12 Feb. 1682

DDKE/HMC/438 Letter from R. Bradshaigh, Jr, to Roger Kenyon: news of Sir Thomas Preston and the earl of Shaftesbury, 19 Feb. 1681–1682

QSB/1/130/68 Petition of Raphe Cocker for pass to take his blind son, who cannot travel more than six miles a day, to London to be cured of the king's evil, 1633–4

QSP/461/7 Manchester: Susanna Dyson, widow, wishes to take her child to London to be touched for the king's evil, 1676–7

QSP/484/12 Penwortham: payment of carrier's bill of £3 11s. taking son of Lambeartt Coward to London, with king's evil, 1678

Shrewsbury, Shropshire Archives
P198/A/1/2 Much Wenlock general register, 1642–98
P281/B/1/1/1 Tong churchwardens' accounts, 1670: Mary Paynton being sent to London to be touched at a cost of 40s.

Taunton: Somerset Archives and Local Studies
DD/SE/45/1/20 Hugh Sexey's Hospital: petition to feoffees for charitable gifts: John Brock's petition re his daughters with scrofula
DD/SE/45/1/34 Hugh Sexey's Hospital: petition to feoffees for charitable gifts: petition of the widow Margarte Drew for relief due to blindness caused by scrofula

Warwick, County Record Office
DRB63/1 Hampton in Arden, parish register, 1599–1732

Winchester, Hampshire Record Office
29M79 Register, 1653–1812, for the parish of West Worldham
32M66/PR4 Register, 1678–1719, for the parish of Selborne
38M85/BC/A15 Packet of general notes concerning Andover's history, sixteenth–twentieth century
60M67/PR4 Register of burials, 1678–1714, for the parish of Andover
63M70/PI6/85b Note, 1686–7, for the parish of Bramley
91M79/PR2 Register, 1678–1795, for the parish of Faccombe
SRO/PR9/1/1 Register, for the parish of South Stoneham
W/E6/8 Winchester account book: accounts of payments out of coffer

Woking, Surrey History Centre
LM/1379/80/1 [Recipe for the cure of the king's evil]
P23/1/1 Records, 1538–1902, for the parish of St Katherine, Merstham
PSH/GU/HT/1/ 1 Records, 1558–1812, for the parish of Holy Trinity, Guildford
PSH/STK/1/1 Records, 1662–1727, for the parish of Stoke
PSH/WIT/1/1 Records, 1653–1771, for the parish of All Saints, Witley

Woodhorn, Northumberland Archives
SANT/BEQ/4/26/133 Record of 133 people touched on 6 Mar. 1667

Worcester, Worcestershire Archive and Archaeology Service
110:155/88 Quarter sessions report, 1688–9

BIBLIOGRAPHY

UNITED STATES

New Haven, Connecticut, Beinecke Library
OSB, MSS 1, box 2, folder 64, Poley newsletters

Washington, DC, Folger Shakespeare Library
MS Folger 266450 Account of the number of people touched by Charles II to cure the king's evil, 8 Jan.–12 July 1683

Washington, DC, National Library of Medicine
MS f115 'King's evil: a collection of items pertaining to the royal touch for the healing of scrofula, 1628–1712'

Newspapers and journals

Adams Weekly Courant
Athenian Gazette
Bristol Weekly Intelligencer
Daily Courant
English Post
Evening Post
Flying Post
General Evening Post
Kingdomes Weekly Intelligencer
London Evening Post
London Gazette
Mercurius Aulicus
Mercurius Elenctius
Mercurius Publicus
Paris Gazette
Parliamentary Intelligencer
Perfect Occurrences
Post
Post Man
The Protestant (Domestic) Intelligence
True Briton

Printed primary sources

The accession, coronation, and marriage of Mary Tudor as related in four manuscripts of the Escorial, ed. and trans. C.V. Malfatti, Barcelona 1956
The accession of Queen Mary: being the contemporary narrative of Antonio de Guaras, a Spanish merchant resident in London, ed. and trans. Richard Garnett, London 1892
An account of the preservation of King Charles II after the Battle of Worcester drawn up by himself, London 1766

229

Alumni oxonienses: the members of the University of Oxford, 1500–1714, ed. J. Foster, Oxford–London 1891

Andrewes, L., *Sermons*, ed. G. M. Story, Oxford 1967

—— *Selected writings*, ed. P. E. Hewison, Manchester 1995

An answer to a scoffing and lying libel put forth and privately dispersed under the title of a wonderful account of the curing of the kings-evil by Madam Fanshaw the duke of Monmouth's sister, London 1681

Anthony, F., *Medicinae chymicae et veri potabilis auri assertio*, London 1610

—— *Apologia Veritatis illucescentis, pro auro potabile*, London 1616

—— *The Apologie, or, Defence of a verity heretofore published concerning a medicine called aurum potabile*, London 1616

Aquinas, T., *Summa theologiae*, ed. R. J. Batten, London 1975

Ashmole, E., *Theatrum chemicum Britannicum*, London 1652

—— *The institution, laws and ceremonies of the Most Noble Order of the Garter*, London 1672

—— *Elias Ashmole: his autobiographical and historical notes, his correspondence and other contemporary sources*, ed. C. H. Joster, Oxford 1967

Aubrey, J., *Miscellanies*, in *Three prose works*, 1–125

—— *Observations*, in *Three prose works*, 305–63

—— *Remains of Gentilisme and Judaisme* (1686–7), in *Three prose works*, 127–304

—— *Remaines of Gentilisme and Judaism* (1686–7), ed. James Britten, London 1881

—— *Miscellanies upon the following subjects collected by John Aubrey Esq*, London 1696

—— *The natural history of Wiltshire*, ed. John Britten, London 1847

—— *Three prose works*, ed. J. Buchanan-Brown, Fontwell 1972

—— *Brief lives*, ed. John Buchanan- Brown, London 2000

Aylmer, J., *An harborrowe for faithful and trewe subiectes, agaynst the late blowne blast, concerning the government of wemmen*, London 1559

Bacon, F.,, *The history of the reign of Henry VII*, ed. R. Lockyer, London 1971

Badger, J., *A collection of remarkable cures of the king's evil, perfected by the royal touch, collected from the writings of many eminent physicians and surgeons and learned men*, London 1748

Baron, W., *Regicides no saints nor martyrs*, London 1700

Baxter, R., *The certainty of the world of spirits*, London 1691

Becket, W., *A free and impartial enquiry into the antiquity and efficacy of touching for the cure of the king's evil*, London 1722

Bentley, W., *Excerpta historica*, London 1833

Birch, *The history of the Royal Society of London For Improving Natural Knowledge*, London 1756–7

Bird, J., *Grounds of grammer penned and published: by Iohn Bird schoolemaster in the citty of Glocester*, Oxford 1639

—— *Ostenta Carolina, or, The late calamities of England with the authors of them*, London 1661

Blackmore, R., *Discourses on the gout, a rheumatism, and the king's evil*, London 1726

Blondel, J., *The strength of imagination in pregnant women examined; and the opinion that marks and deformities in children arise from thence, demonstrated to be a vulgar error,* London 1727

―― *The power of the mother's imagination over the foetus examined,* London 1729

Blount, T., *Boscobel, or, The history of his sacred majesties most miraculous preservation after the battle of Worcester, 3 Sept. 1651,* London 1660

Book of Common Prayer, London 1707

The Booke of Common Prayer, and administrations of the sacraments, London 1633

Boorde, A., *The breviary of healthe,* London 1547; 2nd edn, 1552

―― *The fyrst boke of the introduction of knowledge,* London 1547

―― *The fyrst boke of the introduction of knowledge,* ed. F. J. Furnivall, London 1870

Boswell, J., *Boswell's Life of Johnson,* ed. G. Birkbeck Hill, Oxford 1974

―― *The life of Samuel Johnson,* ed. J. Canning, London 1991

Boyle, R., *Of the reconcileableness of specifick medicines to the corpuscular philosophy to which is annexed a discourse about the advantages of the use of simple medicines,* (London 1685), in *Works of Robert Boyle*

―― *The works of Robert Boyle,* ed. M. Hunter and E. B. Davis, London 1999–2000

Brenchley Rye, W., *England as seen by foreigners in the days of Elizabeth and James the First,* London 1865

Browne, B. C., 'Letter copied by G. E. Lloyd Baker, 24 August 1888 from the letter in his possession at Hardwicke Court, Gloucester', *EHR* v/17 (1890), 120–4

Browne, J., *A compleat treatise of the muscles,* London 1681, 1683

―― *Adenochoiradelogia, or, An atomic–chirurgical treatise of glandules and strumaes, or king's evil swellings,* London 1684

Browne, T., *The letters of Sir Thomas Browne,* ed. G. Keynes, London 1931

Burnet, G., *Some passages of the life and death of John, earl of Rochester who died the 26th of July, 1680,* London 1680

―― *Bishop Burnet's history of his own time: with notes by the earls of Dartmouth and Hardwicke, Speaker Onslow and Dean Swift: to which are added other annotations,* Cambridge 1833

―― *Supplement to the 'History of my own time',* ed. H. C. Foxcroft, Oxford 1902

Calcagnini, C., *Opera,* Basle 1544

Calendar of state papers, domestic series, of the reign of Charles I, 1625–49: preserved in the State Paper Department of Her Majesty's Public Record Office, London 1825–97

Calendar of state papers, domestic series, of the reign of Charles II: preserved in the State Paper Department of Her Majesty's Public Record Office, ed. M. A. Everett Green and others, London 1860–1939

Calendar of state papers, domestic series, of the reign of James I: preserved in the State Paper Department of Her Majesty's Public Record Office, ed. M. A. Everett Green, London 1857–9

Calendar of state papers and manuscripts, relating to English affairs, existing in the archives and collections of Venice: and in other libraries of northern Italy, ed. Rawden Brown, London 1864–1947

Calendar of treasury papers preserved in Her Majesty's Public Record Office, prepared by J. Redington, London 1868–97

Campana di Cavelli, E. R., *Les Derniers Stuarts à Saint-Germain en Laye: documents inédits et authentiques puisés aux archives publique et privées*, Paris 1871

Carr, R., *Epistolae medicinales variis occasionibus conscriptae*, London 1691

Carte, T., *A general history of England*, London, 1747–55

Cartwright, T., *The diary of Dr Thomas Cartwright, bishop of Chester: commencing at the time of his elevation to that see, August M.DC.LXXXVI; and terminating with the visitation of St Mary Magdalene College, Oxford, October M.DC. LXXXVII*, London 1843

Casserius G., *Tabulae anatomicae*, Venice 1627

Catalogue of the collection of playing cards bequeathed to the trustees of the British Museum by the late Lady Charlote Schreiber, comp. F. M. O'Donoghue, London 1901

Catalogue of printed broadsides in the possession of the Society of Antiquaries of London, comp. R. Lemon, London 1866

Cavendish, G., *Life of Wolsey*, London 1885

The ceremonies us'd in the time of King Henry VII for the healing of them that be diseas'd with the kings evil, London 1686

Certain sermons or homilies (1547); and, A homily against disobedience and wilful rebellion (1570): a critical edition, ed. R. B. Bond, Toronto 1987

Chamberlayne, E., *Anglia notitia, or, The present state of England*, London 1670

The character of a coffee-house with the symptomes of a town-wit, London 1673

A choice collection of wonderful miracles, ghosts, and visions, London 1681

The chronicle and political papers of King Edward VI, ed. W. K. Jordan, London 1966

Clifford Fielding, C. M., *Royalist father and Roundhead son, being the memoirs of the first and second earls of Denbigh, 1600–1675*, London 1915

Clowes, W., *A right fruitful and approved treatise for the artificial cure of that malady called in Latin struma*, London 1602

—— *Selected writings of William Clowes*, ed. F. N. L. Poynter, London 1948

Collier, J., *An ecclesiastical history of Great Britain*, London,1708–14

Collins, A., *A discourse of freethinking*, London 1713

The Conway letters: the correspondence of Anne, Viscountess Conway, Henry More, and their friends, 1642–84, ed. M. Hope Nicolson and S. Hutton, Oxford 1992

The correspondence of Nathan Walworth and Peter Seddon of Oxford, and other documents chiefly relating to the building of Ringley Chapel, ed. J. S. Fletcher Manchester 1880

The correspondence of Robert Boyle, ed. M. Hunter, A. Clericuzio and L. M. Principe, London 2001

'Count Lorenzo Magalotti's description of the ceremony of touching for the king's evil, 1669', in A. Browning (ed.), *English historical documents*, London 1953

[De Lamberty, G.], 'Mr T., L. B.', *Memoires de la derniére revolution d'Angleterre*, La Haye 1702

Defoe, D., *Reflections on the late, great revolution in England*, London 1689

—— *A supplement to the advice from the Scandal Club*, No. 3, (London 1704), in *Defoe's Review*, ed. A. W. Secord, New York 1938, i, facsimile bk III

—— *Jure divino*, London 1706

Documentary annals of the reformed Church of England: being a collection of injunc-

tions, declarations, orders, articles of enquiry &c from the year 1546 to the year 1716, ed. E. Cardwell, Oxford 1844

Documents illustrative of the history of the English Church, ed. H. Gee and W. J. Hardy, London 1896

Donne, J., *Donne's sermons, selected passages with an essay by Logan Pearsall Smith*, Oxford 1919

Douglas, D. C. (gen. ed.), *English historical documents*, VIII: *1660–1714*, ed. Andrew Browning, London 1953

Drake, F., *Eboracum, or, The history and antiquities of the city of York, from its original to the present time; together with the history of the cathedral church and the lives of the archbishops*, London 1736

Dunton, J., *The life and errors of John Dunton, citizen of London*, London 1705

Durant, T., *A treatise on the king's evil, setting forth a new theory on that disease; and a new method of curing indurated and ulcerated glands of the neck*, London 1762

Edes, R., *Great Britains resurrection, or, Englands complacencie in her soveraigne King Charles II*, London 1660

Eikon basilike, London 1649

English coronation records, ed. L. G. Wickham Legg, London 1901

Evelyn, J., *The diary of John Evelyn*, ed. E. S. De Beer, Oxford 1955

The Fairfax correspondence: memoirs of the reign of Charles I, ed. G. W. Johnson, London 1848

Fern, T., *A perfect cure for the king's evil, whether hereditary or accidental*, London 1709

Finet, J., *Finetti philoxenis: some choice observations of Sir John Finet Knight*, ed. J. Howell, London 1656

The Flemings in Oxford, ed. J. R. McGrath, Oxford 1904

Forsett, E., *A comparative discourse of the bodies natural and politique*, London 1606

Fuller, T., *The church history of Britain*, London 1655

Fuller, T., *The works of Henry Smith: including sermons, treatises, prayers and poems, with a life of the author*, Edinburgh 1867

Garrison, F. H., 'A relic of the king's evil in the Surgeon General's Library (Washington DC)', *Proceedings of the Royal Society of Medicine* vii (1914), 227–34

Gibbs, J., *Observations of various eminent cures of scrofulous distempers commonly called the king's evil*, London–Exeter 1712

Glanvill, J., *A blow at modern Sadducism*, London 1668

In God's name: examples of preaching in England from the Act of Supremacy to the Act of Uniformity, 1533–1622, ed. J. Chandos, London 1971

Goodall, C., *The Royal College of Physicians of London founded and established by law; as appears by letters patents, acts of parliament, adjudged cases, &c. And an historical account of the college's proceedings against empiricks and unlicensed practisers in every princes reign from their first incorporation to the murther of the royal martr, King Charles the First*, London 1684

Les Grandes Chroniques de France, ed. J. Viard, Paris 1920–53

Graunt, J., *Natural and political observations made upon the Bills of Mortality*, London 1663

Greatrakes, V., *A brief account of Mr Valentine Greatrakes and divers of the strange cures by him lately performed*, London 1666

Gwinne, M., *Aurum non aurum*, London 1611

Hall, J., *Select observations on English bodies*, London 1657

Hearne, T., *Reliquiae Hearnianae: the remains of Thomas Hearne*, ed. P. Bliss, Oxford 1857

Helgaud of Fleury, *Vie de Robert le Pieux*, ed. and trans. R. H. Bautier and G. Labory, Paris 1965

Herrick, R., 'To the king to cure the evil', in *Hesperides, or, The works both humane and divine of Robert Herrick Esq.*, London 1648

Heylyn, P., *Examen historicum, or, A discovery and examination of the mistakes, falsities and defects in some modern histories occasioned by the partiality and inadvertencies of their severall authours*, London 1659

Hippocratic writings, ed. G. E. R. Lloyd (1950), London 1983

His grace the duke of Monmouth honoured in his progress in the west of England in an account of a most extraordinary cure of the kings evil, London 1680

HMC, *Fourth report: the manuscripts of the of the right hon. the earl de la Warr at Knole Park, Co. Kent*, calendared by A. J. Horwood , London 1874

—— *Sixth report of the Royal Commission*, London 1877

—— *Seventh report: the manuscripts of Sir Harry Verney, Bart., at Claydon House, Co. Bucks*, calendared by A. J. Horwood, London 1879

—— *Report of the manuscripts at Wells Cathedral*, London 1885

—— *Twelfth report: the manuscripts of his grace the duke of Rutland K.G., preserved at Belvoir Castle*, London 1889

—— *Report on the manuscripts of Mrs. Frankland-Russell-Astley, of Chequers Court, Bucks*, London 1900

—— *Eighth report: manuscripts of the duke of Marlborough at Blenheim, County Oxford*, London 1907–9

—— *Calendar of manuscripts of the marquess of Bath at Longleat, Wilts.*, London 1908

—— *Report on the manuscripts of the most honourable the marquess of Downshire, preserved at Easthampstead Park, Berkshire*, London 1924–95

Hobbes, T., *Human nature*, London 1650

—— *Leviathan* (1651), ed. C. B. Macpherson, London 1958

Holinshed, R., *Chronicles of England, Scotlande, and Irelande*, London 1577

Howell, T. B., *A complete collection of state trials*, xi, London 1811

Howson, J., *A sermon preached at St. Maries Oxford the 17 day of November, 1602, in defence of the festivities of the Church of England and namely that of her Majesties coronation*, Oxford 1603

The humble petition of divers hundreds of the kings poore subjects, afflicted with that grievous infirmitie, called the kings evill, London 1643

Hume, D., *The history of England, from the invasion of Julius Cæsar to the abdication of James the Second, 1688*, London 1754–61

Hutchinson, L., *Memoirs of the life of Colonel Hutchinson*, ed. C. H. Firth, London 1885

Hyde, E., *The history of the rebellion and Civil Wars in England*, London 1702–4.

Illustrations of British history, biography and manners in the reigns of Henry VIII, Edward VI, Mary, Elizabeth and James I, ed. Edmund Lodge, London 1838

'Inquiries concerning Valentine Greatrakes', *Robert Boyles's 'heads' and 'inquiries'*, ed. M. Hunter (Robert Boyle Project occasional papers i, 2005)

The inventories of St George's Chapel, Windsor Castle, 1384–1667, ed. M. F. Bond, London 1947

The inventory of King Henry VIII: Society of Antiquaries MS 127 and British Library MS Harley 1419, ed. D. Starkey, London 1998

James VI, *The trew law of free monarchies*, Edinburgh 1598

James VI and I, *James VI and I: political writings*, ed. J. P. Sommerville, Cambridge 1994

Johnson, S., *Diaries, prayers and annals*, ed. E. L. McAdam, London 1958

Journal of the House of Commons, London 1830

Journal of the House of Lords, London 1802

A joyful message for al loyall subjects: sent from the kings majesties royall court at Causam, London 1647

Keble J. (ed.), *Reports in the Court of King's Bench from the XII to the XXX year of the reign of Charles II*, London 1685

Knox, J., *First blast of the trumpet against the monstrous regiment of women* (Geneva 1558), in *The works of John Knox*, ed. L. David (1895), New York 1966

Knox, R. and S. Leslie (eds), *The miracles of Henry VI*, London 1923

L'Estrange, H., *The alliance of divine offices*, London 1659

Laurentius, A. (A. Du Laurens), *De mirabili strumas sanadi vi solis Galliae regibus Christianissimus divinitus concessa*, Paris 1609

Letter from a gentleman at Rome to his friend in London, giving some very surprising cures in the kings evil, London 1721

Letter sent into France to the lord duke of Buckingham his grace: of a great miracle wrought by a piece of a handkerchefe, dipped in his majesties bloud, n.a., London 1649

Letters addressed from London to Sir Joseph Williamson while plenipotentiary at the Congress of Cologne in the Years 1673 and 1674, ed. W. D. Christie (Camden Society, 1874)

The letters and diplomatic instructions of Queen Anne, ed. B. Curtis Brown, London 1935

Letters and papers, foreign and domestic, of the reign of Henry VIII, ed. J. S. Brewer and others, London 1862–1932

Liber regie capelle: a manuscript in the Biblioteca Publica, Evora, ed. Walter Ullmann, London 1961

The Life of King Edward: who rests at Westminster, ed. and trans. F. Barlow, London 1962

Lives of Edward the Confessor, ed. H. R. Luard, London 1858

Lloyd, D., *Wonders no miracles or, Mr. Valentine Greatrates gift of healing examined upon occasion of a sad effect of his stroaking, March the 7, 1665, at one Mr. Cressets house in Charter-house-yard*, London 1666

Lodge, E. (ed.), *Illustrations of British history, biography and manners in the reigns of Henry VIII, Edward VI, Mary, Elizabeth and James I*, London 1838

The London diaries of William Nicolson, bishop of Carlisle, 1702–18, ed. C. Jones and G. Holmes, Oxford 1985

The loyal subjects hearty wishes to King Charles the Second, printed for John Andrews, London n.d.

Luttrell, N., *A brief historical relation of state affairs, from September 1678 to April 1714*, Farnborough 1969

Machiavelli, N., *The discourses* (1531), ed. B. Crick and B. Richardson, trans. L. J. Walker, London 2003

Magalotti, L., *Travels of Lorenzo the third, Grand Duke of Tuscany, through England, during the reign of King Charles II* (1669), London 1821

—— *Lorenzo Magalotti at the court of Charles II: his Relazione d' Inghliterra of 1668*, ed. and trans. W. E. Knowles Middleton, Waterloo, ONT 1980

—— *The Manner of his majesties curing the disease, called the king's evil*, London 1679

Manning, O. and W. Bray, *The history and antiquities of the county of Surrey*, London 1804–14

Maskell, W., *Monumenta ritualia ecclesiae Anglicanae*, Oxford 1882

Maxwell, J., *A poem shewing the excellencie of our soveraigne king James his hand*, in *The laudable life and deplorable death of … Prince Henry*, London 1612

Maynwaring, A., *The lives of two illustrious generals, John, duke of Marlborough and Francis Eugene, prince of Savoy*, London 1713

Melville, J., *The autobiography and diary of Mr James Melville, with a continuation of the diary*, ed. R. Pitcairn, Edinburgh 1842

Memoirs of the Verney family during the seventeenth century, ed. F. Verney and M. M. Verney, London 1907

Middlesex county records, ed. J. C. Jeafferson, London, 1886–92

A miracle of miracles: wrought by the blood of King Charles the First, of happy memory, upon a mayd at Detford foure miles from London, who by the violence of the disease called the kings evill was blinde one whole yeere, London 1649

Misson, H. de Valburg, *M. Misson's memoirs and observations in his travels over England*, trans. Mr Ozell, London 1719

Molins, W., *Muskotomia*, London 1648

Morhof, D. G., *Princeps medicus*, Rostock 1665

Morley, J., *An essay on the nature and cure of the king's evil*, London 1760

Morton, T., *A catholike appeale for Protestants*, London 1609

Nichols, J., *Literary anecdotes of the eighteenth century*, London 1812–16

—— *The progresses, processions and magnificent festivities of King James the First, his royal consort, family and court*, London 1828

Nicolas, N. H., *The privy purse expences of king Henry VIII: from November 1520, to December 1532*, London 1827

The obituary of Richard Smyth, secondary of the Poultry Compter London, ed. H. Ellis (Camden Society, 1849)

Occasional thoughts on the power of curing the king's-evil ascribed to the kings of England, London 1748

The office of consecrating cramp rings, used by the Catholick kings of England, London 1694

The offices or prayers to be used at the ceremony of touching for the king's evil, London 1618

Oldmixon, J., *A history of England during the reigns of King William and Queen Mary, Queen Anne and King George I*, London 1735

Palmer, R., *Catalogue of Western manuscripts in the Wellcome Library for the History & Understanding of Medicine: Western manuscripts 5120–6244*, London 1999

Parsons, G., *A little book of rare receipts for the cure of several distempers*, London 1710

Pegge, S., *Curialia miscellanea*, London 1818

Perrinchief, R., *A sermon preached before the honourable House of Commons at St Margaret's Westminster on 7 November*, London 1666

Pepys, S., *The diary of Samuel Pepys*, ed. R. Latham and W. Matthews, London 1970–83

Planché, J. R., *Regal records, or, A chronicle of the coronations of queens regnant of England*, London 1838

Postlethwayt, J., J. Graunt, W. Petty, C. Morris and W. Heberden, *A collection of the yearly Bills of Mortality, from 1657 to 1758 inclusive*, London 1759

Primrose, J., *Popular errors*, London 1651

Privy Council registers preserved in the Public Record Office, London 1967–8

Rawlin, T., *Admonitio pseudo-chymicis, seu, alphabetarium philosophicum*, London 1620

Redesdale, A. B. Freeman-Mitford, Lord, *Memories*, London 1915

Ridley, N., *The works of Nicholas Ridley*, ed. H. Christmas (1843), Cambridge 1988

Roberts, D., *Remarks on the king's evil or scrophula*, London 1791

Rouvroy, Louis de, duc de Saint-Simon, *Memoirs of duc de Saint-Simon, 1710–1715: the bastards triumphant*, ed. and trans. L. Norton, Warwick, NY 2007

St Louis' advice to his son, ed. and trans. D. Munro and G. Clarke Sellery, in *Medieval civilisation*, New York 1910, http://www.fordham.edu/halsall/source/stlouis1.html

Say, W., *Liber regie capelle* (1446), ed. W. Ullmann (Henry Bradshaw Society, 1961)

Scot, R., *The discoverie of witchcraft*, London 1584

A second letter to the lord duke of Buckingham his grace at the court of France, London 1649

Sermons or homilies appointed to be read in churches in the time of Queen Elizabeth, of famous memory, London 1817

Shakespeare, W., *The tragedy of Macbeth*, ed. N. Brooke, Oxford 1994

Shellinks, W., *The journal of William Schellinks' travels in England, 1661–1663*, ed. and trans. M. Exwood and H. L. Lehmann, London 1993

Slaughter, Thomas P. (ed.), *Ideology and politics on the eve of the Restoration: Newcastle's advice to Charles II*, Philadelphia 1984

[Sloane, H.], *Magic and mental disorder: Sir Hans Sloane's memoir of John Beaumont*, ed. M. Hunter (Robert Boyle Project, 2011)

Smith, H., *The works of Henry Smith*, ed. T. Fuller, Edinburgh 1867

'Some observations of the effects of touch and friction', *Philosophical Transactions* (1665–78), i. 206–9

Stapleton, 'A brief summary of the wardrobe accounts of the tenth, eleventh and fourteenth years of King Edward II', *Archaeologia* xxvi (1836), 318–45

Strickland, *The lives of the seven bishops committed to the Tower in 1688*, London 1866

Stuart Royal Proclamations, I: Royal proclamations of King James I, 1603–1625, ed. J. F. Larkin and P. L. Hughes, Oxford 1973

Stuart Royal Proclamations, II: Royal proclamations of King Charles I, 1625–1646, ed. J. F. Larkin and P. L. Hughes Oxford 1983

Stubbe, H., *The miraculous conformist, or, An account of severall marvallous cures performed by the stroaking of the hands of Mr Valentine Greatrakes*, Oxford 1666

A summary of occurrences relating to the miraculous preservation of our late sovereign lord, King Charles II, London 1688

Swift, J., 'Memoirs relating to that change which happened in the queen's ministry in the year 1710', in *The prose works of Jonathan Swift: historical and political tracts – English*, ed. T. Scott, London 1901

—— *Journal to Stella*, ed. H. Williams, Oxford 1948

T. A., ΧΕΙΡΕΞΟΚΗ: *the excellency or handy-work of the royal hand*, London 1665

Tailor, J., *Tailors travels from London to the Isle of Wight, with his returne, and occasion of his journey*, London 1648

Toland, J., *Amyntor, or. A defence of Milton's life*, London 1699

Tooker, W., *Charisma sive donum sanationis*, London 1597

A true and wonderful account of a cure of the kings-evil, by Mrs Fanshaw, sister to … the duke of Monmouth, London 1681

Tudor royal proclamations, ed. P. L. Hughes and J. F. Larkin, New Haven 1964–9

Turner, D., *De morbis cutaneis: a treatise of diseases incident to the skin*, London 1714

—— *The art of surgery*, London 1722

Vergil, P., *Anglia historia*, London 1555

—— *Polydore Vergil's English history*, ed. H. Ellis, London 1846

Verney letters of the eighteenth century from the MSS at Claydon House, ed. M. M. Verney, London 1930

Vickers, W., *A brief account of a specifick remedy for the curing of the king's evil*, London 1709

Voltaire, *The age of Louis XIV*, trans. M. P. Pollack, London 1926

Warton, T., *The life and literary remains of Ralph Bathurst*, Oxford 1761

Weldon, A., *The court and character of King James I*, London 1650

The Wentworth papers, 1705–1739: selected from the private and family correspondence of Thomas Wentworth, Lord Raby, created in 1711 earl of Strafford, ed. J. J. Cartwright, London 1883

Whiston, W., *Memoirs of the life and writings of Mr. William Whiston*, London 1753

White, T., *A treatise on struma or scrofula*, London 1784

Wicquefort, A. van, *A relation in form of a journal, of the voyage and residence which the most excellent and most mighty Prince Charles the II of Great Britain, &c. hath made in Holland, from the 25 of May, to the 2 of June, 1660*, trans. W. Lower, The Hague, 1660

Wilmot, J., *The letters of John Wilmot, earl of Rochester*, ed. Jeremy Treglow, Oxford 1980

—— *The complete works*, ed. F. H. Ellis, London 1994

Wilson, A., *The history of Great Britain, being the life and reign of King James the First*, London 1653

Wiseman, R., *Several chirurgical treatises*, London 1676

—— 'Treatise IV: Of the king's evil', in Wiseman, *Several chirurgical treatises*, 245–312.

Wood, A. *Athenae Oxonienses*, ed. Philip Bliss, London 1813–20

—— *The life and times of Anthony à Wood, antiquary, of Oxford, 1632–1695*, ed. A. Clark, Oxford 1891

Wordsworth, C. (ed.), *The manner of the coronation of King Charles the First* (Henry Bradshaw Society, 1892)

Yonge, J., *Medicaster medicatus, or, A remedy for the itch of scribbling*, London 1685

Secondary sources

Adamson, J., 'The making of the *ancién regime court*, 1500–1700', in Adamson, *The princely courts of Europe*, 7–41

—— 'The Tudor and Stuart courts, 1509–1714', in Adamson, *The princely courts of Europe*, 95–117

—— (ed.), *The princely courts of Europe, 1500–1700* (1999), London 2000

Alford, S., *Kingship and politics in the reign of Edward VI*, Cambridge 2002

Allen, D., 'An admission ticket to the ceremony of touching?', *Numismatic Chronicle* 5th ser. xviii (1938), 292–4

Andrews, W., *The doctor in history, literature, folklore etc*, Hull–London 1896

Anglo, S., *Images of Tudor kingship*, London 1992

Anon., 'The royal cure for the king's evil', *British Medical Journal* ii (1899), 1234–5

Archibald, M., 'Coins and medals', in McGregor, *Sir Hans Sloane*, 150–66

Arnold, F. H., 'Sussex certificates for the royal touch', *Sussex Archaeological Collections* xxv (1873), 204–12

Arnold, J. H., *What is medieval history?*, Cambridge 2008

Asch, R. G., *Sacral kingship between disenchantment and re-enchantment: the French and English monarchies, 1587–1688*, New York–Oxford 2014

Aston, M., *England's iconoclasts*, I: *Laws against images*, Oxford 1988

Aylmer, G. E., *Rebellion or Revolution? England, 1640–1660*, Oxford 1986

Backhouse, J., 'Queen Mary's manual for blessing cramp rings and touching for the evil: the rituals of the royal healing ceremonies, written and illuminated for Mary I (1553–58)', in J. Browne and T. Dean, *Westminster Cathedral: building of faith*, London 1995, 200–2

Backscheider, P., *Daniel Defoe: his life*, London 1989

—— 'Defoe, Daniel (1660?–1731)', *ODNB*

Baine, R. M., *Daniel Defoe and the supernatural*, Athens, GA 1969

Bak, J. M. (ed.), *Coronations: medieval and early modern monarchic ritual*, Berkeley 1990

Baker, P., 'Rhetoric, reality and the varieties of Civil War radicalism', in J. Adamson (ed.), *The English Civil War: conflict and contexts, 1640–1649*, Basingstoke 2009

Baldwin, D., *The Chapel Royal, ancient and modern*, London 1990

Barlow, F., *Edward the Confessor*, New Haven 1970

—— 'The king's evil', *EHR* xcv (1980), 3–27

—— *The Norman Conquest and beyond*, London 1983

Barry, J., 'The Society for the Reformation of Manners, 1700–5', in J. Barry and K. Morgan (eds), *Reformation and revival in eighteenth-century Bristol*, Stroud 1994, 1–62

Bayne, C. G., 'The coronation of Queen Elizabeth', *EHR*, xxii (1907), 650–73

Benedict, J., 'Rosewell, Thomas (1630–92)', *ODNB*

Bernard, G., 'The Church of England, 1529–1640', *History* lxxv (1990), 183–206

Berry, H., *Gender, society and print culture in late-Stuart England*, Aldershot 2003

—— 'Dunton, John (1659–1732)', *ODNB*

Bertelli, S., *The king's body: sacred rituals of power in mediaeval and early modern Europe*, trans. R. Burr Litchfield, University Park, PA 2001

Bickersteth, J. and R. W. Dunning, *Clerks of the Closet in the royal household*, Stroud 1991

Blaen, T., *Medicinal jewels, magical gems: precious stones in early modern Britain*, Crediton 2012

Blanning, T. C. W., *The culture of power and the power of culture: old regime Europe, 1660–1789*, Oxford 2002

Bloch, M., *L'Ile de France*, Paris 1913, trans. as *The Ile de France*, London 1971

—— *Les Rois thaumaturges: étude sur le caractère surnaturel attribué a la puissance royale particulièrement en France et en Angleterre*, Strasburg–Paris 1924, trans. by J. E. Anderson as *The royal touch: sacred monarchy and scrofula in England and France*, London 1973; trans. into Italian as *Il re taumaturghi*, Turin, 1973

—— *La Société féodale*, Paris 1939, 1940, trans. L. A. Manyon as *Feudal society*, London 1961

—— *The historian's craft*, trans. Peter Putnam (1954), Manchester 1992

Bolvig, A. and P. Lindles (eds), *History and images: towards a new iconography*, Turnhout 2003

Bonner, C., 'Magical amulets', *Harvard Theological Review* xxxix/1 (1946), 25–54

Bossy, J. 'The mass as a social institution, 1200–1700', *P&P* c (Aug. 1983), 29–61

—— *Christianity in the West, 1400–1700*, Oxford 1985

Bostridge, I., *Witchcraft and its transformations,1650 to 1750*, Oxford 1997

Bowie, F., *The anthropology of religion: an introduction*, Oxford 2006

Bramwell, B., *Atlas of clinical medicine*, Edinburgh 1892–6

Braudel, F., *La Mediterranee et le monde mediterraneen, a l'epoque de Philippe II*, Paris 1949, trans. by S. Reynolds as *The Mediterranean and the Mediterranean world in the age of Philip II*, London 1972–3

—— 'Bloch, Marc', in David. L. Sills (ed.), *The international encyclopaedia of the social sciences*, ii, New York 1968, 92–5

Breathnach, C. S., 'Robert Boyle's approach to the ministrations of Valentine Greatrakes', *History of Psychiatry* x (1999), 87–109

Briggs, A. and P. Burke, *A social history of the media, from Gutenberg to the internet*, Cambridge 2005

Broad, J., 'Denton, William (*bap.* 1605, *d.* 1691)', ODNB

Brockliss, L. and C. Jones, *The medical world of early modern France*, Oxford 1997

Brogan, S., 'The royal touch', *History Today* lxi (Feb. 2011), 46–52.

Brooke, J. and I. Maclean (eds), *Heterodoxy in early modern science and religion*, Oxford 2005

Brown, T. M., 'The College of Physicians and the acceptance of iatromechanism in England, 1665–1695', *Bulletin of the History of Medicine* xliv/1 (1970), 12–30

—— 'Medicine in the shadow of *Principia*', *Journal of the History of Ideas* xlviii/4 (1987), 629–48

Buc, P., 'David's adultery with Bathsheba and the healing power of Capetian kings', *Viator* xxiv (1993), 101–20

Bucholz, R. O., '"Nothing but ceremony": Queen Anne and the limitations of royal ritual', *JBS* xxx/3 (1991), 288–323

—— *The Augustan court: Queen Anne and the decline of court culture*, Stanford, CA 1993

Bull, M. (ed.), *France in the central Middle Ages*, Oxford 2002

Burgess, G., *Absolute monarchy and the Stuart constitution*, London–New Haven 1996

Burguière, A., *The Annales School*, trans. J. M. Todd, Ithaca–London 2009

Burke, P., *Popular culture in early modern Europe*, London 1978

—— 'Sacred rulers, royal priests: rituals of the early modern popes', 'Rituals of healing in early modern Italy', and 'The repudiation of ritual in early modern Europe', in P. Burke, *The historical anthropology of early modern Italy*, Cambridge 1987, 168–82, 223–38

—— *The French historical revolution: the Annales School, 1929–1989*, Cambridge 1990

—— *The fabrication of Louis XIV*, New Haven 1992

—— and A. Briggs, *A social history of the media, from Gutenberg to the internet*, Cambridge 2005

Burns, J. H. and M. Goldie (eds), *The Cambridge history of political thought, 1450–1700*, Cambridge 1991

Burrow, J. A., *Gestures and looks in medieval narrative*, Cambridge 2002

Burt, S., 'The Societies for the Reformation of Manners: between John Locke and the Devil in Augustan England', in R. D. Lund (ed.), *The margins of orthodoxy: heterodox writing and cultural response, 1660–1750*, Cambridge 1995, 149–69

Butler, J., *Gender trouble*, London 1990

Butler, M., 'The invention of Britain and the early Stuart masque', in M. Smuts (ed.), *The Stuart court and Europe: essays in politics and political culture*, Cambridge 1996, 65–85

Cain, T., 'Herrick, Robert (*bap.* 1591, *d.* 1674)', ODNB

Carlton, C., *Charles I, the personal monarch*, London 1983

—— *Archbishop William Laud*, London 1987

Carpenter, D., 'The meetings of kings Henry III and Louis IX', in M. Prestwich, R. Britnell and R. Frame (eds), *Thirteenth Century England, X: Proceedings of the Durham Conference 2003*, Woodbridge 2005, 1–30

—— 'King Henry III and Saint Edward the Confessor: the origin of the cult', *EHR* cxxii (2007), 865–91

Challis, C. E., *The Tudor coinage*, Manchester 1978

Chambers, R., *History of the rebellion in Scotland in 1745, 1746*, Edinburgh 1827

Champion, J., *The pillars of priestcraft shaken: the Church of England and its enemies, 1660–1730*, Cambridge 1992

Cheney, C. R. and M. Jones (eds), *A handbook of dates: for students of British history*, Cambridge 2000

Cherry, J., 'Healing through faith: the continuation of medieval attitudes to jewellery into the Renaissance', *Renaissance Studies* xv/2 (2001), 154–71

Chrimes, S. B., *Henry VII*, London 1972

Clark, J. C. D., *English Society, 1668–1832: ideology, social structure and political practice during the ancient regime*, Cambridge 1985

Clark, K., *Daniel Defoe: the whole frame of nature, time and providence*, Basingstoke 2007

Clark, O. W., 'Charming for the king's evil', *Folk-Lore* vi/2 (1895), 205

Clark, S., 'King James' *Daemonologie*: witchcraft and kingship' in S. Anglo (ed.), *The damned art: essays in the literature of witchcraft*, London 1977, 156–81

—— 'Inversion, misrule and the meaning of witchcraft', *P&P* lxxxvii (May 1980), 98–127

—— *Thinking with demons*, Oxford 1997

Claydon, T., *William III and the godly revolution*, Cambridge 1996

—— *William III*, Harlow 2002

—— 'William III and II (1650–1702)', *ODNB*

Clegg, C. S., 'Holinshed, Raphael (*c.* 1525–1580?)', *ODNB*

Coiro, A. B., 'Herrick's *Hesperides*: the name and the frame', *English Literary History* lii/2 (1985), 311–36

—— *Robert Herrick's Hesperides and the emblematic book tradition*, Baltimore 1988

Colbert-Rhodes, R., 'Emile Durkheim and the historical thought of Marc Bloch', *Theory and Society* v/1 (1978), 45–73

Collins, S. L., *From divine cosmos to sovereign state: an intellectual history of consciousness and the idea of order in Renaissance England*, Oxford 1989

Cook, H. J., 'Living in revolutionary times: medical change under William and Mary', in Bruce T. Moran (ed.), *Patronage and institutions: science, technology and medicine at the European court, 1500–1750*, Rochester, NY 1991, 111–35

—— 'Good advice and little medicine: the professional authority of early modern English physicians', *JBS* xxxiii (1994), 1–31

Cooper, T., rev. S. Bakewell, 'Butler, William (1535–1618)', *ODNB*.

Copeman, W. S. C., *Doctors and disease in Tudor times*, London 1960

Corns, T. N., 'Evans, Arise [Rhys, Rice] (*b. c.*1607, *d.* in or after 1660)', *ODNB*

Corp, E., *A court in exile: the Stuarts in France, 1689–1718*, Cambridge 2004

—— *The Stuarts in Italy: a royal court in permanent exile*, Cambridge 2011

Coward, B., *The Stuart age*, London 1994

Cox, J. C., *The parish registers of England*, London 1910

Craig, J., *The Mint: a history of the London Mint from A.D. 287 to 1948*, Cambridge 1948

Crawfurd, R., *The king's evil*, Oxford 1911

—— 'The blessing of cramp-rings: a chapter in the history of the treatment of epilepsy', in C. Singer (ed.), *Studies in the History and Method of Science*, i, Oxford 1917, 165–87

Cruikshanks, E., *The Glorious Revolution*, Basingstoke 2000

Curtis, T. C. and W. A. Speck, 'The societies for the Reformation of Manners: a case study in the theory and practice of moral reform', *Literature & History* iii (1976), 45–64

Cutten, G. B., *Three thousand years of mental healing*, London 1911

Davies, J., *The Caroline captivity of the Church: Charles I and the re-moulding of Anglicanism, 1625–41*, Oxford 1992

Davidson, L., T. Hitchcock, T. Keirn and R. Shoemake (eds), *Stilling the grumbling hive*, Stroud 1992

Davis, E., 'The Psalms in Hebrew medical amulets', *Vetus Testamentum* xlii (1992), 173–8

Davis, N. Z., 'Women on top', in N. Z. Davis, *Society and culture in early modern France*, Stanford, CA 1975, 124–51

—— 'The sacred and the body social in sixteenth-century Lyon', *P&P* xc (Feb. 1981), 40–70

Day, W. G. (ed.), *Catalogue of the Pepys Library at Magdalene College, Cambridge: the Pepys ballads*, Cambridge 1987

De Krey, G., *Restoration and revolution in Britain*, Basingstoke 2007

Dear, P., 'Miracles, experiments and the ordinary course of nature', *Isis* lxxxi/4 (1990), 663–83

Delumeau, J., *Le Péché et La peur*, Paris 1983, trans. E. Nicholson as *Sin and fear: the emergence of a Western guilt culture, 13th–18th centuries*, New York 1990

Doran, J., *London in the Jacobite times*, London 1877

Doran, S. and C. Durston, *Princes, pastors and people: the Church and religion in England, 1529–1689*, London 1991

Douglas, M., *Purity and danger: an analysis of the concepts of pollution and taboo*, London 1966

—— *Evans-Pritchard*, Glasgow 1980

Dow, F. D., *Radicalism in the English Revolution*, Oxford 1985

Drummond, J. C., *The Englishman's diet*, London 1940

Duffy, E., 'Valentine Greatrakes, the Irish stroker: miracle, science and orthodoxy in Restoration England', in K. Robbins (ed.), *Religion and humanism* (Studies in Church History xvii, 1981), 251–73

—— *The stripping of the altars: traditional religion in England, 1400–1580*, London 1992

Eccleshall, R., *Order and reason in politics: theories of absolute and limited monarchy in early modern England*, Oxford 1978

Eisenstein, E., *The printing press as an agent of change: communication and cultural transformations in early modern Europe*, Cambridge 1979

—— *The printing revolution in early modern Europe*, Cambridge 1983

Ellenzweig, S., *The fringes of belief: English literature, ancient heresy, and the politics of freethinking, 1660–1760*, Stanford, CA 2008

Elmer, P., *The miraculous conformist: Valentine Greatrakes, the body politic, and the politics of healing in Restoration Britain*, Oxford 2013

Engell, I., *Studies in divine kingship in the ancient Near East*, Oxford 1967

Ettlinger, E., 'Documents of British superstition in Oxford', *Folklore* liv/1 (1943), 227–49

Evans, J., *Magical jewels of the Middle Ages and Renaissance, particularly in England*, Oxford 1922

Evans-Pritchard, E. E., *Theories of primitive religion*, Oxford 1965

Farquhar, H., 'Royal charities, I: Angels as healing-pieces for the king's evil', *BNJ* xii (1916), 39–135

—— 'Royal charities, II: Touchpieces for the king's evil', *BNJ* xiii (1917), 95–163

—— 'Royal charities, III: Continuation of touchpieces for the king's evil: James II to William III', *BNJ* xiv (1918), 88–120

—— 'Royal charities, IV: Conclusion of touchpieces for the king's evil: Anne and the Stuart princes', *BNJ* xv (1919), 141–84

Febvre, L., *Le Problèm de l'incroyance au XVIe siècle: la religion de Rabelais* (1942), trans. by B. Gottheb of *The problem of unbelief in the sixteenth century: the religion of Rabelais*, Cambridge, MA 1982

Fincham, K. (ed.), *The early Stuart Church*, Basingstoke 1993

Figgis, J. N., *The divine right of kings* (1896), Gloucester, MA 1970

Finaly, R., *Parish registers: an introduction*, Norwich 1981

Fink, C., *Marc Bloch: a life in history*, Cambridge 1989

Finley-Crosswhite, A., 'Henri IV and the diseased body politic', in M. Gosman,

A. MacDonald and A. Vanderjagt (eds), *Princes and princely culture, 1450–1650*, Leiden 2003), i. 131–46

Fitzpatrick, B. L., 'Rivington family (per. *c*.1710–*c*.1960)', *ODNB*

Foister, S., *Holbein in England*, London 2006

Forbes, T. R., *Chronicle from Aldgate: life and death in Shakespeare's London*, New Haven 1971

Force, J. E., *William Whiston: honest Newtonian*, Cambridge 1985

Fowler, A., *Robert Herrick*, London 1982

Fox, A., *Oral and literate culture in England*, Oxford 2000

—— and D. Wolf (eds), *The spoken word: oral culture in England, 1500–1850*, Manchester 2002

Frank, R. G., Jr, *Harvey and the Oxford physiologists: scientific ideas and social interaction*, Los Angeles 1980

Frazer, J. G., *The golden bough: a study in magic and religion* (1922), abridged edn, London 1929

French, R. K., 'Scrofula', in K. F. Kiple, *Cambridge historical dictionary of disease*, Cambridge 1993, 292–4

Friedman, S., *Marc Bloch, sociology and geography: encountering changing disciplines*, Cambridge 1996

Fulcer, A. B., 'Charming for the king's evil', *Folk-Lore* vii/3 (1896), 295

Furdell, E. L., *The royal doctors, 1485–1714: medical personnel at the Tudor and Stuart courts*, New York 2001

—— 'Profit or principle? Religion, publishing, and medicine', in Furdell, *Publishing and medicine*, 74–92

—— *Publishing and medicine in early modern England*, New York 2002

—— 'Boorde, Andrew (*c*.1490–1549)', *ODNB*

Gadd, I., 'Newcomb, Thomas, the elder (1625x7–81)', *ODNB*

Garnier, F., *Le Langage de l'image au moyen âge*, Paris 1982–9

Gascoigne, J., ' "The wisdom of the Egyptians" and the secularisation of history in the age of Newton', in S. Gaukroger (ed.), *The uses of antiquity*, Boston 1991, 171–212

Gaskill, M., *Crime and mentalities in early modern England*, Cambridge 2000

Geertz, C., 'Centres, kings and charisma: symbolics of power', in C. Geertz, *Local knowledge: further essays in interpretative anthropology*, New York 1983, 121–46

Geertz, H., 'An anthropology of religion and magic, I', *Journal of Interdisciplinary History* vi (1975), 71–89

Gettings, F., *Dictionary of occult, hermetic and alchemical sigils*, London 1981

Giacomini, M. P., *Sir Richard Blackmore and the Bible*, Lanham, MD 2007

Giuseppi, M. S., *Guide to the contents of the Public Record Office*, London 1963–8

Globe, A., *Peter Stent, London printseller, circa 1642–1665: being a catalogue raisonné of his engraved prints and books with an historical and bibliographical introduction*, Vancouver 1985

Gluckman, L. K., 'The royal touch and the Maori equivalent', *Adler Museum of the History of Medicine* vi/1 (1980), 6–10

Goldie, M., 'The Hilton Gang: terrorising dissent in 1680s London', *History Today* xlvii (Oct.1997), 26–32

—— 'Restoration political thought', in Lionel K. J. Glassey (ed.), *The reigns of Charles II and James VII and II*, London 1997, 12–35

Goldsmith, M. M., 'Public virtue and private vices', *Eighteenth-Century Studies* ix (1976), 477–510

Grafton, A., *Cardano's cosmos: the worlds and works of a Renaissance astrologer*, London 1999

Green, E., 'On the cure by touch, with some notes on some cases in Somerset', *Proceedings of the Bath Natural History and Antiquarian Field Club* v (1883), 74–98

Greenblatt, S., 'Shakespeare and the exorcists', in S. Greenblatt, *Shakespeareann negotiations*, Los Angeles 1988, 94–128

Greene, T. M., 'Magic and festivity at the Renaissance court: the 1987 Josephine Waters Bennett Lecture', *Renaissance Quarterly* xl (1987), 636–59

Greenleaf, W. H., *Order, empiricism and politics: two traditions of English political thought, 1500–1700*, Oxford 1964

Gregg, E., 'Was Queen Anne a Jacobite?', *History* lvii/191(1972), 358–75

—— *Queen Anne*, New Haven 2014

Gregori, F., 'Blackmore, Sir Richard (1654–1729)'

Grell, P. O. and A. Cunningham (eds), *Religio medici: medicine and religion in seventeenth-century England*, Aldershot 1996

—— *Medicine and religion in Enlightenment Europe*, Aldershot 2007

Griffiths, A., *The print in Stuart Britain*, London 1998

Grzybowski, S. and E. A. Allen, 'The history and importance of scrofula', *The Lancet*, 2 Dec 1995, 1472–4

Guerrini, A., 'Isaac Newton, George Cheyne and the "Principia Medicinae"', in R. French and A. Wear (eds), *The medical revolution of the 17th century*, Cambridge 1989, 222–45

—— 'Newtonianism, medicine and religion', in Grell and Cunningham, *Religio medici*, 293–312

Gunn, S. J., 'Henry VII (1457–1509)', *ODNB*

Gunther, R. T., *Early science in Oxford*, I: *Chemistry, Mathematics, Physics and surveying*, Oxford 1923

Gusmer, C. W., *The ministry of healing in the Church of England: an ecumenical liturgical study*, Great Watering 1974

Guthrie, N., 'Johnson's touch-piece and the "charge of fame": personal and public aspects of the medal in eighteenth-century Britain', in J. C. D. Clark and H. Erskine-Hill (eds), *The politics of Samuel Johnson*, London 2012, 90–111.

Hageman, E. H., *Robert Herrick: a reference guide*, Boston 1983

Haigh, C., *The reign of Elizabeth I*, London 1984

—— *The English Reformation revised*, Cambridge 1987

—— *English Reformations: religion, politics and society under the Tudors*, Oxford 1993

—— 'The taming of the Reformation: preachers, pastors and parishioners in Elizabethan and early Stuart England', *History* lxxxv (2000), 572–88

Halket, S. and J. Laing, J., *Dictionary of anonymous and pseudonymous English literature*, Edinburgh 1926–62

Hall, J., *Illustrated dictionary of symbols in eastern and western art*, London 1994

Hallam, E. M., 'Royal burial and the cult of kingship in France and England, 1060–1330', *Journal of Medieval History* viii (1982), 359–80

—— and J. Everard, *Capetian France, 987–1328*, London 2001

Handley, S., 'Carte, Thomas (*bap.* 1686, *d.* 1754)', *ODNB*

Harding, V., 'The population of London, 1550–1700: a review of the published evidence', *London Journal* xv (1990). 111–28

Harley, D., 'Spiritual physic, providence and English medicine, 1560–1640', in O. P. Grell and A. Cunningham (eds), *Medicine and the Reformation*, London 1993, 101–17

Harman, P. M., *The culture of nature in Britain*, New Haven–London 2009

Harris, J., S. Orgel and R. Strong (eds), *The king's Arcadia: Inigo Jones and the Stuart masque*, London 1973

Harris, T., *London crowds in the reign of Charles II*, Cambridge 1987

—— (ed.), *Popular culture in England, c.1500–1850*. London 1995

Haton, R., *George I: elector and king*, London 1978

Hearn, K., 'Merchant clients for the painter Jan Siberechts', in M. Galinou (ed.), *City merchants and the arts, 1670–1720*, Wetherby 2004, 83–92

Hedeman, A. D., *The royal image: illustrations of the Grandes Chroniques de France, 1274–1422*, Berkeley 1991

Heiman, P. M., '"Nature is a perpetual worker": Newton's aether and 18th-century natural philosophy', *Ambix* xx (1973), 1–25

Hembry, P., *The English spa, 1560–1815: a social history*, London 1990

Henry, J., *The scientific revolution and the origins of modern science*, Basingstoke 2008

Hill, C., *The world turned upside down*, London 1972

Hollaender, E., *Wunder, Wundergerbert und Wundergestalt in Einblattdrucken des fünfzehnten bis achtzehnten Jahr hunderts*, Stuttgart 1921

Holmes, G. S., *Augustan England: professions, state and society, 1680–1730*, London 1982

—— *British politics in the age of Anne*, London 1987

Hopper, S., *To be a pilgrim: the medieval pilgrimage experience*, Stroud 2002

Hoppit, J., *A land of liberty? England, 1689–1727*, Oxford 2000

Horrox, R. and W. M. Ormond (eds), *A social history of England, 1200–1500*, Cambridge 2006

Hudson, W., *The English deists:studies in early Enlightenment*, London 2009

Hunt, A., *The drama of coronation*, Cambridge 2008

Hunter, M., *John Aubrey and the realm of learning*, New York 1975

—— *Science and Society in Restoration England*, Cambridge 1981

—— 'The problem of "atheism" in early modern England', *Transactions of the Royal Historical Society* 5th ser. xxxv (1985), 135–57

—— *Establishing the new science: the experience of the early Royal Society*, Woodbridge 1989

—— 'Science and the English public', in M. Hamilton-Phillips and R. P. Maccubbin (eds), *The age of William III and Mary II: power, politics and patronage, 1688–1702*, Williamsburg 1989, 165–70

—— *The Royal Society and its Fellows, 1660–1700*, 2nd edn, Oxford 1994

—— *Science and the shape of orthodoxy: intellectual change in late seventeenth-century Britain*, Woodbridge 1995

—— 'The witchcraft controversy and the nature of free thought in Restoration England: John Wagstaffe's *The question of witchcraft debated* (1669)', in Hunter, *Science and the shape of orthodoxy*, 286–307

—— *The occult laboratory: magic, science and second sight in late seventeenth-century Scotland*, Woodbridge 2001

—— *Editing early modern texts: an introduction to principles and practice*, London 2008

—— *Boyle: between God and science*, New Haven 2009

—— 'Boyle et la surnaturel', in Myriam Dennehy and Charles Ramond (eds), *La Philosophie naturelle de Robert Boyle*, Paris 2009, 213–36

—— 'Scientific change: its setting and stimuli', in B. Coward (ed.), *A companion to Stuart Britain* (2003), Chichester 2009, 214–29

—— 'The Royal Society and the decline of magic', *Notes and Records of the Royal Society* lxv (Jan. 2011), 103–19

—— (ed.), *Printed images in early modern Britain: essays in interpretation*, Farnham 2010

—— and D. Wootton (eds), *Atheism from the Reformation to the Enlightenment*, Oxford 1992

Hunter, R. A. and I. Macalpine, 'John Bird on "Reckets" (London, 1661)', *Journal of the History of Medicine* xiii/3 (1958), 397–403

Huppert, G., 'The Annales School before the *Annales*', *Review* i (1978), 215–19

Hussey, E. L. *On the epidemic small-pox in Oxford in 1854–5*, London 1860

—— 'On the cure of scrofulous diseases attributed to the royal touch', *Archaeological Journal* x (1883), 187–211

Hutton, R., *Charles II: king of England, Scotland and Ireland*, Oxford 1989

—— *The rise and fall of Merry England: the ritual year, 1400–1700*, Oxford 1994

Jackson, R. A., *Vive le roi! A history of the French coronation from Charles V to Charles X*, Chapel Hill 1984

Jacob, E. F., 'Review of Marc Bloch's *Les Rois thaumaturges*', *EHR* xl (1925), 267–70

Jacob, J. R., *Robert Boyle and the English Revolution: a study in social and intellectual change*, New York 1977

Jenner, M., 'The roasting of the rump: scatology and the body politic in Restoration England: a reply', *P&P* cxcvi (Aug. 2007), 273–86

Johnson, R., *Saint Michael the archangel in medieval English legend*, Woodbridge 2005

Johnstone, H., 'Poor-relief in the royal households of thirteenth-century England', *Speculum* iv/2 (1929), 149–67

Jones, M., *The print in early modern England*, London 2010

Jordan, W. C., *Louis IX and the challenge of the crusade: a study in rulership*, Princeton 1979

Jordan, W. K., *Edward VI: the young king: the protectorship of the duke of Somerset*, London 1968

—— *Edward VI: the threshold of power: the dominance of the duke of Northumberland*, London 1970

Kalman Gluckman, L., *The royal touch in England: a theory of origin derived from observations in the New Zealand Maori*, Wellington, NZ 1971

Kantorowicz, E. H., *The king's two bodies: a study in mediaeval political theology*, Princeton 1957

Kaplan, B. B., 'Greatrakes the Stroker: the interpretation of his contemporaries', *Isis* lxxii/2 (1982), 178–85

Kassell, L., 'The economy of magic in early modern England', in M. Pelling and S. Mandelbrote (eds), *The practice of reform in health, medicine and science, 1500–2000: essays for Charles Webster*, Aldershot 2005, 43–57

Keay, A., *The magnificent monarch: Charles II and the ceremonies of power*, London 2008

Keeble, N. H., *The literary culture of Nonconformity*, Leicester 1987

—— *The Restoration: England in the 1660s*, Oxford 2002

Kenyon, J. P., *Revolution principles: the politics of party, 1689–1720*, Cambridge 1977

Kenyon, R. L., *The gold coins of England*, London 1884

Keynes, G., *The life of William Harvey*, Oxford 1966

King, E., *Medieval England, 1066–1485*, Oxford 1988

Kiple, K. F., 'Scrofula: the king's evil and struma Africana', in K. F. Kiple (ed.), *Plague, pox and pestilence in London*, London 1997, 44–9

Kisby, F., '"When the king goeth a procession": chapel ceremonies and services, the ritual year, and religious reforms at the early Tudor court, 1485–1547', *JBS* xl (2001), 44–75

Kishlansky, M., 'Charles I: a case of mistaken identity', *P&P* clxxxix (Nov. 2005), 41–80

Klaniczay, G., The *uses of supernatural power: the transformation of popular religion in medieval and early modern Europe*, Cambridge 1990

Klein, L., 'Coffeehouse civility, 1660–1714: an aspect of post-courtly culture in England', *Huntingdon Library Quarterly* lix (1997), 30–51

Knighton, C. S. and R. Mortimer (eds), *Westminster Abbey reformed, 1540–1640*, Aldershot 2003

Koldeweij, A. M., 'Lifting the veil on pilgrim badges', in J. Stopford (ed.), *Pilgrimage explored*, York 1999, 161–88

Koziol, G., *Begging pardon and favour: ritual and political order in early medieval France*, Ithaca 1992

—— 'England, France, and the problem of sacrality in twelfth-century ritual', in T. N. Bisson (ed.), *Cultures of power: lordship, status and process in twelfth-century Europe*, Philadelphia 1995, 124–48

Kunz, G. F., *Rings for the finger*, London 1917

Lacey, A., *The cult of King Charles the martyr*, Woodbridge 2003.

Lake, P., 'Calvinism and the English Church', *P&P* cxiv (Feb. 1987), 32–76

Landouzy, L., *Le Toucher des ecrouelles: l'Hôpital Saint-Marcoul: la mal du roi*, Paris 1907

Larner, C., 'James VI and I and witchcraft', in Alan G. R. Smith (ed.),*The reign of James VI and I*, London 1973, 74–90

Lee, M., Jr, *Great Britain's Solomon: James VI and I in his three kingdoms* Urbana, IL 1990

Lee, S., 'Becket, William (1684–1738)', rev. Michael Bevan, *ODNB*

Lévi-Bruhl, L., *La Mentalité primitive*, Paris 1922, trans. L. A. Clare as *Primitive mentality*, London 1923

Levin, C., '"Would I could give you help and succour": Elizabeth I and the politics of touch', *Albion* xxi/2 (1989), 191–205

—— *'The heart and stomach of a king': Elizabeth I and the politics of sex and power*, Philadelphia 1994

Levine, P., *The amateur and the professional: antiquarians, historians and archaeologists in Victorian England, 1838–1886* , Cambridge 1986

Levy Peck, L. (ed.), *The mental world of the Jacobean court*, Cambridge 1991

Lister, J., 'The royal touch', *New England Journal of Medicine* (1953), 197–8

Loach, J., *Edward VI*, ed. G. Bernard and P. Williams, New Haven 1999

Loschky, D. J., 'The usefulness of England's parish registers', *Review of Economics and Statistics* xlix/4 (1967), 471–9

Love, H., 'Sedley, Sir Charles, fifth baronet (*bap*. 1639, *d*. 1701)', *ODNB*

Lovejoy, A. J., *The great chain of being: a study of the history of an idea*, New York 1960

Löwe, J. A., 'Tooker, William (1553/4–1621)', *ODNB*

Lyle, I., 'Bernard, Charles (*bap*. 1652, *d*. 1710)', *ODNB*

—— 'Browne, John (1642–1702/3)', *ODNB*

Lyon, B., 'Marc Bloch: historian', *French Historical Studies* xv/2 (1987), 195–207

Macaulay, T. B., *The history of England from the accession of James II* (1848–55), London 1898

MacCulloch, D., *Thomas Cranmer: a life*, New Haven 1996

—— *Tudor Church militant: Edward VI and the Protestant Reformation*, London 1999

—— *Reformation: Europe's house divided*, London 2004

McCullough, P. C., *Sermons at court: politics and religion in Elizabethan and Jacobean preaching*, Cambridge 1998

MacDonald, M., *Witchcraft and hysteria in Elizabethan London: Edward Jorden and the Mary Glover case*, London 1991

MacDonald Ross, G., 'The royal touch and the Book of Common Prayer', *Notes and Queries* n.s. xxx (1983), 433–5

MacGregor, A., 'The life, character and concerns of Sir Hans Sloane', in MacGregor, *Sir Hans Sloane*

—— 'Medieval and late antiquities', in MacGregor, *Sir Hans Sloane*, 150–66

—— (ed.), *Sir Hans Sloane: collector, scientist, antiquary, founding father of the British Museum*, London 1994

McGregor, J. F. and B. Reay, *Radical religion in the English Revolution*, Oxford 1984

McKeith, R., 'Samuel Johnson's childhood illnesses and the king's evil', *Medical History* x/4 (1966), 386–99

McKeon, M., *Politics and poetry in Restoration England: the case of Dryden's annus mirabilis*, London 1975

McKerrow, R. B., *A dictionary of printers and booksellers in England, Scotland and Ireland, and of foreign printers of English books, 1557–1640*, London 1910

McLaughlin, E., *Parish registers*, Solihull 1986

McShane, A., 'The gazet in metre, or, The rhiming newsmonger: the English broadside ballad as intelligencer: a new narrative', in J.W. Koopmans (ed.), *News and politics in early modern Europe (1500–1800)*, Dudley, MA 2005, 131–50

—— 'Typography matters: branding ballads and gelding curates in Stuart England', in J. Hinks and C. Armstrong (eds.), *Book trade connections from the seventeenth to the twentieth centuries*, London 2008, 19–44

—— '"Ne sutor ultra crepidam": political cobblers and broadside ballads in late seventeenth-century England', in P. Fumerton and A. Guerrini (eds), *Ballads and broadsides, 1500–1800*, Aldershot 2010, 207–28

—— 'Broadsides and ballads from the beginnings of print to 1660', in J. Raymond (ed.), *The Oxford history of popular print culture, I: Britain and Ireland to 1660*, Oxford 2011

—— *Political broadside ballads of seventeenth-century England: a critical bibliography*, London 2011

Marsh, C., *Popular religion in sixteenth-century England*, London 1998

Marshall, A., 'The Westminster magistrate and the Irish stroker: Sir Edmund Godfrey and Valentine Greatrakes: some unpublished correspondence', *HJ* xl (1997), 499–505

Marshall, P., *Reformation England, 1480–1642*, London 2003

Mendle, M., *Dangerous positions: mixed government, the estates of the realm, and the answer to the XIX propositions*, Tuscaloosa, AL 1985

Merrick, J., *The desacralisation of the French monarchy in the eighteenth century*, Baton Rouge 1990

Miller, J., *Popery and politics in England, 1660–88*, Cambridge 1973

—— *James II: a study in kingship*, London 1978

—— *The Glorious Revolution*, London 1983

—— *Charles II*, London 1991

—— *A brief history of the English Civil Wars*, London 2009

Mintz, S. I., *The hunting of Leviathan*, Cambridge 1962

Mitchell, D. (ed.), *Goldsmiths, silversmiths and bankers: innovation and the transfer of skill*, London 1995

Mollenauer, L. W., *Strange revelations: magic, poison and sacrilege in Louis XIV's France*, Philadelphia 2007

Monod, P. K., *Jacobitism and the English people, 1688–1788*, Cambridge 1989

—— *The power of kings: monarchy and religion in Europe, 1589–1715*, New Haven 1999

—— *Solomon's secret arts: the occult in the age of Enlightenment*, New Haven 2013

Morman, F. W., *Robert Herrick: a biographical and critical study*, London 1910

Morrill, J. and J. Walter, 'Order and disorder in the English Revolution', in J. Morrill (ed.), *The nature of the English Revolution*, London 1993, 359–91

Morris, G. C. R., 'A portrait of Thomas Hollier, Pepys's surgeon', *Annals of the Royal College of Surgeons of England* lxi (1979), 224–9

——'Hollier, Thomas (*bap.* 1609, *d.* 1690)', *ODNB*

Mortimer, R., *Angevin England, 1154–1258*, Oxford 1994

Muir, E., *Ritual in early modern Europe*, 2nd edn, Cambridge 2005

Munk, W., *The roll of the Royal College of Physicians of London*, London 1878

Murray, I. G., 'Clowes, William (1543/4–1604)', *ODNB*

Nederman, C. J. and K. Langdon (ed.), *Medieval political theory: the quest for the body politic, 1100–1400*, London 1993

Nicholls, C., 'On the obsolete custom of touching for the king's evil', *Home Counties Magazine* xiv (1912), 112–22

Normand, L., and G. Roberts, *Witchcraft in early modern Scotland: James VI's Demonology and the North Berwick witches*, Exeter 2000

North, M., 'Ignoto in the age of print: the manipulation of anonymity in early modern England', *Studies in Philology* xci/4 (1994), 390–416

Novak, M. E., *Daniel Defoe: master of fictions*, Oxford 2001

—— 'Defoe's political and religious journalism', in J. Richetti (ed.), *The Cambridge companion to Daniel Defoe*, Cambridge 2008, 25–44

O'Connell, S., *The popular print in England*, London 1999

O'Higgins, J., *Anthony Collins: the man and his works*, The Hague 1970

Ogg, D., *England in the reign of William III*, Oxford 1955

Ollard, R., *The escape of Charles II*, London 1986

Ormrod, W. M., 'The personal religion of Edward III', *Speculum* lxiv (1989), 849–77

Owen, E., 'The Croes Nawdd', *Y Cymmrodor* xliii (1932), 13–17

Pady, D. S., 'The medico-psychological interests of King James I', *Clio Medica* xix (1984), 22–31

Paine, S., *Amulets: sacred charms of power and protection*, Rochester, VT 2004

Parish H. and W. G. Naphy (eds), *Religion and superstition in Reformation Europe*, Manchester 2002

Parry, G., 'Wilson, Arthur (*bap.* 1595, *d.* 1652)', *ODNB*

Patterson, W. B., *King James VI and I and the reunion of Christendom*, Cambridge 1997

Paul, H. N., *The royal play of Macbeth*, New York 1950

Pavitt, W. T., *The book of talismans, amulets, and zodiacal charms*, London 1914

Peerless, B., 'The Queen Anne prayer book: a touch of the "king's evil"', *Lancing College Journal* (1982)

Peristiany, J. G. and J. Pitt-Rivers (eds), *Honour and grace in anthropology*, Cambridge 1999

Pettigrew, T. J., 'The royal gift of healing', in his *On superstitions connected with the history and practice of medicine and surgery*, London 1844

Phillips, B., 'The prevalence and alleged increase of scrofula', *Journal of the Statistical Society of London* ix/2 (1846), 152–7

Phillips, J. E., Jr, 'The background of Spencer's attitude toward women rulers', *Huntington Library Quarterly* v (1941), 5–32

Pierce, H., *Unseemly pictures: graphic satire and politics in early modern England*, London 2008

Pincus, S., *1688: the first modern revolution*, New Haven 2009

Plomer, H. R., *A dictionary of the booksellers and printers who were at work in England, Scotland and Ireland from 1641 to 1667*, London 1907

—— and others, *A dictionary of the printers and booksellers who were at work in England, Scotland and Ireland: from 1668 to 1725*, London 1922

Porter, R., *English society in the eighteenth century*, London 1982

—— 'The patient's view: doing medical history from below', *Theory and Society* xiv/2 (1985), 175–98

—— *Mind forg'd manacles: a history of madness in England from the Restoration to the Regency*, London 1987

—— *The popularization of medicine, 1650–1850*, London 1992

—— 'The people's health in Georgian England', in Tim Harris (ed.), *Popular culture in England, c. 1500–1850*, London 1995, 124–42

—— *The greatest benefit to mankind: a medical history of humanity from antiquity to the present*, London 1997

—— *Enlightenment: Britain and the creation of the modern world*, London 2000

—— *Bodies politic: disease, death and doctors in Britain, 1650–1900*, London 2001

—— (ed.), *The medicinal history of water and spas*, London 1990

Porterfield, A., *Healing in the history of Christianity*, Oxford 2005

Potter, D. (ed.), *France in the later Middle Ages*, Oxford 2002

Prestwich, M., 'The piety of Edward I', in W. M. Ormrod (ed.), *England in the thirteenth century: proceedings of the 1984 Harlaxton symposium*, Woodbridge 1985, 120–8

—— *Edward I* (1988), New Haven 1990

Prochaska, F. K., *Philanthropy and the hospitals of London: the King's Fund, 1897–1990*, Oxford 1992

Rawcliffe, C., *Medicine and society in late medieval England*, Stroud 1999

Raymond, J., *News, newspapers, and society in early modern Britain*, London 1999

Redworth, G., *The prince and the infanta: the cultural politics of the Spanish match*, New Haven 2003

Renwick Riddell, W., 'The king's evil and high treason', *Journal of the American Institute of Criminal Law and Criminology* xix/4 (1929), 545–50

Richard, J., *Saint Louis: crusader king of France*, trans. Jean Birrell, Cambridge 1992

Richards, J., '"His nowe majestie" and the English monarchy: the kingship of Charles I before 1640', *P&P* cxiii (Nov. 1986), 70–96

Ridley, J., *The life and times of Mary Tudor*, London 1973

Riley, P. F., *A lust for virtue: Louis XIV's attack on sin in seventeenth-century France*, Westport, CN 2001

Robinson, B., *The Royal Maundy*, London 1977

—— *Silver pennies and linen towels: the story of Royal Maundy*, London 1992

Robinson, F. E., *Trinity College*, London 1898

Rogers, P., 'Oldmixon, John (1672/3–1742)', *ODNB*

—— 'Johnson, Samuel (1709–84)', *ODNB*

Rolleston, J. D., rev. H. C. G. Matthew, 'Crawfurd, Sir Raymond Henry Payne (1865–1938)'

Roper, J. (ed.), *Charms and charming in Europe*, London 2004

Rowse, A. L., 'The coronation of Queen Elizabeth I', *History Today* iii (May 1953), 301–10

Ruiz, T. F., 'Unsacred monarchy: the kings of Castile in the late Middle Ages', in S. Wilentz (ed.), *Rites of power: symbolism, ritual and politics since the Middle Ages*, Philadelphia 1999, 109–44

Russell, C., 'Divine rights in the early seventeenth century', in J. Morrill, P. Slack and D. Woolf (ed.), *Public duty and private conscience in seventeenth-century England: essays presented to G. E. Aylmer*, Oxford 1993, 101–20

Sainty, J. C. and R. O. Bucholz, *Officials of the royal household 1660–1837*, I: *Department of the Lord Chamberlain and associated offices*, London 1997–8

Scalingi, P. L., 'The sceptre or the distaff: the question of female sovereignty, 1516–1607', *The Historian* xli (1978), 59–75

Schaffer, S., 'Natural philosophy and public spectacle in the 18th century', *History of Science* xxi (1983), 1–43

—— 'Newton's comets and the transformation of astrology', in P. Curry (ed.), *Astrology, science and society: historical essays*, Wolfeboro, NH 1987, 219–43

—— 'The consuming flame: electrical showmen and Tory mystics in the world of goods', in J. Brewer and R. Porter (eds), *Consumption and the world of goods*, London 1993, 489–526

—— 'Regeneration: the body of natural philosophers in Restoration England', in C. Lawrence and S. Shapin (eds), *Science incarnate: historical embodiments of natural knowledge*, London 1998, 83–120

Schaich, M. (ed), *Monarchy and religion: the transformation of royal culture in eighteenth-century Europe*, Oxford 2007

Schneidmüller, B., 'Constructing identities in medieval France', in M. Bull (ed.), *France in the central Middle Ages*, Oxford 2002, 15–42

Schramm, P. E., A history of the English coronation, trans. L. G. Wickham Legg, Oxford 1937

Schwoerer, L. G., 'The coronation of William and Mary, April 11, 1689', in L. G. Schwoerer (ed.), The Revolution of 1688–89: changing perspectives, Cambridge 1992, 107–30

Scribner, R. 'Oral culture and the diffusion of Reformation ideas', in his Popular culture and popular movements in Reformation Germany, London 1987, 49–70

Shapin, S. and S. Shaffer, Leviathan and the air pump: Hobbes, Boyle and the experimental life, Princeton 1985

Sharpe, K., 'The image of virtue: the court and household of Charles I, 1625–1642', in D. Starkey (ed.), The English court, London 1987, 226–60

—— Politics and ideas in early Stuart England, London 1989

—— The personal rule of Charles I, New Haven 1992

—— Selling the Tudor monarchy: authority and image in sixteenth-century England, London 2009

—— Image wars: promoting kings and commonwealths in England, 1603–1660, New Haven 2010

—— Rebranding rule: the restoration and revolution monarchy, 1660–1714, New Haven 2013

Shaw, J., Miracles in Enlightenment England, New Haven 2006

Sheppard, E., Memorials of St James's Palace, London 1894

Shoemaker, R. B., 'Reforming the city: the Reformation of Manners campaign in London, 1690–1738', in Davidson, Hitchcock, Keirn and Shoemaker, Stilling the grumbling hive, 99–120

Shonhorn, M., Defoe's politics: parliament, power, kingship and Robinson Crusoe, Cambridge 1991

Siraisi, N. G., The clock and the mirror: Girolamo Cardano and Renaissance magic, Princeton 1997

Slack, P., 'Mirrors of health and treasures of poor men: the uses of the vernacular medical literature of Tudor England', in C. Webster (ed.), Health, medicine and mortality in the sixteenth century, Cambridge 1979, 237–73

Sloan, A. W., English medicine in the seventeenth century, Durham 1996

Smith, H., ' "Last of all the heavenly birth": Queen Anne and sacral queenship', History of Parliament xxviii/1 (2009), 137–49

Smuts, R. M., Court culture and the origins of a royalist tradition in early Stuart England, Philadelphia 1987

Smyth, A., Autobiography in early modern England, Cambridge 2010

Snobelen, S. D., 'Whiston, William (1667–1752)', ODNB

Solomon, H. M., Sir Richard Blackmore, Boston 1980

Sommerville, J. P., Politics and ideology in England, 1603–1640, London 1986

—— 'James I and the divine right of kings: English politics and continental theory', in Levy Peck, Mental world, 55–70

Sommerville, M., Sex and subjection: attitudes to women in early modern society, London 1995

Sowerby, S., Making toleration: the repealers and the Glorious Revolution, Cambridge, MA 2013

Sparrow Simpson, W., 'On the forms of prayer recited "At the healing" or touching for the king's evil', Journal of the Archaeological Association xxvii (1871), 282–307

Speck, W. A., *Reluctant revolutionaries: Englishmen and the Revolution of 1688*, Oxford 1988

Spurr, J., *The Restoration Church of England, 1646–1689*, New Haven 1991

—— 'The Church, the societies and the moral revolution of 1688', in J. Walsh, C. Haydon and S. Taylor (eds), *The Church of England c. 1689–c. 1833: from toleration to Tractarianism*, Cambridge 1993, 127–42

—— *England in the 1670s: this masquerading age*, Oxford 2000

Stark, W., *The sociology of religion: a study of Christendom*, London 1966

Starkey, D., 'Representation through intimacy: a study in the symbolism of monarchy and court office in early modern England', in I. Lewis (ed.), *Symbols and sentiments: cross-cultural studies in symbolism*, London 1977, 187–224

—— *Elizabeth: apprenticeship*, London 2000

Steggle, M., 'Bathurst, Ralph (1619/20–1704)', *ODNB*

Steneck, N. H., 'Greatrakes the stroker: the interpretation of historians', *Isis* lxxii/2 (1982), 161–77

Stewart, L. R., *The rise of public science: rhetoric, technology and natural philosophy in Newtonian Britain, 1660–1750*, Cambridge 1992

Stirling, K., 'Rereading Marc Bloch: the life and works of a visionary', *Modernist History Compass* v/2 (2007), 525–38

Stobart, A., '"Lett her refrain from all hott spices": medicinal recipes and advice in the treatment of the king's evil in seventeenth-century south-west England', in M. DiMeo and S. Pennell (eds), *Reading and writing recipe books, 1550–1800*, Manchester 2013, 203–24

Stocking, G. W., *Victorian anthropology*, London 1987

Straka, G., 'The final phase of divine right theory in England, 1688–1702', *EHR* lxxvii (1962), 638–58

Strong, R., *Van Dyck: Charles I on horseback*, New York 1972

—— *The cult of Elizabeth*, London 1977

—— *Artists of the Tudor court: the portrait miniature rediscovered,1520–1620*, London 1983

—— *Gloriana: the portraits of Elizabeth I*, London 1987

—— *Coronation: a history of kingship and the British monarchy*, London 2005

Sturdy, D. J., 'The royal touch in England', in H. Duchhardt, R. A. Jackson and D. J. Sturdy (eds), *European monarchy: its evolution and practice from antiquity to modern times*, Stuttgart 1992, 171–84

Summers, C. J., 'Herrick's political poetry: the strategies of his art', in R. B. Rollin and J. M. Patrick (eds), *'Trust to Good Verses': Herrick tercentenary essays*, Pittsburgh 1978, 171–83

—— 'Herrick's political counterplots', *Studies in English Literature, 1500–1900*, xxv/1 (1985), 165–82

Sutherland, C. H. V., *Gold: its beauty, power and allure*, London 1969

Sutherland, J., *The Restoration newspaper and its development*, Cambridge 1986

Sweet, R., *Antiquaries: the discovery of the past in eighteenth-century Britain*, London 2004

Symonds, H., 'Charles I, the trials of the pyx, the mint marks and the mint accounts', *Numismatic Chronicle* 4th ser. x (1910), 380–98

—— 'Mint marks and denominations of the coinage of James I as disclosed by the trials of the pyx', *BNJ* n.s. ix (1912), 207–27

Symons, J., 'Pettigrew, Thomas Joseph (1791–1865)', *ODNB*

Tambiah, S. J., *Magic, science, religion, and the scope of rationality*, Cambridge 1990

Tanner, J. R., *English constitutional conflicts of the seventeenth century*, London 1928

Tate, W. E., *The parish chest: a study of the parochial administration in England*, Cambridge 1951

Taylor, L. J. and others (eds), *Encyclopedia of medieval pilgrimage*, Leiden–Boston 2010

Tennant, W. C., 'Croes Naid', *National Library of Wales Journal* (1951–2), 102–15

Theilmann, J. M., 'The miracles of king Henry VI of England', *Historian* xlii/3 (1980), 456–71

Thomas, K., *Religion and the decline of magic: studies in popular beliefs in sixteenth and seventeenth century England* (1971), London 1997

Thomas, P. W., 'Charles I of England: the tragedy of absolutism', in A. G. Dickens (ed.), *The courts of Europe*, London 1977, 191–212

Thompson, C. J. S., *Royal cramp and other medycinable rings*, London 1921

Tout, T. F. (ed.), *The place of the reign of Edward II in English history*, Manchester 1914

Toynbee, M. R., 'Charles I and the king's evil', *Folk-Lore* lxi/1 (1950), 1–14

Troost, W., *William III: the stadholder-king*, trans. J. C. Grayson, Aldershot 2005

Turrell, J. F., 'The ritual of royal healing in early modern England', *Anglican and Episcopal History* lxviii/1 (1999), 3–36

Twining, L., *Symbols and emblems of early and medieval Christian art*, London 1885

Tyake, N., *Anti-Calvinists: the rise of English Arminianism*, Oxford 1990

Vincent, N., *The holy blood: King Henry III and the Westminster blood relic*, Cambridge 2006

Walker, D. P., *Spiritual and demonic magic: from Ficino to Campanella*, London 1958

—— 'Valentine Greatrakes, the Irish stroker and the question of miracles', *Mélanges sur la literature de la Renaissance á la mémoire de V. L. Saulnier*, Geneva 1984, 343–56

—— 'The cessation of miracles', in I. Merkeland and A. G. Debus (eds), *Hermeticism and the Renaissance: intellectual history and the occult in early modern Europe*, Cranberry, NJ 1988, 111–24

Waller, R. D., 'Lorenzo Magalotti in England, 1668–9', *Italian Studies* ii (1939), 49–56

Wallis Budge, E. A., *Amulets and superstitions*, London 1930

Walsham, A., *Providence in early modern England* (1999), Oxford 2001

—— 'Miracles in post-Reformation England', in K. Cooper and J. Gregory (eds), *Signs, wonders, miracles: representations of divine power in the life of the Church* (Studies in Church History xli, 2005), 273–306.

—— 'Recording superstition in early modern Britain: the origins of folklore', in S. A. Smith and A. Knight (eds), *The religion of fools? Superstition past and present*, Oxford 2008, 178–206

—— 'The Reformation and "The disenchantment of the world" reassessed', *HJ* li/2 (2008), 497–528

—— 'Skeletons in the cupboard: relics after the English Reformation', in A. Walsham (ed.), *Relics and remains* (*P&P* supplement v, 2010), 121–43

—— *The reformation of the landscape: religion, identity and memory in early modern Britain and Ireland*, Oxford 2011

Walter, J., 'The impact on society: a word turned upside down?', in J. Morrill (ed.), *The impact of the English Civil War*, London 1991, 104–22

Waterton, Edmund, 'On a remarkable incident in the *Life* of St Edward the Confessor, with notices of royal cramp rings', *Archaeological Journal* xxi (1864), 103–13

Watt, T., *Cheap print and popular piety*, Cambridge 1991

Wear, A., A. K. French and I. M. Lone (eds.), *The medical Renaissance of the sixteenth century* (1985), Cambridge 1987

Wear, A. (ed.), *Health and healing in early modern England: studies in social and intellectual history*, Farnham–Burlington, Vᴛ 1998

—— *Knowledge and practice in English medicine, 1550–1680*, Cambridge 2000

Webb, D., *Pilgrims and pilgrimage in the medieval west*, London 1999

—— *Medieval European pilgrimage, c. 700–c. 1500*, Basingstoke 2002

Weber, H., 'The monarch's sacred body', in H. Weber, *Paper bullets: print and kingship under Charles II*, Lexington, Kʏ 1996, 50–87

Weber, M., *From Max Weber: essays in sociology*, ed. and trans. H. H. Gerth and C. Wright Mills, London 1947

—— *The sociology of religion*, Boston 1993

Wedgwood, C. V., *The trial of Charles I*, London 1964

Weisner, M., *Women and gender in early modern Europe*, Cambridge 1993

Werrett, S., 'Healing the nation's wounds: royal ritual and experimental philosophy in Restoration England', *History of Science* xxxviii/4 (2000), 377–99

Westfall, Richard S., *Never at rest: a biography of Isaac Newton*, Cambridge 1980

Wheeler, S., 'Medicine in art: Henry ɪv of France touching for scrofula, by Pierre Firens', *Journal of the History of Medicine and Allied Sciences* lviii/1 (2003), 79–81

White, F. V., 'Anthony, Francis (1550–1623)', *ODNB*

White, P., 'The rise of Arminianism reconsidered', *P&P* ci (Nov. 1983), 34–54

Whitet, T. D., 'John Badger, Apothecaryite', *Pharmaceutical Historian* iii/1 (1973), 2–4

Whiting, J. R. S., *A handful of history*, Dursley, Glos. 1978

Wigelsworth, J. R., *Deism in Enlightenment England: theology, politics, and Newtonian public science*, Manchester 2009

Willets, I. E., 'John Knight and the king's healing', *Journal of the Royal Society of Medicine* lxxxvii (1994), 756–7

Willis, D., 'The monarch and the sacred: Shakespeare and the ceremony for the healing of the king's evil', in L. Woodbridge and E. Berry (eds), *True rites and maimed rites: ritual and anti-ritual in Shakespeare and his age*, Urbana–Chicago 1992, 147–67

Wilson, H., *The court wits of the Restoration*, Princeton 1948

—— *The court wits of the Restoration: an introduction*, London 1967

Wilson, H. A., 'The coronation of Queen Elizabeth', *EHR* xxiii (1908), 87–91

Wilson, P. K., '"Out of sight, out of mind?": the Daniel Turner–James Blondel dispute over the power of the maternal imagination', *Annals of Science* xlix (1992), 63–85

—— 'Daniel Turner and the art of surgery in eighteenth-century London', *Journal of the Royal Society of Medicine* lxxxvii (1994), 781–85

—— 'Turner, Daniel (1667–1741)', *ODNB*

Woolf, N., 'The sovereign remedy: touch-pieces and the king's evil', *BNJ* xlix (1980 for 1979), 99–121

—— 'The sovereign remedy: touch-pieces and the king's evil, ii', *BNJ* l (1981 for 1980), 91–116

—— *The medallic record of the Jacobite movement*, London 1988

Woolgar, C. M., *The senses in late medieval England*, New Haven 2006

Wootton, D., 'Lucien Febvre and the problem of unbelief in the early modern period', *Journal of Modern History* lx (1988), 695–730

Wormald, J., 'James vi and i: two kings or one?', *History* lxviii (1983), 187–209

—— 'James vi and i, *Basilicon doron* and *The trew law of free monarchies*: the Scottish context and the English translation', in Levy Peck, *Mental world*, 36–54

Wright, P., *The story of royal Maundy*, London 1990

Würzbach, N., *The rise of the English street ballad*, trans. G. Walls, Cambridge 1990

Zaller, R., 'Breaking the vessels: the desacralisation of monarchy in early modern England', *Sixteenth-Century Journal* xxix/3 (1998), 757–78

Internet Resources

Bucholz, R. O., *The database of court officers, 1660–1839*, <http://www.luc.edu/history/fac_resources/bucholz/DCO/DCO.html>

Louis, St, *St Louis' advice to his Son*, in *Medieval civilisation*, ed. and trans. D. Munro and G. Clarke Sellery, New York 1910, <http://www.fordham.edu/halsall/source/stlouis1.html>

Oxford dictionary of national biography, ed. H. C. G. Mathew and B. Harrison, Oxford 2004, <http://www.oxforddnb.com>

The return of the king: an anthology of English poems commemorating the restoration of Charles II, ed. Gerald MacLean, <http://etext.virginia.edu/etcbin/toccer-new2?id=MacKing.xml&images=images/modeng&data=/texts/english/modeng/parsed&tag=public&part=teiHeader>

Robert Boyle Project (online hub of Boyle studies, offering various resources, including the occasional papers), < http://www.bbk.ac.uk/boyle/>

Unpublished dissertations

Brogan, S., 'The royal touch in early modern England: its changing rationale and practice', PhD, London 2011

Dixon-Smith, S., 'Feeding the poor to commemorate the dead: the *pro anima* almsgiving of King Henry iii of England, 1227–72', PhD, London 2002

McShane, A., '"Rime and reason": the political world of the broadside ballad, 1640–1689', PhD, Warwick 2004

Index

[Page numbers in bold indicate an illustration]

052454=64

INDEX